Replacement Parts

Replacement Parts

The Ethics of Procuring and Replacing Organs in Humans

Arthur L. Caplan, James J. McCartney,
Daniel P. Reid, Editors

Georgetown University Press / Washington, DC

Library of Congress Cataloging-in-Publication Data

Replacement parts : the ethics of procuring and replacing organs in humans / Arthur L. Caplan, James J. McCartney, Daniel P. Reid, editors.
      pages cm
   Includes bibliographical references and index.
         Summary: The supply of human organs in the United States continues to lag behind demand. By any objective standard the public policy of "encouraged volunteerism," established with the adoption of the Uniform Anatomical Gift Act in 1968, has failed. How should the United States and the health care community address this ongoing scarcity? What strategies would be both morally acceptable and effective? Noted bioethicist Arthur Caplan and his coeditors have brought together seminal essays and articles from the most significant literature in the fields of medicine, policy, philosophy and religion to help analyze and assess these questions. Caplan's introductory essay explains why present policies are inadequate, and succeeding sections of the book address the following issues: the determination of death and the "dead donor rule"; the morally divisive case of anencephalic infants as organ donors; the sale of cadaveric or live organs; strategies for increasing the number of available organs, including the market; and how some organ seekers, such as Apple's Steve Jobs, "game the system" by creating advantageous circumstances for organ donation.
ISBN 978-1-62616-235-8 (hc : alk. paper) — ISBN 978-1-62616-236-5 (pb : alk. paper) — ISBN 978-1-62616-237-2 (eb)
   1. Donation of organs, tissues, etc.—Moral and ethical aspects. 2. Procurement of organs, tissues, etc.—Moral and ethical aspects. 3. Transplantation of organs, tissues, etc.—Moral and ethical aspects. 4. Allocation of organs, tissues, etc.—Moral and ethical aspects. I. Caplan, Arthur L., editor. II. McCartney, James J., editor. III. Reid, Daniel P., editor
   RD129.5.R47 2015
   174.2'97954—dc23

                              2015007446

16 15   9 8 7 6 5 4 3 2 First printing

Printed in the United States of America

Cover design by Anne C. Kerns, Anne Likes Red, Inc. Cover image by Corbis/Media Bakery.

Dedication

I want to thank my colleagues in the Division of Medical Ethics and in the School of Medicine at NYU Langone Medical Center for their encouragement. In putting together this volume, I also want to thank my wife, Meg, who showed her usual tolerance of my working just a few evenings and weekends to get this done.

—Arthur L. Caplan

I wish to thank my faculty colleagues in the Department of Philosophy at Villanova University for the support and friendship they have shown me for more than twenty-five years. I also wish to dedicate this work to all the law students, graduate students, and undergraduate students I have taught and mentored at Villanova and elsewhere.

—James J. McCartney

For those teachers who fostered and supported my natural curiosity, thank you. And for my friends and family, thank you for your patience and understanding while I was working on this volume.

—Daniel P. Reid

Contents

Contents

Acknowledgments

The authors wish to specifically acknowledge the following people, also acknowledging that many others have been very helpful and supportive as we have constructed this volume:

- Kathryn Fogarty, who has researched and organized the biographical material of all authors and editors.
- Nikolaus Fogle and other members of the Falvey Memorial Library staff at Villanova University who have procured and reviewed clean .pdf documents for conversion to Word, and have generally provided assistance whenever it has been requested.
- Kathryn Murphy, who worked as a summer intern for editor James McCartney and researched and collected some of the original articles considered for this book.
- Billy Alfano, for his assistance in Italian translations.
- Many individuals who worked with all the editors to help us reduce permissions costs for this volume.
- The staff of Georgetown University Press, specifically Richard Brown and Milica Cosic, for their continual help and support throughout the process of creating this volume.
- The contributors and publishers of the texts in this volume, for granting us permission to republish their works.

Introduction

Arthur L. Caplan

Present Policies Regarding Organ Procurement Are Inadequate

Why does the supply of organs lag behind demand? There are many reasons for believing that current systems of organ procurement are not as efficient as they could be in obtaining organs from cadaver sources. In the United States the prevailing, long-standing public policy is one of "encouraged voluntarism." This policy was established when states began adopting the Uniform Anatomical Gift Act in 1968 (Caplan, 1984; DeVita and Caplan, 2007). The United States as well as Canada, the United Kingdom, Denmark, Australia and many other nations rely on altruistic donation reinforced by ongoing public education campaigns to obtain cadaver donors. In Israel and Singapore priority in access to transplants is an additional incentive to be a donor (Quigley, 2012; Chandler, 2005). Individuals may use donor cards to make their wish to donate all or some organs after their death. In some parts of the world and many states in the United States, computer registries of donors or objectors facilitate organ donation.

Public surveys show support for organ donation in the United States at levels not reflected in actual donor rates (Mayo Clinic, 2013). Some who wished to be organ donors are missed. A few are not identified as such at the time of death by health care personnel. In other cases, while families in the United States do not have the legal standing to veto a signed request to donate by a deceased relative, in practice they are almost always accorded that right.

Why Has "Encouraged Voluntarism" Fallen Short?

There are many reasons why the policy of encouraged voluntarism has not produced as many organs for transplant as might be expected. Many people still do not carry a donor card or other written directive specifying the disposition of their bodies when they die. Often people do not discuss their wish to donate with their family, partners, or friends. Rates of donation among the poor are low. Computer registries help but they are no substitute for discussions about donation prior to death. Many people are loath to contemplate their own death, much less make plans for the disposition of their bodies. This means that many people are not going to fill out a donor card just as they are not going to make out a will, buy a funeral plot, or complete an advance directive concerning the kind of medical care they would like to have if they become incompetent (Caplan, 1984).

The fact that health care has in recent years become increasingly centralized in large and impersonal institutions undermines trust between patients and health care providers. It is very difficult to trust in the good intentions of strangers. Some people are afraid that if they carry a donor card, they may not receive the aggressive medical care they might need so that others can be given their organs. Still others believe that only the rich can get transplants and so see no reason to act as donors.

The failure to secure higher rates of compliance with respect to written directives and the mistrust of hospitals and health care providers are, however, only part of the explanation for low rates of organ procurement. The reality in the United States, Canada, Germany, the UK, and many other nations is that when the subject of donation is raised, it is done with the presumption that the family of the deceased must decide to opt into donation. It may be possible to obtain a higher rate of donation simply by changing the philosophy underlying requests to donate from an "opt in" approach to an "opt out" approach (Caplan, 2014). Still other nations such as China are willing to execute "prisoners" to obtain a steady supply of organs—a grossly unethical approach to obtaining organs (Caplan, 2012; Wang, 2010). There is some enthusiasm for using markets to increase the cadaver supply (Davis, 2009; Hughes, 2009; Jaycox, 2012; Kerstein, 2009; Lawlor, 2011; Slabbert, 2012; Taylor, 2009). And some argue that the pool of prospective donors should be expanded by relaxing the "dead donor rule"—the requirement that death be pronounced prior to organ

retrieval. Proposals have included adding those who are absolutely terminally ill, including anencephalic babies, to including those who are not brain-dead but pronounced dead on the basis of cardiac failure, to those who are irreversibly comatose or minimally conscious (Kirkpatrick, Beasley, and Caplan, 2010).

Should the Definition of Death Be Changed?

Most donated organs now come from people declared dead on the basis of neurological criteria—the absence of brain activity. Brain death typically occurs after cardiopulmonary death, the cessation of a heartbeat and breathing, unless the person is put on a ventilator or other life-prolonging technology. One way to expand the pool of deceased donors is to allow patients or their surrogates to request removal of life-prolonging procedures and then to include them for possible transplantation when they have been declared dead by cardiopulmonary criteria. This recommendation was made by a panel of the Institute of Medicine in 2006.

Donation after circulatory determination of death (DCDD) has become more common around the world, but the practice is controversial. First, it is medically more complex than donation after brain death because of the risk of organs being harmed by oxygen deprivation. Second, there is ethical concern that DCDD will lead to substandard health care at the end of life—for example, inadequate morphine in the effort to avoid harming the organs. The Institute of Medicine report recommends ethical guidelines already used in Europe, such as preventing the organ recovery team from being the ones to decide when to discontinue cardiopulmonary resuscitation.

Others argue that brain death itself is not

a clear, bright line. By acknowledging that fact and relaxing the standard for taking organs, the potential pool of donors could be greatly expanded. But any policy that relaxes the dead donor rule is sure to provoke controversy among those worried that the living and especially the disabled would be killed in order to benefit others (Smith, Rodriguez-Arias, and Ortega, 2012).

Getting More Organs—Markets?

Two basic strategies have been proposed to provide incentives for people to sell their organs when they die. One strategy is simply to permit organ sales in the United States by changing the National Organ Transplant Act (NOTA), the 1986 federal law that bans organ sales. Then, individuals would be free to broker contracts with persons interested in selling at prices mutually agreed upon by both parties (Lawlor, 2011; Slabbert, 2012). The other strategy is to create a regulated market in which the government would act as the purchaser of organs—setting a fixed price and enforcing conditions of sale (Lawlor, 2011; Matas, 2006). Both proposals have drawn heated ethical criticism.

Would markets really work in the United States or other economically advanced nations to increase organ supply? It is hard to imagine many people in wealthy countries eager to sell their organs upon their death who do not now donate them. In fact, even if compensation is relatively high, few will agree to sell. Polls show that the disincentive to cadaver donation has more to do with aesthetic, emotional, or religious concerns than a lack of payment. That has been the experience with markets in human eggs for research purposes and paid surrogacy in the United States, with prices escalating through the roof and still relatively

few sellers. If there is already a fear of premature pronouncement of death to obtain organs, enacting market incentives for cadaver donation is likely to exacerbate this fear (DeVita and Caplan, 2007).

Perhaps living persons can be induced to sell non-vital organs. In fact, the United States now obtains more kidneys for transplant from those who donate a kidney to a friend or a family member than from cadaver sources. However, markets that incentivize living persons have their own ethical problems.

One problem is that only kidneys are likely to be available in a living seller market. Hearts will obviously not be. Lungs and liver involve such risky procurement surgery that they are not likely to attract sellers. Another moral challenge is that only the poor and very desperate will want to sell their body parts. If you need money, you might sell your kidney to try to feed your family or to pay back a debt. This may be a "rational" decision, but that does not make it a matter of free choice. Talk of individual rights and autonomy is hollow if those with no options must "choose" to sell their organs to purchase life's necessities (Caplan and Prior, 2009; Jaycox, 2012; Kerstein, 2009; Lawlor, 2011; Taylor, 2009). Choice requires options as well as information and some degree of freedom.

Major religious traditions oppose payment on the grounds that persons do not own but are, rather, the stewards of their bodies (Caplan and Prior, 2009; Caplan, 2014). Payment also introduces risks concerning the quality of organs obtained. And payment may give persons an inducement to kill or take organs from others to pay debts.

Another very important ethical challenge to proposals to permit markets is that selling organs, even in a tightly regulated market, violates the ethics of medicine. The core ethical norm of the medical profession is the principle Do No Harm. The only morally defensible way to remove an organ from someone is if the donor chooses to undergo the harm of surgery solely to help another and if there is sufficient medical benefit to the recipient. The creation of a market puts medicine and nursing in the position of removing body parts from people solely to abet those people's interest in securing compensation (Caplan, 2004; Caplan, 2014). In a market, even a regulated one, doctors and nurses would be using their skills to help people harm themselves for money. The resulting distrust and loss of professional standing may be too high a price to pay for a gamble that living sellers who want their kidneys removed for sale may possibly help increase the organ supply (Tan, Marcos, and Shapiro, 2008).

Default to Donation

If public opinion surveys can be trusted, most Americans are willing to serve as donors when they die. The problem is that encouraged voluntarism using donor cards does not seem to fully tap this powerful sentiment. There is another way of modifying existing practice that would respect the dignity and value of individual choice while at the same time holding out the prospect of increasing the number of organs obtained from cadaver sources. It requires a shift in the ethical presumptions that prevail about organ donation.

If public policy were to be modified to a default that presumes people do want to be donors, this might have a positive impact on donation rates. Some nations, such as France, Austria, Belgium, and Spain, have legislated versions of presumed consent with a consequent positive impact on their cadaver donor rates (Abadie and Gay, 2006; Byk, 2009; Neades, 2009).

A policy of default to donation addresses many of the failings of the current approach to cadaver organ procurement. It allows opting out of cadaver donation while allowing the view of the majority toward donation to set policy.

There are two main worries about shifting to a default-to-donation policy in the United States, the UK, Canada, and other nations. One is that forcing a choice will lead to many more people opting out than currently do. This has not been seen in nations with default-to-donation policies. The other is simple resistance to the shift toward donation for fear that objections will not be accurately tracked. The increasing use of computer registries may help buffer this concern.

Toughening Encouraged Voluntarism— Charity to Obligation?

For many years, the rhetoric in educating the public has emphasized charity. People are constantly being urged through public service advertisements in magazines, in newspapers, and on radio and television to "make the gift of life." What is interesting about "gift" to urge organ donation is that the moral force of such language is not particularly strong. Gifts are a form of charity. Most moral theories recognize a strong moral obligation, or duty, not to harm others. But few theories posit the existence of an obligation or duty to give gifts to other people. Gift-giving behavior is viewed as morally laudable, but it is not often seen as mandatory.

The question raised by using "gift" in this context is whether society really wants to view organ donation in this way. One answer is to examine the ways in which positive obligations, or duties, to aid other people are usually generated. Some duties to help others arise as a result of particular roles or jobs in society.

Firefighters, parents, and nurses all have special duties to render positive aid to others even when helping requires sacrifice and potential risk. Another way in which duties to help others can arise is through the act of contracting or promising. I can voluntarily promise to help someone else if the need should arise and can be blamed for my failure to do so under the appropriate circumstances (Caplan, 1998).

Neither of these arguments for positive obligations is applicable to the situation with respect to cadaver organ donation. Unless I have promised to donate an organ to another and try to renege on my promise, there would seem to be no ground for saying that I ought to be an organ donor in any sense stronger than pure charity.

There is, however, another way in which duties to help others can go beyond exceptional cases of charity or gift-giving. If it is possible for someone to do a great deal of good for another person without facing the prospect of a great deal of risk or even inconvenience, and if there is a strong likelihood of benefit for the recipient, then a duty exists that is stronger than the relatively weak obligations associated with supererogatory acts. If, for example, a strong swimmer can save the life of a drowning child merely by swimming twenty feet out into a calm lake, it would seem morally reprehensible and blameworthy for the swimmer not to do so. Indeed, it would seem odd to describe such a rescue as a charitable act, heroism, or even a gift from the swimmer to the drowning child (Caplan, 1998). Is donation after death closer to an obligation of this sort? If it is true that many can be helped by an increase in the supply of organs, and if it is also true that the dead can suffer no harm by using their tissues and organs for transplantation, then is it correct to describe a decision to donate as a gift that is praiseworthy if offered but not blameworthy if withheld? Or as an obligation that is both? Unless one holds religious views about the need to try to insure an intact body post-mortem, it is hard to see how the ability to help others could overcome a reluctance to donate. Perhaps, shifting the rhetoric of donation to duty rather than gift would increase the supply of cadaver organs (Veatch, 2002).

Dealing with Scarcity—Equity in Transplantation

The trust that is essential for public support is a product of a key ethical value: equity. The values of altruism and autonomy—the foundations of organ procurement—rest on the presumption that organs, which are given freely, voluntarily, and altruistically, will be distributed in a fair and impartial manner to those in need. Any policies, practices, or activities that suggest otherwise imperil the entire enterprise of voluntary and altruistic organ donation. There is sufficient evidence of inequity in the allocation of organs to raise doubts about the fairness of the existing system. If inequity is perceived, then trust is imperiled and donation will be adversely impacted.

The ever-present news stories of families desperately seeking funds, begging for money to pay for transplants in many nations, leave an especially bitter taste in the mouths of a public that expects altruism. If organs are requested from the rich and poor alike but given primarily to the rich, how can we expect the public to support transplantation policies?

An impressive number of papers have appeared in the past few years in professional journals maintaining that women, the elderly, the physically and mentally disabled, and minorities are not represented in the ranks of those receiving transplants to the extent that they could and should be (Reese, 2007).

Policies that give priority of access to patients on artificial heart assist devices (LVADs), or to those who require multiple organ transplants or retransplantation, leave plenty of room for doubt about what values are being used to allocate scarce organs. The tolerance of multiple listing (Sanaei, 2010)—or going to more than one transplant center to be wait-listed—by those who can afford to do so and thus gain access to a larger share of the organ donor pool, a strategy that Steve Jobs and Lou Reed used to obtain livers, is blatantly unfair. Explicit policies at some centers, which exclude some categories of patients from the prospective recipient pool because they have a history of crime, drug abuse including marijuana, or simply because they have a mental disability, give further reason for doubt about equity in the allocation of organs.

In addition, that so many hospitals and medical centers have rushed into the transplant field raises legitimate doubts about the fairness of the system for distributing organs and tissues. The competition between transplant centers to secure organs is certainly not in the public interest, especially when distribution is partly based on geography and there is little unmet need for access to a center in the United States in terms of program availability. The impression that the allocation of organs is based on bias, prejudice, favoritism, greed, geography or ability to command publicity is enough to weaken public confidence that the system is equitable. Flat rates for cadaver organ donation may reflect skepticism about the fairness for rationing what is given.

Is It Fair to Give Everyone in Need an Equal Chance to Get a Transplant?

In order to know whether the distribution of organs in the United States is fair and equitable, it is not sufficient to look at data on who did and did not get transplanted in any given year. This information is necessary but not sufficient for evaluating the fairness of the distribution. All that any pattern of distribution proves is that there may be reason for concern about inequity. The underrepresentation of minorities, the poor, the disabled, or the elderly in the ranks of transplant recipients might be unfortunate, but it might not be unfair.

To know whether the distribution of organs is fair, it is necessary to know the pattern of need for transplants. If every person is at equal risk of end stage organ failure, or if those who actually suffer organ failure of various kinds represent a microcosm of the overall American population or any national population, then any deviation from this average in the distribution of organs gives reason for concern about fairness.

A final assessment of the equity of the distribution of organs will depend on an examination of the criteria and rules (or lack thereof) being followed by transplant centers. It might be fair to give men more organs than women or whites fewer organs than blacks if the allocation were based on a set of criteria and rules that men and women and blacks and whites could all agree are fair, even if the rules work to the disadvantage of some persons or groups (Veatch, 2002).

In asking what criteria, policies, and procedures are used to allocate organs, it is tempting to seek the answer by examining what happens to a particular organ that is donated or what decisions are made on any given day in the case of a particular transplant program. But looking only at such situations conveys a very misleading impression of how allocation decisions are actually made.

The question of who gets organs is a

function of numerous factors: how many transplant programs there are, how many organ donors there are, what standards exist for evaluating the suitability of organs for transplant, how far organs and tissues can be shipped without damage, whether a person has health insurance or not, and a host of other variables. The fairness of organ allocation cannot be understood simply by watching what various surgeons or transplant centers actually do when they have the opportunity to transplant a donated organ. Transplant centers, and the surgeons who administer particular organ transplant programs within them, need to deal only with those patients who have actually made it through their doors. But many potential recipients never appear on any center's waiting list. Sometimes this is due to a failure to refer patients who are perceived as noncompliant. In other instances, the transplant team may not want to attempt a risky or novel form of transplant and may not accept a referral (deSante and Caplan, 2014). The most important ethical decisions about allocation take place long before an organ actually arrives to be used at a particular transplant center.

Justice and Rationing Scarce Organs for Transplantation

There is no consensus about what constitutes fair distribution with respect to scarce resources. There are theories of justice that would direct resources to those most likely to benefit from them, to those who are seen as most deserving, to those who are seen as likely to make the greatest social contribution in the future, to those willing to pay the highest price for them, to those who have the greatest responsibility for nurturing the lives of others, to those likely to enjoy the highest quality of life, or through a random system of allocation such as a lottery.

In health care, a strong case can be made for following a policy that maximizes the number of lives saved. Of course these lives must be of minimally decent quality since merely maintaining biological function in a body is not a standard of quality of life that most people deem worthy of medical resources. The criteria used to determine rationing schemes must be linked to the effectiveness of the resource, since the same standards may not be appropriate when one is trying to decide who gets access to a resource known to save lives, such as heart transplants, as against granting access to resources whose effectiveness is poor or uncertain, such as pancreas transplants, intestinal transplants, and lung transplants for children.

If a form of transplantation works, then it would seem that efficacy in the saving of life should drive allocation. After all, those who give organs say they do so to save lives. Those who transplant say they do so to save lives. And the reason organ transplantation has special status as a noncommodity in Western societies is that the goal of making the gift of an organ available is to save lives. If the goal is to save lives, then giving organs to the sickest persons who need them is not necessarily the best way to achieve this goal. There must be more attention paid in the future in transplant allocation policies in the United States and other nations to outcomes as well as need and urgency (Reese and Caplan, 2011).

The current set of criteria in the United States reflects a complex set of moral considerations including sensitivity to the need for efficacy shown in weighting biological factors and moving pediatric patients to the head of many organ waiting lists, fairness exhibited in giving preference for prior donation as well as to waiting time, justice in permitting some of those with no access in their home nations to enter the system from foreign nations, and deservingness in allowing the better off greater access through multiple listing and to wealthy foreigners who constitute the majority of non-US recipients. While much is made of the weight given to waiting time, no single value governs the current system of rationing.

Proponents of change in rationing criteria to give more weight to efficacy make their case based on the waste in lives and life years lost created by too much emphasis on waiting time (Hippen, Thistlethwaite, and Ross, 2011; Reese et al., 2010; Reese and Caplan, 2011). To improve survival with a transplant, a system of rules weighted toward "survival matching" could be used. This means allocating the highest-quality kidneys to the candidates with the highest-estimated post-transplant survival and allocating the remaining organs so that candidates receive the highest priority that are within ten to fifteen years, older or younger, of the donor's age (Reese and Caplan, 2011).

It is true that the current ability to forecast graft and recipient survival is far from perfect (Hippen et al., 2011). But evidence for meaningful survival is not so deficient that it could not be invoked in a general way to help guide the more effective use of the scarce supply of organs. More to the point, criticism about the limits of current prognostication variables such as age, weight, or comorbidity to predict who will do the best with a transplant does not meet the criticism that the system does not give sufficient weight to efficacy. It is merely an argument for more research toward getting evidence to achieve that end (Reese et al., 2010).

The case for moving toward more efficacy in rationing makes ethical sense relative to distributing other scarce, valuable resources.

In rationing situations, saving the most lives and the greatest number of quality life years is a strategy that is followed in rescue scenarios or when facing public health emergencies (Reese et al., 2010). Giving the greatest weight to efficacy also seems consistent with what donors intend. Shifting toward efficacy defined as both increasing the odds of saving lives and saving the most life years, while not the exclusive value for rationing, would seem to make the most moral sense in confronting limited resources. Shifting public policy to expand those limited resources and minimize scarcity is a powerful requirement in any situation where rationing exists including transplantation.

The aim of this current book is to present some select articles that will stimulate discussion on many of the topics presented above. Most articles have an extensive set of notes or references that should serve as an excellent bibliography for those pursuing one or more of these issues.

References

Abadie A, Gay S. (2006). The impact of presumed consent legislation on cadaveric organ donation: A cross-country study. *Journal of Health Economics* 25: 599–620.

Byk C. (2009). The European protocol on organ transplant: key issues. *Journal International De Bioethique* 20(3): 119–33.

Caplan AL. (1984). Organ procurement: it's not in the cards. *Hastings Center Report* 14 (October): 6–9.

Caplan AL, Coehlo DH, eds. (1998). *The Ethics of Organ Transplants*. New York: Prometheus.

Caplan AL, Prior C. (2009). *Trafficking in organs, tissues and cells and trafficking in human beings for the purpose of the removal of organs*. Joint Council of Europe/United Nations Study, Strasbourg.

Caplan AL. (2014). It is not morally acceptable to buy and sell organs for human transplantation, in: Caplan AL, Arp R, eds., *Contemporary Debates in Bioethics*. Wiley: 59–67.

Caplan AL. (2004). Transplantation at any price? *American Journal of Transplantation* 4(12): 1933–34.

Caplan, AL. (2012). Editorial position on publishing articles on human organ transplantation. *Journal of Clinical Investigation*. doi: 10.1172/JCI61904

Caplan AL, deSante, J. (2015). Can any system of rationing withstand the plea of a ten-year-old girl? in: Caplan AL, McCartney JJ, Reid DP, eds., *Replacement Parts*. Georgetown University Press.

Chandler JA. (2005). Priority systems in the allocation of organs for transplant: should we reward those who have previously agreed to donate? *Health Law Journal* 13. SSRN: http://ssrn.com/abstract=849644

Davis F, Crowe S. (2009). Organ markets and the ends of medicine. *Journal of Medicine and Philosophy* 34(6): 586–605.

DeVita M, Caplan AL. (2007). Caring for organs or for patients? Ethical concerns about the Uniform Anatomical Gift Act. *Annals of Internal Medicine* 147: 876–879.

Hippen BJ, Thistlethwaite JR, Ross LF. (2011). Risk, prognosis and unintended consequences in kidney allocation. *New England Journal of Medicine*: 1285–1287.

Hughes, P. (2009). Constraint, consent, and well-being in human kidney sales. *Journal of Medicine and Philosophy* 34(6): 606–631.

Jaycox, MP. (2012). Coercion, autonomy, and the preferential option for the poor in the ethics of organ transplantation. *Developing World Bioethics* 12(3):135–147.

Kerstein S. (2009). Autonomy, moral constraints, and markets in kidneys. *Journal of Medicine and Philosophy* 34(6): 573–585.

Kirkpatrick J, Beasley KD, Caplan AL. (2010). Death is just not what it used to be. *Cambridge Quarterly of Health Care Ethics* 19(1): 7–16.

Lawlor R. (2011). Organ sales needn't be exploitative (but it matters if they are). *Bioethics* 25(5): 250–259.

Matas A. (2006). Why we should develop a regulated system of kidney sales: A call for action! *Clinical Journal of the American Society of Nephrology* 1(6): 1129–1132.

Mayo Clinic News Network. (2013). Mayo Clinic poll shows half of Americans would consider donating a kidney to a stranger. April 17. http://newsnetwork.mayoclinic.org/discussion/mayo-clinic-poll-shows-half-of-americans-would-consider-donating-a-kidney-to-a-stranger/.

Neades B. (2009). Presumed consent to organ donation in three European countries. *Nursing Ethics: An International Journal for Health Care Professionals* 16(3): 267–282.

Quigley M. (2012). Organ donation & priority points in Israel: an ethical analysis. *Transplantation* 93(10): 970–973. doi: 10.1097/TP.0b013e31824e3d95

Reese P, Oyedeji A, Grossman R. (2007). Race and Living Kidney Donors. *Transplantation* 83(8): 1139.

Reese P, Abt PL, Bloom RD, Karlawish J, Caplan AL. (2010). Should we use age to ration health care? The case of kidney transplantation. *Journal of the American Geriatrics Society* 58(10): 1–7.

Reese PR, Caplan AL. (2011). Better off living—the ethics of the new UNOS proposal for allocating kidneys for transplantation. *Clinical Journal of the American Society of Nephrology* 9: 2310–2312.

Sanaei A. (2010). Multiple listing in kidney transplantation. *American Journal of Kidney Diseases* 55(4): 717–725. doi: 10.1053/j.ajkd.2009.11.022

Slabbert M. (2012). This is my kidney, I should be able to do with it what I want: towards a legal framework for organ transplants in South Africa. *Medicine and Law* 31(4): 617–640.

Smith MJ, Rodriguez-Arias D, Ortega I. (2012). Avoiding violation of the dead donor rule. *American Journal of Bioethics* 12(6): 15–17.

Tan HP, Marcos A, Shapiro R, eds. (2008). *Living Donor Organ Transplantation*. McGraw-Hill.

Taylor JS. (2009). Autonomy and organ sales, revisited. *The Journal of Medicine and Philosophy* 34(6): 632–648.

Veatch R. (2002). *Transplantation Ethics*. Georgetown University Press.

Wang M. (2010). Organ donation by capital prisoners in china: reflections in Confucian ethics. *Journal of Medicine and Philosophy* 35(2): 197–212.

The Dead Donor Rule, the Determination of Death, and Organ Transplantation from (Almost?) Cadavers

James J. McCartney

Replacement Parts starts with an introduction that provides a major overview of the ethical issues dealing with organ transplantation. Part I then deals with the interrelated themes of the dead donor rule, the determination of death, and organ transplantation from cadavers (or, as some of the authors in this part suggest, almost cadavers). The first two chapters are related. Koppelman suggests, for reasons of respect for autonomy and maximizing organ donation, that in the situation of organ donation from willing dying donors, the dead donor rule can and should at times be rejected. McCartney is opposed to this position, arguing that respect for persons is more than respect for autonomy and also includes protection of the vulnerable. McCartney also suggests that if the dead donor rule was known to be abandoned, fewer people rather than more would be willing to be organ donors.

The Truog et al. and Chaten chapters both argue against the dead donor role. Truog et al. argue first, in a way similar to Koppelman, that dying persons should be allowed to donate organs before death. But they also hold that brain death is not really the death of the person because it does not destroy the "integrative capacity" of the person, and that by adopting brain death as a criterion for determination of death in the law, we have effectively abandoned the dead donor rule. Truog et al. hold that this is ethically acceptable. These authors also raise questions about organ donation after cardiac death and question whether the irreversible standard of the law for determining cardiac death has really been met. Chaten argues that the dead donor rule consistently impedes physicians in fulfilling their primary duty to act for the good of their prospective donor patients, which compromises the virtue of fidelity. And he holds that it also weakens many other virtues necessary for physicians to provide excellent end-of-life care. He believes that as admirable as the dead donor rule is in theory, it provides many ethical conflicts for health care professionals in practice.

Chiong argues that, while the whole-brain criterion of death is roughly correct, the conceptual framework that its advocates have appealed to is deeply philosophically flawed. He provides a rigorous philosophical defense of what seems to be position two of the white paper of the President's Commission for the Study of Ethical Problems in Medicine and Biomedical and Behavioral Research, *Defining Death: Medical Legal and Ethical Issues in the Determination of Death* (see the Shewmon chapter below).

Magnus et al. and the chapter by Karol

Wojtyła (Pope John Paul II) both justify the acceptance of brain death. Magnus et al. emphasize that dying is a process and that denying that brain death is an important marker in that process would cause untold confusion and great legal uncertainty if it were abandoned at this point. Their argument is more pragmatic than conceptual, and they hold that it is very difficult to determine conceptually exactly when death occurs during the process of dying and that the determination of death using the criterion of whole-brain death provides a measurable and irreversible step in that process that should continue to be accepted in the law. Wojtyła seems to accept this approach since he holds that the death of the person is an event that no scientific technique or empirical method can identify directly and that the "criteria" for ascertaining death used by medicine today should not be understood as the technical-scientific determination of the exact moment of a person's death, but as a scientifically secure means of identifying the biological signs that a person has indeed died. However, he also holds that the determination of death should be a "moral" certainty and accepts brain death because in total brain death a person has lost "integrative capacity," which may mean something different in the Catholic tradition from what authors such as Truog or Shewmon mean by this phrase.

Shewmon has been a pioneer in showing that total brain failure does not destroy the body's "integrative capacity" as he understands it, and his chapter provides a history of the development of the concept of "brain death," utilizing the White Paper of the President's Council on Bioethics cited above. He holds that this paper is in many respects a refreshing, thoughtful, and comprehensive reexamination of this complex topic. His arguments agree with the section of the paper that argues that total brain failure does not indicate a person has died. These arguments are significant in that they provide justification for those like Shewmon who believe that organs should not be removed from those declared brain dead until respiration and circulation have irreversibly ceased. But they also provide justification for Truog and others to argue that the dead donor rule is a legal and ethical fiction.

Bernat's chapter raises many practical, ethical, and legal issues raised by controlled donation after cardiac (circulatory) death (CDCD) including treatment of donors before death to enhance organ viability, informed consent issues, and the importance of the decision of a patient (or a surrogate) to have life-sustaining therapy withheld always to remain independent of and unconnected to the decision to donate organs.

Wilkinson and Savulescu's provocative chapter is very strong. They conclude that organ conscription would have the greatest potential to increase the numbers of organs available for transplantation, though it would come at the cost of patient and family autonomy. If organ conscription were not acceptable, the alternative that would have the greatest potential in terms of organ numbers would be organ donation euthanasia.

The final article by Zeiler et al. discusses ethical questions related to controlled and uncontrolled non-heart-beating donation. It argues that certain preparative measures, such as giving anticoagulants, should be acceptable before patients are dead; however, when they have passed a point where further curative treatment is futile, they are in the process of dying and they are unconscious. Further, the chapter discusses consequences of technological developments based on improvement of a chest compression apparatus used today to make mechanical heart resuscitation possible.

The chapters in this part raise many important issues that relate to cadaveric (or almost cadaveric) organ donation. Most of the chapters have extensive notes or references that can be used for further study. The exception to this is the Wilkinson and Savulescu chapter in which there are no notes, but those interested in their arguments should consult their full text, which provides a great many very helpful references.

Chapter 1

The Dead Donor Rule and the Concept of Death

Severing the Ties That Bind Them

Elysa R. Koppelman

Abstract

One goal of the transplant community is to seek ways to increase the number of people who are willing and able to donate organs. People in states between life and death are often medically excellent candidates for donating organs. Yet public policy surrounding organ procurement is a delicate matter. While there is the utilitarian goal of increasing organ supply, there is also the deontologic concern about respect for persons. Public policy must properly mediate between these two concerns. Currently the dead donor (dd) rule is appealed to as an attempt at such mediation. I argue that given the lack of consensus on a definition of death, the dd rule is no longer successful at mediating utilitarian and deontologic concerns. I suggest instead that focusing on a particular person's history can be successful.

Advances in medical technology have enabled us to isolate and separate the three main components thought to be central to death—components that previously seemed to happen almost simultaneously. While one's brain, heart, and breathing used to stop functioning within moments of each other, advances in technology have enabled us to maintain the functions of some even though others have been lost. These suspended states have called into question our previous ideas about life and death. While people in PVS (permanent vegetative state) or who satisfy the criteria for brain death do not appear to fit our previous conceptions of death, neither do they fit our previous conceptions of living. Through technological advances we have created slippery areas between life and death. Or, perhaps more accurately, we have extended these states, enabling their discovery and forcing us to deal with them. Should we mourn for the patient in PVS? Should her marriage be dissolved? Can we take organs from her?

There is currently an organ shortage. While the number of patients awaiting transplants continues to increase, the number of organ donors remains virtually unchanged. The transplant community continually seeks ways to increase the number of people who are willing and able to donate organs. People in states between life and death are often medically excellent candidates for donating organs. Basic body functions can be maintained, keeping organs fresh. And taking organs from these patients will increase the organ supply. Yet public policy surrounding organ procurement is a delicate matter. While there is the utilitarian goal of increasing the organ supply, there is also the deontologic concern about respect for persons. The end of increasing the organ supply is a good one. But the goodness of the end does not justify using *any* means to achieve that end. Potential donors should not be treated as mere means to the end of organ procurement. We should not harm potential donors in the name of utilitarian goals, but we would harm potential donors by failing to treat them with respect.

We can thus characterize the concerns of the organ transplant community as the attempt to reconcile or mediate the utilitarian goal with deontological considerations about respect for persons. The question that needs to be answered is this: how can we successfully temper efforts to foster the utilitarian goal without at the same time significantly undermining that goal? Currently, decisions about harvesting organs are made according to a principle called the dead donor rule (dd rule), which tempers the utilitarian goal of increasing the organ supply on the basis of a distinction between life and death. According to the dd rule it is immoral to kill patients by taking their organs. This means that living persons cannot donate vital organs and cannot donate nonvital organs if doing so would lead to death. Advocates of the dd rule seem to suggest that life gives people a particular moral and social status that creates expectations or obligations to treat them in certain ways (even if they request to be treated differently). It is inappropriate to mourn for those who are still living. Marriages between two living people cannot be dissolved unless both parties have a voice. Increasing the organ supply by using living people only as a means is unacceptable.

If the dd rule is correct, then our definition of death has important policy implications, for the circumstances under which a person is declared dead will determine the circumstances under which her organs can be removed. This supposed connection between time of death and moral/social dilemmas has driven discussions about the meaning and criteria of death and has grounded those discussions in pragmatic concerns. Many theorists tried to "build consensus against competing concepts" of death. What had become slippery, they reasoned, needed to be regrasped. And this attempt to find consensus was given a public spin. Finding consensus was first seen as a means of "protecting physicians against the public's fear of organ thieves". But with the advent of the autonomy movement, definitions and criteria of death were "heralded as a means of protecting the public against futile and callous medical intervention" (Pernick 1999).

The attempt to develop a consensus definition of death was unsuccessful largely because this effort was entangled with other social and moral agendas. Many theorists believe that this discussion became not a matter of regrasping the definition of death in order to resolve moral and social dilemmas, but rather a matter of resolving moral and social dilemmas by playing with the definition of death. Consensus about the definition of death has not been reached, leaving questions about the moral status of removing organs in many cases unresolved—at least for those who advocate the dd rule.

The moral status of taking organs from patients who fall in these states eludes us for two reasons. First, the dd rule seems to establish an important connection between determinations of death and organ procurement that renders a conclusive definition of death vastly important for determining the moral status. However, second, the concept of death is elusive, so a conclusive definition cannot be found. The dilemmas that appear to be associated with determinations of death (like organ procurement) need to be resolved in another way. There are two main approaches to this policy problem: one may either adhere to the dd rule, with its focus on the distinction between life and death, and decide how public policy should deal with the lack of consensus, or one may rethink the dd rule and sever the connection between determinations of death and organ procurement (at least in some cases). In the remainder of this paper I discuss each of these options. I argue that the dd rule can no longer successfully mediate the utilitarian goal with deontologic considerations for patients in these suspended states, because the focus of the rule is misguided. I conclude by arguing that the apparent necessary connection between death and organ procurement is not as necessary as dd rule advocates seem to think. I suggest that by focusing instead on a particular patient's history, true respect can be given to potential organ donors without undermining efforts to at least sustain the current number of organ donors.

Lack of Consensus, Public Policy, and the Dead Donor Rule

Many theorists, such as Charo and Veatch, recognize that a definitive definition is not necessary for a sensible policy. They argue that an appreciation of the concept's ambiguity—not a quest for a conclusive definition of death—should influence policy. Can the dd rule be part of a sensible policy? There are two main ways in which the ambiguity of death can influence a public policy in which determinations of death play a central role. One is to recognize the ambiguity and embrace it. The other is to "acknowledge and discard it" (Charo 1999). Veatch supports the former view. Charo supports the latter.

Veatch and Charo both believe that death is an ambiguous concept because it is not a purely biological concept. Death is a "social, normative issue" that is influenced by "religion, metaphysics, and values" (Veatch 1999); it is a concept that is intimately tied with social or political goals (Charo 1999). Death has moral, religious, and political connotations making its extension something not purely empirical, but laden with feelings, values, and beliefs. Because of this belief about the nature of death, these theorists claim that a single moment is insufficient to justify all social and moral concerns that seem to be connected with death for all people. Both theorists share the intuition that lies behind the dd rule, claiming that we need moments of death, both socially and psychologically, but they argue that these moments differ among individuals and cultures.

Charo argues that for public policy it seems far easier to recognize and then disregard the ambiguity of death than to embrace it. She questions whether the general public can handle the ambiguity and subtle nuances needed to make personal decisions about the meaning of death. Public acceptance, she writes, "is far easier to gain by urging people to focus on a single, simple, seemingly self-evident truth." What the public needs are "simple rules that are accessible to common sense and common experience." The public has accepted "legal fictions" in the past, Charo points out, because their acceptance resolves moral or social problems in a way that exemplifies presumptions about "the hierarchy of values to be upheld in any particular situation in which they are implicated." The same approach might work for public policy surrounding death. Given the difficulties in reaching consensus on a medical definition of death, law can be used to create fictions.

For example, we have accepted the legal fiction of considering persons who have been missing for a certain amount of years as dead. Although the real status of the missing person is unknown, we have agreed to accept a set of somewhat arbitrary facts as grounds for acting as if the person is dead. We deem it reasonable to act this way in agreed-upon circumstances in part because doing so allows us to uphold certain values we believe to be important. Likewise, Charo argues, we might get the public to agree that patients in PVS can be considered dead for the purpose of resolving marital concerns. This is because some values that marriage reflects are not being met if one partner is in PVS, and the public believes that these values are important enough to outweigh any rights the PVS patient might have in this area.

Determinations of death seem to be connected to many moral and social acts. But since there is no consensus about death for all moral and social acts, Charo suggests that we accept a different point for each moral and social act that depends on death as a legal fiction and that we do so in the name of upholding important social values. Each point at which we consider a patient dead for a particular purpose needs to be easily accepted and understood by the public.

Can we use this concept of legal fiction to resolve the problem of applying the dd rule in light of our lack of consensus about death? Perhaps, it might be argued, we already have. States have adopted brain death as a kind of legal fiction. But as Charo notes, the adoption of brain death into state law has not been completely successful. While this approach has succeeded at the legislative level and has made organ procurement possible, it has failed to succeed completely at the emotional level. This failure, in part, accounts for the resistance encountered to expansion of the legal

definition of death to encompass other non-sentient states.

Why have brain death laws not been successful at the emotional level? Legal fictions work best when they go along with societal thought. They work best when they fit a kind of common-sense reality constructed by similar ontological and/or moral commitments. They work best when there is public consensus on the conditions under which it is reasonable to perform the moral or social act in question and agreement on how to determine whether those conditions obtain. As Charo puts it, legal fictions must be "simple, seemingly self-evident truths that are accessible to common sense and common experience."

The legal fiction of considering missing persons dead for resolving marital concerns is successful because there is widespread agreement that the alternative, which is to require that the spouses of missing persons put their lives on hold indefinitely, is unacceptable. There is agreement about the hierarchy of values upheld in this situation; there is a common-sense reality constructed from similar moral commitments; and there is agreement on the facts under which it is reasonable to consider a person dead for this purpose and on the evidence required to prove that those facts obtain. The public has reached a kind of consensus.

The problem with the legal concept of brain death is that there is no consensus on the state of affairs under which it would be reasonable to act as if the person were dead for certain purposes, such as removing organs or withdrawing life support. There is no common-sense reality; there is no common experience. We cannot get the public to "focus on a single, simple, self-evident truth," because there are too many alternative ontological and moral commitments—commitments that carry with them strong emotions because they are often tied intimately to one's identity or worldview. And it seems consensus is unlikely given the social, political, and normative nature of the concept of death. Legal fictions might be a good idea in some cases, but it is unlikely that they will work here. Recognizing and then disregarding the ambiguity of death simply has not been successful. So how can advocates of the dd rule respond to the fact that brain death has not been completely accepted by the public as a legal fiction?

The contrary approaches—discarding and embracing ambiguity—are reflected in a discussion on the Critical Care Medicine-Listserv (CCM-L) concerning how to approach the parents of a brain-dead child about organ donation.[1] Should you

A. tell parents that their child is dead and that the organs are being kept functioning by artificial means; or
B. tell the parents that their child is brain-dead and then explain what that means?

Aviel Roy-Shapira, who posted this question, wrote that arguments for A focused on the claim that the message of death should be unambiguous (that is, the ambiguity should be downplayed or masked) and that arguments for B. emphasized that the ambiguity cannot be masked, that "the family cannot believe a direct statement of death, seeing their beloved all rosy, with a regular heart rate on the monitor."

Many healthcare professionals downplay the ambiguity of death. Consider some of the responses to the Listserv question. One respondent wrote, "When the diagnosis [of brain death] is made I tell the family that the patient is dead, not brain-dead. [Previous discussions with the family] usually allows them to understand that even though the heart is still beating, the patient is dead." Another wrote that families need "to be treated firmly and compassionately but they do not need ambivalence." Yet another suggested that professionals never use the term *life support,* because it will "confuse relatives and can be seized on by cranks."

Downplaying the ambiguity of death is problematic. With this approach people can make decisions, but the decisions are already stacked. Getting people to adopt legal fictions by downplaying the ambiguity is clearly a means of convincing them that they are being treated with respect, but the respect is not real. Acknowledging peoples' ability to make rational choices generates true respect. Hiding what one believes to be the truth from decision makers makes this less a legal fiction and more a noble lie. We should be asking the public if it is willing to extend or revise its definition of death and if so, under what conditions. We should not be coercing people by downplaying the ambiguity and thereby denying the public the opportunity to share in the decision, because such actions represent a breach of true respect for persons. Those who take this paternalistic approach imply that most of us lack the ability to reason and need the legal system (with the help of healthcare professionals) to reason for us.

The alternative is to acknowledge the ambiguity of death and to embrace it; that is, be candid about it and let the public embrace it. This is Veatch's position. He suggests that we must tolerate pluralism in the definition and criteria of death. Given the social, normative nature of death, Veatch claims that picking any one definition as policy amounts to imposing one set of religious or moral views on everyone else. For pragmatic reasons, Veatch suggests that society choose a default definition of death. Nevertheless, death would really mean "being in a condition that an individual or culture believes is appropriate for engaging in death-associated behaviors." An individual should be free to disagree with the default position. If society chooses whole brain death as the default definition, Orthodox Jews, who rely essentially on respiratory function to determine death, should be free to disagree on the basis of their religious, moral, or social beliefs.

Veatch's view, we might think, would increase the willingness of people to participate in organ donation. People value the autonomy that Veatch's view seems to embrace. Surely if people were given a say in what it means to die they might be more willing to participate in organ donation. For example, this approach could allow parents to donate the organs of anencephalic infants. Valuing autonomy (as opposed to merely paying it lip service) is admirable. Yet embracing autonomy as Veatch suggests faces two problems.

First, should we be willing to accept just any proposed definition of death? To do so, it seems, would be wrongheaded. While valuing autonomy is admirable, we cannot value it at the expense of other concerns. Surely we would want to limit the definitions that any given person or culture can invoke. Veatch's proposal requires finding a way to limit what individuals can do in the service of their agendas. Second, for individuals to have a real choice about the meaning of death, they must have information about the ambiguous character of death. Without adequate information, there is no true choice. So this approach would require revealing ambiguities about the

nature of death to the public: ambiguities that have been downplayed or masked. The choice to participate in the organ donation process depends largely on trust. The question, then, is whether revealing the ambiguities of death to the public now, after a long history of masking the ambiguities, would undermine that trust. I believe it would. Publicizing the ambiguities might undermine the utilitarian goal of the organ transplant community by making people vividly aware of previous attempts to diminish the ambiguities. The public might well perceive that they have been lied to and denied adequate information with which to make informed choices.

One justification of the dd rule is that it fosters people's trust in the organ transplant community. By assuring the public that its rights will be protected, the utilitarian goal can ultimately be achieved. Veatch's proposed policy, if we were really concerned about the free choice of individuals, could undermine one of the reasons for adopting the dd rule in the first place. As Fost points out, "exposing the ambiguities of the current ways in which death is defined risks a public reaction that could adversely affect the fragile trust necessary for more traditional forms of organ donation" (Fost 1999).

Rethinking the Dead Donor Rule

Clearly the dd rule, with its focus on defining death, cannot successfully mediate the concerns of the organ transplant community. By truly treating people with respect within the confines of the dd rule, we risk compromising the utilitarian goal. But attempting to protect the utilitarian goal seems to work only by breaching respect for persons. This brings us to the third, and best, alternative for dealing with this problem—to rethink the dd rule. As Youngner, Arnold, and DeVita (1999) write, "Perhaps our society can accept a frank discussion about relaxing the dd rule in borderline cases better than it can tolerate efforts by the transplant community to minimize or ignore uncertainty and disagreement [about the concept of death] within the scholarly community."

At least one study suggests that healthcare professionals might be willing to do so. A questionnaire was given to transplant physicians, clinical coordinators, and medical and nursing students. It was found that 60% supported procuring organs from anencephalic and "higher brain-dead" patients, while 75% did not support procuring organs from non-heart-beating donors unless the patient was declared brain-dead before procurement began. This study suggests that current recommendations to increase organ donation by looking to non-heart-beating organ donation might be misguided and that we might look instead to anencephalic infants and those in PVS. At the very least, the author of this study claims, further ethical discussion and analysis are warranted (DuBois 1999).

I would like to further the discussion by suggesting that the focus of the dd rule is misguided. The rationale behind the dd rule is to ensure that potential organ donors are respected, because disrespecting persons is a kind of harm. But an adequate understanding of respect for persons is not achieved by making a distinction between life and death. The point of death does not mark the point at which a person can no longer be harmed. It is not life itself that entitles one to respect, but something else. The mere focus on the distinction between life and death is misguided. The dd rule seems to be missing something.

Fost rightly recognizes that there is an important connection between a particular patient's rationality or ability to set ends and using her as a means. As Kant has shown, we use people as a means only when we fail to recognize them as subjects, as people who have the ability to reason and set ends. Treating a person as a means is degrading and disrespectful only if doing so violates her ability to set ends.

Something like this idea causes some theorists to suggest that one reason for claiming that the dd rule is not applicable to patients in slippery states is that people in at least many of these states lack any interests at all. The rationale behind the dd rule, they claim, is to ensure respect for persons and this is accomplished by assuring that the ends (or interests) of potential donors are not threatened (Fost). And since people in at least many of these states lack any ends (interests) at all, the dd rule is not applicable to them. They argue, "ethical concerns about using people as mere means do not apply to persons who due to absence of cortical function lack interests altogether" (Robertson 1999). Furthermore, they claim, there is no ethical or legal obligation to aggressively treat these patients. The proponents of the dd rule, they argue, are misguided. It is not life itself that gives one moral and social status, but the ability to set ends and the ability to reason. Since people who are brain-dead or who are in PVS clearly lack this ability, they are surely not being harmed if organs are removed.

But this line of argument is also misguided. The fact that a patient is brain-dead or in PVS does not mean that she has no interests or ends. Clearly there is a sense in which there are still ends in such situations; what is absent is the person's awareness of her own ends. As Nagel argues, most harms and goods befall a person "identified by his history and his possibilities, rather than merely by his categorical state of the moment" (Nagel 1993). Consider Nagel's case of a man who is betrayed by his friends and ridiculed behind his back. Can we really say that as long as he never finds out (as long as he never suffers) he has not been injured? Some utilitarians argue that this man is harmed because he will be unhappy if he finds out about the betrayal. But this position cannot be correct, for it does not allow for an adequate explanation of why the discovery of betrayal causes suffering. Betrayal is not bad because it makes us unhappy. Rather, the discovery of betrayal makes us unhappy because it is bad to be betrayed (Nagel). Furthermore, we consider people who have no chance of discovering betrayal at all as being harmed. A person whose reputation has been ruined by lies after she died is harmed. And a person suffers misfortune if the executor of his will ignores his ends (Nagel).

Clearly, not all things we regard as good or bad are so because we are in a certain condition at a certain time. And if people who have already died can be harmed, then people who are unaware of having any ends can be harmed too. In fact, proponents of the dd rule probably recognize this and might even claim that people who are unaware of current ends are even more susceptible to harm and need greater protection. The dd rule, then, cannot be modified or rejected on the basis of the claim that certain patients lack current ends or an awareness of them.

Proponents of the dd rule claim that life itself gives patients a particular moral and social status that renders different treatment of patients with non–fully functioning brains immoral. Critics of the dd rule argue that it is current interests (a fully functioning brain) that give patients a particular moral and social status and this justifies different treatment of patients whose brains are not fully

functioning. What both sides fail to realize is that a clear line between these two groups of patients cannot be drawn. This is because both sides fail to recognize that more often than not we need to know a person's history to tell whether she is harmed.

Nagel explains this idea eloquently. He argues, "While [a] subject can be exactly located in a sequence of places and times, the same is not necessarily true of the goods and ills that befall him." Nagel examines the case of an intelligent person who suffers a brain injury that reduces him to the condition of a contented infant. We would certainly consider this a fairly substantial misfortune for the person. Yet we cannot really say that a contented infant is unfortunate. In fact, as long as his basic desires are satisfied, he is quite content. Rather, "the intelligent adult who has been *reduced* to this condition is the subject of the misfortune."

While the man with the brain injury does not mind his condition and is content, we still understand the claim that he has suffered a misfortune. The view that because he is content we have no reason to pity him now rests on a mistaken assumption about the "temporal relation between a subject of a misfortune and the circumstances that constitute it" (Nagel). If we limit our focus to the person he is now, we cannot find the misfortune. Yet if we widen our focus to include the person he was and the person he could now be had there been no accident, the idea that he has suffered misfortune makes sense. Nagel shows us here that being unaware of current interests or ends does not indicate that a person cannot be harmed. Such a person can be harmed because there are many evils "that depend on a contrast between the reality and the possible alternatives. A man is the subject of good and evil as much because he has hopes that may or may not be fulfilled, or possibilities that may or may not be realized, as because of his capacity to suffer and enjoy."

What this really shows, in part, is that a person can be harmed not only if she is used as a mere means but also if she is not treated as an end. Most harms or evils that befall a person do so because there is a lack of focus on her as a subject—as someone who can reason and who can formulate rational ends. The person whose will is not followed is harmed because her specified ends are not fulfilled—ends that in this case have outlived her.

Given this, the very ideas that underlie the dd rule are sometimes violated in our attempt to apply it. One reason for the dd rule is to ensure respect for persons. But proponents of the dd rule are misguided about the nature of respect. They claim that respecting persons amounts to not using them as a mere means. But, clearly, respect has a positive aspect also—to treat persons as ends. Some critics of the dd rule have realized this, but they, too, are misguided about the true nature of respect. The mere fact that a person is unaware of her ends does not mean that our obligation to treat her as an end disappears. When we think about respect and harm, we should not focus solely on a particular moment of time but rather on a span of time.

If a person has previously indicated that she wants to donate organs and has decided in an advance directive to forgo life-sustaining treatment if in PVS or if brain-dead, then denying her the opportunity to donate in a way that has the best chance for success is a harm. Denying her this is a form of disrespect. It is a lack of focus on her as a subject—as a person who has used her ability to reason to formulate rational ends. In this case applying the dd rule with the misguided notion of harm that informs it actually disrespects what the rule

was designed to protect. By applying the dd rule, we are failing to help patients achieve the fate that best fulfills their personhood. And this failure, especially given the implications of medical progress, reflects a moral cowardice and an abdication of our common humanity. By changing our focus we will realize that life and death distinctions are not always compatible with respect for persons. This, I think, will allow us to change from the dead donor rule to a "respect for donor" rule. Where a patient has an advance directive, taking organs from her while she is in a slippery state does not harm the donor and might, in fact, benefit her.

Of course, we must be fairly certain that changes to the dd rule will bring more benefit than harm to persons and to the transplant community (see Robertson). Thus we must ask, does this proposed change of focus from life versus death to respect versus harm successfully temper utilitarian efforts to increase the organ supply without at the same time undermining those very efforts? I have argued that if the public really understands the nature of harm and respect, then it would realize that the dd rule focuses on the wrong question. Because this notion of harm (and its corresponding notion of respect) is immersed in a notion of autonomy— something the general public easily understands and embraces as having value—it is something the public can understand and accept. One might argue that, practically speaking, not many people will insert such a donor clause in an advance directive. This might be true. Significantly *increasing* the organ supply under these considerations would certainly require some new and additional policies. But giving true respect to persons should be given priority. Furthermore, unlike with some suggestions of applying the dd rule under the life versus death criteria, giving deontologic considerations this kind of priority will surely not undermine the utilitarian goal. Changing policy for potential donors in suspended states will satisfy the main concern of the organ transplant community—it will successfully temper efforts to increase the organ supply by deontological concerns without simultaneously undermining that goal.

Without an advance directive we would have to rely on the family's understanding of the patient's history. These kinds of decisions are very complex and so are subject to error. In the absence of advance directives indicating a desire to donate, it seems we must take the default position and not allow organs to be removed from patients in these states. This is not to say that I reject surrogate decision making in other contexts. Rather, I am claiming that for the change to public policy that I am suggesting, surrogate decision making should not be allowed—at least initially. People are comfortable with surrogate decision making because they trust that their surrogate will make good decisions. But part of this trust may come from the idea that our surrogates tend to follow certain norms to which the majority of people surrounding us adhere. What we would want generally coincides with what we take to be the norm. Taking organs from these patients is not currently a norm and so might not be something patients would have even entertained as a possible choice their surrogate would have made on their behalf. Once the public clearly understands the changes to the dd rule, we may rethink this caveat.

Critics might wonder whether advance directives are even reliable indicators of the patient's goals and values. Are advance directives a reliable way to honor the life projects of a person who can no longer act on her own? This is precisely Dworkin's (1994) worry when she considers advance directives of patients with Alzheimer's. But an important distinction must be made between patients with Alzheimer's and patients in slippery states. In the Alzheimer's case patients go through phases where there is awareness that interests are still present. To use Nagel's words, patients with Alzheimer's still have categorical states of the moment and so are still capable of experiencing pleasure and pain. The concern about advance directives in this case is a concern about whether patients can adequately predict what it would be like to be a person with dementia. To make good decisions about how our future self should be treated, we must understand what these categorical states of the moment will be like. And we must have a reliable way of evaluating what we think these states would be. Cases in which a person's advance directive appears to conflict with what her later self expresses seem to indicate that these predictions might not always be correct. In these cases the crucial question is whether an advance directive must be followed when experiential interests that seem to indicate otherwise still exist. But slippery states represent a different kind of case, one where there are no new or different interests that can conflict with the advance directive. There is no categorical state of the moment.

One might claim that the differences I cited between patients with Alzheimer's and patients in slippery states are not relevant. As with the Alzheimer's case, it may be argued, patients might not adequately predict what it might be like for them to be in such a state. But this doesn't seem right. There isn't really anything that being in such a state is like, for being in such a state is like being in no state at all. And while this might be hard to imagine, we don't have to worry about making erroneous predictions as we do in the Alzheimer's case where new interests and desires are capable of being formed. There is no conflict between what the patient expressed in the advance directive and her present experiential state. Of course there might be conflict between what the patient expressed in her advance directive and the desires of her family. But this is rarely a reason to treat a person differently from how she wants to be treated. The right to autonomy, at least in some cases, should survive our ability to exercise it. Clearly, suspended states exemplify just such a case.

Will this position lead us down a slippery slope? Why limit this to patients in these states? What's to stop us from allowing a perfectly healthy person to donate a vital organ? The answer to these questions, I believe, lies with Kant. Kant holds that treating people as ends is an obligation only if their goals or projects are rational or moral. Surely it can be argued that the end of giving vital organs when not in a suspended state is almost always irrational or immoral, while the end of giving vital organs when in such a state is not. While Kant argued against suicide to relieve one's own suffering, he left open the question of whether suicide to save one's country or to escape impending madness was immoral. Ending one's life in a suspended state by donating organs seems to be more analogous to committing suicide to save one's country or to escape impending madness. There seems to be nothing irrational or immoral about that. Yet ending one's life by donating vital organs if one is not in such a state does seem immoral. Doing so, one could argue, violates the categorical imperative as it fails to celebrate or recognize one's humanity.

There seems to be nothing wrong with following an advance directive to remove organs from a person in a suspended state. Changing our focus from a distinction between life and death to respect versus harm will help us to understand that this is the case. Of course, successfully changing policy depends on "medical, ethical, *and* social conditions and perceptions" (Robertson 1999). And these conditions are not quite right yet. But working toward getting these conditions right so that the dd rule can be reformulated should be our immediate goal. The first step toward achieving this goal is to help the public to understand that the discussion between defenders and critics of the dd rule is focused on the wrong question. The question "is the patient in this suspended state alive or dead?" is misguided. The answer to this question is "it does not matter." What does matter is the particular patient's history. What matters is knowledge of her life, her values, and her ends. This is where our focus should lie, for this is how we show respect for a person no matter what state she is in. If the goal behind policy is, at least in part, to assure potential donors that they will be respected, then understanding the relationship between a person's history and respect is what is essential.

Note

1. CCM-L archives, including sources for passages quoted in this essay, are available from: http://ccm-1.med .edu.

References

Charo, R. A. 1999. Dusk, dawn, and defining death: Legal classifications and biological categories, in *The definition of death: Contemporary controversies,* ed. S. J. Youngner, R. M. Arnold, and R. Shapiro, 277–92. Baltimore: The Johns Hopkins Press.

DuBois, J. M. 1999. Ethical assessments of brain death and organ procurement: A survey of transplant personnel in the U.S. *Journal of Transplant Coordination* 9:210–17.

Dworkin, R. 1994. *Life's dominion: An argument about abortion, euthanasia, and individual freedom.* New York: Vintage Books.

Fost, N. 1999. The unimportance of death. In *The definition of death: Contemporary controversies,* ed. S. J. Youngner, R. M. Arnold, and R. Shapiro, 161–78. Baltimore: The Johns Hopkins Press.

Nagel, T. 1993. Death. In *The metaphysics of death,* ed. J. M. Fischer, 63–72. Stanford: Stanford University Press.

Pernick, M. S. 1999. Brain death in a cultural context: The reconstruction of death, 1967–1981. In *The definition of death: Contemporary controversies,* ed. S. J. Youngner, R. M. Arnold, and R. Shapiro, 3–33. Baltimore: The Johns Hopkins Press.

Robertson, J. A. 1999. The dead donor rule. *Hastings Center Report* (November–December 1999):6–14.

Veatch, R. 1999. The conscience clause: How much individual choice in defining death can our society tolerate? In *The definition of death: Contemporary controversies,* ed. S. J. Youngner, R. M. Arnold, and R. Shapiro, 137–60. Baltimore: The Johns Hopkins Press.

Youngner, S. J., R. M. Arnold, and M. A. DeVita. 1999. When is dead? *Hastings Center Report* 29(6):14–21. Winter 2003, Volume 3, Number 1.

Chapter 2

The Theoretical and Practical Importance of the Dead Donor Rule

James J. McCartney

In her article "The Dead Donor Rule and the Concept of Death: Severing the Ties that Bind Them" Elysa R. Koppelman claims to be concerned about both the utilitarian goal of increasing the organ supply as well as the deontologic concern about respect for persons (Koppelman 2002). While her concern may be genuine, I will try to show that her solution—abrogating the dead donor rule and focusing instead on particular persons' histories and interests—is misguided because respect for persons is much more than respect for personal autonomy, and because introducing ambiguity about death will make people even more reluctant to donate organs, thus destroying her utilitarian goal.

In 1979 the National Commission for the Protection of Human Subjects of Biomedical and Behavioral Research issued *The Belmont Report* (The National Commission 1979). This report was one of the first (and best, in my opinion) to articulate principles that were applicable not only for research involving human subjects, but also for bioethical issues in general. The Commission's first principle, respect for persons, is described thus:

> Respect for persons incorporates at least two ethical convictions: first, that individuals should be treated as autonomous agents, and second, that persons with diminished autonomy are entitled to protection. The principle of respect for persons thus divides into two separate moral requirements: the requirement to acknowledge autonomy and the requirement to protect those with diminished autonomy. (The National Commission 1979, 4–5)

This latter dimension, the requirement to protect those with diminished autonomy, appears to be the basis and grounding for the dead donor rule since those who are dying could easily be exploited and killed in order to achieve some admittedly worthwhile utilitarian goal (harvesting more organs). But Koppelman would argue that some who are dying are in a slippery or suspended state between life and death, and would further argue that death itself is an ambiguous concept, a position she believes other philosophers have ably shown. Thus she holds that the focus on life versus death, the basis for the dead donor rule, is misguided; and that we should focus instead on respect versus harm, not realizing that if respect is understood as broadly as it is presented in *The Belmont Report*, it is respect for human life which is at issue, not respect for personal autonomy, and the harm which the dead donor rule wants to protect against is homicide committed for the sake of a benefit for someone else and possibly even for the person herself if she has chosen it beforehand. Koppelman does understand that autonomy has its limits; however, she seems to forget that public policy in the U.S. and just about everywhere else limits that autonomy when one wishes to take one's own life or have someone else take it for him (even States that allow physician aid in dying do not allow beneficent homicide!).

This approach to public policy assumes, of course, that death is not as ambiguous as she claims. In an article published in the *Hastings Center Report* in 1998, James L. Bernat provides many persuasive arguments in defense of the whole-brain concept of death (Bernat 1998). In this article he claims that this understanding of death "now has reached a degree of societal acceptance rare for bioethical issues, one that has been sufficient for nearly all jurisdictions in the United States . . . " (Bernat 1998, 14).

What is meant by the "whole-brain concept of death"? To me it indicates that an individual organism of the human species no longer exists who recently did exist (death as event), and that this has been determined by the clinical observation that all the brain, including the brain stem, has irrevocably ceased functioning. While using the criterion of "an individual organism of the human species" as a basis for human life raises many questions at the beginning of life as I have tried to demonstrate elsewhere (McCartney 2002), I believe it raises few questions at the end of life.

I accept that the process of dying is indeed laden with many value-judgments and cultural norms and taboos, but I agree with Bernat that death itself is a biological event which can be determined more or less accurately using clinical criteria—the whole brain death criterion or cardiopulmonary criteria. Thus

it is more accurate to say that the individual has died, and that this has been determined by the appropriate clinical criteria. With this in mind, I always encourage physicians to sign a death certificate when whole-brain death has been determined—before organs are removed and even while other organ and organ systems are functioning more or less in tandem with the assistance of technology.

Pope John Paul II, leader of the Roman Catholic Christian community, has often spoken of the 'culture of death" which marks contemporary Western society. This fact notwithstanding, he has recently taught:

> (The) criterion of brain death 'consists in establishing, according to clearly determined parameters commonly held by the international scientific community, the complete and irreversible cessation of all brain activity (in the cerebrum, cerebellum, and brain stem). This is considered the sign that the individual organism has lost its integrative capacity' (Furton 2002, 455–456 and fn. #2)

This, it seems to me, is the conviction of many in our society and it is reflected in brain death statutes in the various States. Even states like New Jersey and New York accept this understanding of death, although they allow individuals to set stricter standards for determination of death (cardiopulmonary criteria) who, for religious reasons, disagree that the determination of whole-brain death is adequate to show that the organism has died.

If whole-brain death is as broadly accepted as Bernat claims, it would seem that Koppelman's solution could be opposed on strictly utilitarian grounds. What good would be gained by allowing a few people who want to donate vital organs while they are still alive to do so under the rubric of 'respect for persons,' if this would prevent the vast majority of organ donors, who want to be declared dead before vital organs are removed, from considering the possibility of organ donation at all? And while I do agree with Koppelman's laudable goal of increasing organs available for donation, I disagree with her solution on both theoretical and practical grounds as I have tried to briefly demonstrate and show.

References

Koppelman, E. 2002. The dead donor rule and the concept of death: severing the ties that bind them. *The American Journal of Bioethics* 3(1): 1–9 (2003).

The National Commission for the Protection of Human Subjects of Biomedical and Behavioral Research. 1979. *The Belmont Report: Ethical Principle and Guidelines for the Protection of Human Subjects of Research*. DHEW Publication No. (OS) 78-0112; available on line at <http://ohsr.od.nih.gov/mpa/belmont.php3>.

Bernat, J. 1998. A defense of the whole-brain concept of death. *Hastings Center Report* 28(2):14–23.

McCartney, J. 2002. Embryonic stem cell research and respect for human life: philosophical and legal reflections. *Albany Law Review* 65(3):597–624.

Furton, E. 2002. Brain death, the soul, and organic life. *The National Catholic Bioethics Quarterly* 2(3): 455–470.

Chapter 3

The Dead-Donor Rule and the Future of Organ Donation

Robert D. Truog, Franklin G. Miller, and Scott D. Halpern

The ethics of organ transplantation have been premised on "the dead-donor rule" (DDR), which states that vital organs should be taken only from persons who are dead. Yet it is not obvious why certain living patients, such as those who are near death but on life support, should not be allowed to donate their organs, if doing so would benefit others and be consistent with their own interests.

This issue is not merely theoretical. In one recent case, the parents of a young girl wanted to donate her organs after an accident had left her with devastating brain damage. Plans were made to withdraw life support and to procure her organs shortly after death. But the attempt to donate was aborted because the girl did not die quickly enough to allow procurement of viable organs. Her parents experienced this failure to donate as a second loss; they questioned why their daughter could not have been given an anesthetic and had the organs removed before life support was stopped. As another parent of a donor child observed when confronted by the limitations of the DDR, "There was no chance at all that our daughter was going to survive. . . . I can follow the ethicist's argument, but it seems totally ludicrous."[1]

In another recent case described by Dr. Joseph Darby at the University of Pittsburgh

Medical Center, the family of a man with devastating brain injury requested withdrawal of life support. The man had been a strong advocate of organ donation, but he was not a candidate for any of the traditional approaches. His family therefore sought permission for him to donate organs before death. To comply with the DDR, plans were made to remove only nonvital organs (a kidney and a lobe of the liver) while he was under anesthesia and then take him back to the intensive care unit, where life support would be withdrawn. Although the plan was endorsed by the clinical team, the ethics committee, and the hospital administration, it was not honored because multiple surgeons who were contacted refused to recover the organs: the rules of the United Network for Organ Sharing (UNOS) state that the patient must give direct consent for living donation, which this patient's neurologic injury rendered impossible. Consequently, he died without the opportunity to donate. If there were no requirement to comply with the DDR, the family would have been permitted to donate all the patient's vital organs.

Allegiance to the DDR thus limits the procurement of transplantable organs by denying some patients the option to donate in situations in which death is imminent and donation is desired. But the problems with the DDR go deeper than that. The DDR has required physicians and society to develop criteria for declaring patients dead while their organs are still alive. The first response to this challenge was development of the concept of brain death. Patients meeting criteria for brain death were originally considered to be dead because they had lost "the integrated functioning of the organism as a whole," a scientific definition of life reflecting the basic biologic concept of homeostasis.[2] Over the past several decades, however, it has become clear that patients diagnosed as brain dead have not lost this homeostatic balance but can maintain extensive integrated functioning for years.[3] Even though brain death is not compatible with a scientific understanding of death, its wide acceptance suggests that other factors help to justify recovery of organs. For example, brain-dead patients are permanently unconscious and cannot live without a ventilator. Recovery of their organs is therefore considered acceptable if organ donation is desired by the patient or by the surrogate on the patient's behalf.

More recently, to meet the ever growing need for transplantable organs, attention has turned to donors who are declared dead on the basis of the irreversible loss of circulatory function. Here again, we struggle with the need to declare death when organs are still viable for transplantation. This requirement has led to rules permitting organ procurement after the patient has been pulseless for at least 2 minutes. Yet for many such patients, circulatory function is not yet irreversibly lost within this timeframe — cardiopulmonary resuscitation could restore it.

So a compromise has been reached whereby organ procurement may begin before the loss of circulation is known to be irreversible, provided that clinicians wait long enough to have confidence that the heart will not restart on its own, and the patient or surrogate agrees that resuscitation will not be attempted (since such an attempt could result in a patient's being "brought back to life" after having been declared dead).

Reasonable people could hardly be faulted for viewing these compromises as little more than medical charades. We therefore suggest that a sturdier foundation for the ethics of organ transplantation can be found in two fundamental ethical principles: autonomy and nonmaleficence.[4] Respect for autonomy requires that people be given choices in the circumstances of their dying, including donating organs. Nonmaleficence requires protecting patients from harm. Accordingly, patients should be permitted to donate vital organs except in circumstances in which doing so would harm them; and they would not be harmed when their death was imminent owing to a decision to stop life support. That patients be dead before their organs are recovered is not a foundational ethical requirement. Rather, by blocking reasonable requests from patients and families to donate, the DDR both infringes donor autonomy and unnecessarily limits the number and quality of transplantable organs.

Many observers nevertheless insist that the DDR must be upheld to maintain public trust in the organ-transplantation enterprise. However, the limited available evidence suggests that a sizeable proportion of the public is less concerned about the timing of death in organ donation than about the process of decision making and assurances that the patient will not recover —concerns that are compatible with an ethical focus on autonomy and nonmaleficence.[5]

Although shifting the ethical foundation of organ donation from the DDR to the principles of autonomy and nonmaleficence would require creation of legal exceptions to our homicide laws, this would not be the first time we have struggled to reconcile laws with the desire of individual patients to die in the manner of their own choosing. In the 1970s, patients won the right to have ventilator use and other forms of life support discontinued, despite physicians' arguments that doing so would constitute unlawful killing. Since that time, physicians have played an active role in decisions about whether and when life support should be withdrawn, and the willingness of physicians to accept this active role in the dying process has probably enhanced, rather than eroded, the public trust in the profession.

Our society generally supports the view that people should be granted the broadest range of freedoms compatible with assurance of the same for others. Some people may have personal moral views that preclude the approach we describe here, and these views should be respected. Nevertheless, the views of people who may freely avoid these options provide no basis for denying such liberties to those who wish to pursue them. When death is very near, some patients may want to die in the process of helping others to live, even if that means altering the timing or manner of their death. We believe that policymakers should take these citizens' requests seriously and begin to engage in a discussion about abandoning the DDR.

The views expressed are those of the authors and do not necessarily reflect the policy of the National Institutes of Health, the Public Health Service, or the Department of Health and Human Services. Disclosure forms provided by the author are available with the full text of this article at NEJM.org.

From the Departments of Anesthesia and of Global Health and Social Medicine, Harvard Medical School, and the Department of Anesthesiology, Perioperative and Pain Medicine, Boston Children's Hospital—both in Boston (R.D.T.); the Department of Bioethics, National Institutes of Health, Bethesda, MD (F.G.M.); and the Departments of Medicine, Biostatistics and Epidemiology, and Medical Ethics and Health Policy, and the Fostering Improvement in End-of-Life Decision Science (FIELDS) program—all at the University of Pennsylvania, Philadelphia (S.D.H.).

Notes

1. Sanghavi D. When does death start? New York Times Magazine. December 16, 2009 (http://www.nytimes.com/2009/12/20/magazine/20organ-t.html?pagewanted =all& _r=0).

2. Bernat JL, Culver CM, Gert B. On the definition and criterion of death. Ann Intern Med 1981;94: 389–94.

3. Shewmon DA. Chronic "brain death": meta-analysis and conceptual consequences. Neurology 1998; 51: 1538–45.

4. Miller FG, Truog RD. Death, dying, and organ transplantation: reconstructing medical ethics at the end of life. New York: Oxford University Press, 2012.

5. Siminoff LA, Burant C, Youngner SJ. Death and organ procurement: public beliefs and attitudes. Kennedy Inst Ethics J 2004;14:217–34.

Chapter 4

The Dead Donor Rule: Effect on the Virtuous Practice of Medicine

Frank C. Chaten

Abstract

Objective: The President's Council on Bioethics in 2008 reaffirmed the necessity of the dead donor rule and the legitimacy of the current criteria for diagnosing both neurological and cardiac death. In spite of this report, many have continued to express concerns about the ethics of donation after circulatory death, the validity of determining death using neurological criteria and the necessity for maintaining the dead donor rule for organ donation. I analyzed the dead donor rule for its effect on the virtuous practice of medicine by physicians caring for potential organ donors.

Results: The dead donor rule consistently impedes physicians in fulfilling their primary duty to act for the good of their prospective donor patients. This compromises the virtue of fidelity. It also weakens many other virtues necessary for physicians to provide excellent end-of-life care.

Conclusions: The dead donor rule, while ethically powerful in theory, loses its force during translation to the bedside. This is so because the rule mandates simultaneous life and death within the same body for organ donation, a biological status that is inherently contradictory. The rule should be rejected as an ethical norm governing vital organ transplantation at the end of life. Its elimination will strengthen the doctor–patient relationship and foster trustworthiness in organ procurement.

The dead donor rule (DDR) maintains that it is illicit to procure vital organs from donors until after they have been declared dead. Put another way, organ retrieval cannot cause death.[1] Because donors must be declared dead prior to procurement, the DDR requires precise definitions of death. The rule and these definitions have served together as two ethical pillars for organ procurement since the 1960s. The President's Council on Bioethics reaffirmed the importance of the DDR and the legitimacy of current criteria for determining both neurological and circulatory death in 2008.[2] In spite of this report, many physicians and ethicists continue to express deep concerns about both pillars.[3, 4, 5] Franklin Miller and Robert Truog argue that the DDR can be retired, justifying this by minimal donor harm and valid consent.[6]

What has not been discussed, however, is how the DDR performs when translated from ethical scholarship in the conference room to intensive care practice at the bedside. Alan Cribb suggests that 'the virtue-theory tradition of philosophical ethics seems to be relatively well suited to the challenges of translation. By focusing on the character of agents and in particular on the cultivation and exercise of virtues, this tradition offers some account of the 'how' of ethics, that is, how can and should we shape individuals and social institutions if we want to bring about ethically desirable states of affairs?'[7] I will argue that the DDR should be rejected as an absolute moral norm governing vital organ transplantation at the end of life because its translation into clinical practice leads physicians to compromise many virtues essential to the excellent practice of medicine. Eliminating the DDR will strengthen the doctor–patient relationship and foster trustworthiness in organ procurement, both essential requirements to advance the lifesaving goals of organ transplantation.

The DDR and the Virtuous Practice of Medicine

Edmund Pellegrino, MD, has emphasized several virtues of the excellent physician.[8] If the DDR is a sound moral norm for organ transplantation, it should promote these virtues in physicians and the medical community as a whole. But it does not.

Fidelity

Fidelity is pursuing patients' best interests, not taking advantage of their vulnerability and avoiding conflicts of interest. Physicians serve their patients' best interests by promoting their overall good, not merely the restoration of their bodily health.[9] This is true especially at the end of life when physicians are unable to restore physical health. The goal of healing extends three steps beyond the physical to the good of the whole person.

- *The patient's perception of the good* considers the unique values of each patient and how that patient perceives his or her own good. Physicians promote this by respecting autonomy.

For those who donate under brain death criteria and those who die quickly enough to donate after terminal extubation under donation after circulatory death (DCD) protocols, the DDR allows physicians to promote their patient's autonomy. But the rule frustrates physicians in this duty if prospective DCD donors do not die quickly enough following terminal extubation. These patients die without their choice of organ donation respected.

- *The good for humans* is assessed by the same standard for all simply because of their common humanity. Respect and human dignity are entrenched at this level.

Proponents of the DDR emphasize respect and dignity when arguing for its necessity. John Robertson declares that 'the dead donor rule is a centerpiece of the social order's commitment to respect for persons and human life.'[10] The DDR in theory is consistent with respect. But its application often leads doctors away from respect. This is true in both neurological and circulatory death situations. For patients with irreversible apneic coma, it sometimes forces physicians to impose confusing and culturally or religiously unacceptable definitions of death. In these situations, the DDR merely cultivates a veneer of respect, one that is superficial and contingent upon the family's acquiescence to a medico-technical definition of death.

In its 1981 report, the President's Commission for the Study of Ethical and Biomedical and Behavioral Research avoided defining death using cultural or religious values because it was too impractical in the formulation of law.[11] While commissions can avoid defining death using religious and cultural values, bedside clinicians sometimes cannot. Far from disappearing, discomfort with non-traditional definitions of death has simply relocated from the conference room to the bedside. Equating brain death with death of the human being requires that patients accept a Western dualistic philosophy.[12] Many people do believe that irreversible apneic coma constitutes death. But in spite of the fact that most governments and major religions throughout the world endorse brain death, some families still define death using deeply held religious and cultural beliefs. This remains an issue at the bedside, perhaps more so in the globalized world of the 21st century than ever before. I recently cared for a Muslim child whose parents rejected the concept of brain death. They interpreted Islam's definition of death as the absence of respiration regardless of whether the respiration was provided by a ventilator or not.

Physicians do not show deep respect for patients when death is declared irrespective of the family's religious, cultural or intuitive understandings. Physicians hold the trump card; current laws usually force families to accept the medico-technical view of death. This is not to argue that patients and families should decide for themselves when they are dead. But the traditional cardiorespiratory determination of death is most respectful of the most patients because it avoids conflicting with religious and cultural beliefs.

Disrespect to DCD donors is unavoidable. The DDR compels physicians to place patients under a 'death watch' to await and then time a cardiopulmonary arrest. This practice damages donor organs.[13, 14] Sometimes these organs will not even be accepted as gifts by the recipient's transplant surgeon. Donors entrust a part of themselves to their physicians for safekeeping. The DDR then requires them to damage this gift. In no other area of medical practice do physicians knowingly damage something and then implant it into a patient. It is hard to see respect in this practice.

Proponents of the DDR argue that it promotes respect because it assures that humans are not used as the 'mere means' to another's ends, claiming that this is moral only after death.[15] This argument undermines the ethical basis of living donor transplantation. It is integral to the nature of organ transplantation that the donor is used as the means for the health of the recipient. People who donate blood, stem cells, a kidney or parts of their livers are all being used as the means to other's ends. Consent determines that while the donor must be the means to another's good ends, they are not the mere means. Choosing to use oneself or to being used as a means to another's ends is not immoral. It is the essence of helping. As Heubel and Biller-Andorno write, 'But to help . . . means to make oneself a means to another person's end. Only rational beings have the capacity to do this.'[16] When physicians deny patients the opportunity to help as much as they are able, they reduce their humanity as rational human beings. This is the case for all donors under today's DCD protocols, the ones who donate less healthy organs and those precluded from donating at all because they do not die quickly enough.

Perhaps proponents of the DDR believe that physicians are forbidden to participate in actions that cause their patients to be used as the means to other patients' ends. But when the good of patients includes using themselves as the means for others, fidelity requires their physicians to act as their agent because their overall good is at the center of the doctor–patient relationship. The rule in theory promotes respect for humans as humans, but its translation to the bedside leads to practices that do not.

- *The spiritual good* refers to how humans give ultimate meaning to their lives.

While some may donate because they consider their organs as simply spare parts, useless to them when they die (or are just about to die), many other patients donate because they consider organ donation consistent with their ultimate good. Organ procurement organizations stress altruism and the spiritual good when urging people to donate both while they are living and after a determination of their deaths.

But the DDR does not promote the spiritual good of many potential organ donors when DCD protocols prevent them from donating because they did not die quickly enough. However, it must be recognized that some patients may believe that it is unethical to donate vital organs before death and that such an action would be tantamount to suicide. These patients could still be provided an opportunity to donate under DCD protocols if they wished. Fidelity is compromised in current donation practice because physicians often are unable to fulfill their duty to serve all of the interests of dying patients.

Fidelity also requires avoiding conflicts of interest. While the DDR may appear to assist physicians in avoiding the conflict between serving their patients' good and society's need for organs, in reality it is irrelevant. This tension has been debated since the early years of organ transplantation and has not been resolved under the DDR. This was recognized when the ad hoc committee of the Harvard Medical School proposed a neurological definition of death in 1968. A British physician wrote, 'But even if the jurists achieve a new and acceptable meaning for the term "death" the problem remains. It is this: both

profession and public fear that the recipient's doctors, in the interests of their patient, may exert pressure on the donor's doctors and that the result may be that life-supporting treatment is withdrawn, or even refused, earlier than might otherwise have happened.'[17] The new fear is that the system set in place by the DDR may exert pressure on the donor's doctors to declare death earlier than might otherwise have happened. Indeed, this concern underlies the current debate over DCD, the DDR's offspring for this generation.

This is vividly illustrated by cases of heart transplantation from infant DCD donors. In order to salvage viable hearts, a Colorado DCD protocol reduced the interval between pulselessness and declaring death to just over 1 min.[18] If the same heart that drove the circulation in the donor could function in a new body, the donor's circulatory function could not have been irreversibly lost. The DDR has not protected patients from the conflict between their physician's fidelity and society's need for organs. Rather, it has enticed physicians to tinker with the limits of declaring death and in so doing claim that the ethical tension has been resolved.

One strategy to minimize this conflict is to decouple the discussion of the determination of brain death or the discussion about the decision to terminally withdraw mechanical ventilation and the later conversation about organ donation. This strategy admits that the ethical tension is not relieved by donation under the DDR and decoupling would continue in its absence. Patients would still need to be diagnosed with irreversible apneic coma before they would be eligible to donate under neurological criteria. Physicians and families would still hold the same discussions about withdrawal of life support when it no longer serves the best interests of the patients and then discuss organ donation. But these conversations would be infused with more honesty without the DDR.

Intellectual Honesty

Pellegrino writes, 'Acknowledging when one does not know something and being humble enough to admit ignorance is a virtue of healing. Knowing when to say 'I do not know' is a virtue counseled by sources as different as the Babylonian Talmud and Galileo.'[19] The DDR compromises intellectual honesty because the medical profession does not know when death occurs with enough certainty to support the transplantation enterprise, yet attempts to do so anyway.

Regardless of whether or not one accepts the validity of the current definitions of death, it seems hard to argue that the most truthful information physicians can give to a family with a loved one who meets current criteria for brain death is that he or she is in an irreversible apneic coma and will never wake up or breathe again, not that he or she is dead. For a family whose mother has chosen withdrawal of mechanical ventilation under a DCD protocol, the most truthful information is not that she is dead after 2, 5 or 10 min of pulselessness. If death is irreversible, as the public assumes and the Uniform Determination of Death Act (UDDA) requires,[20] it is premature to declare her dead. Rather, the most accurate information is that her heart likely could be restarted and that physicians do not know what neurological function might remain at the time of organ retrieval. Physicians practicing under current DCD protocols are misleading families with a diagnosis of death because this opinion rests upon a covert substitution of a permanent condition (will not be resuscitated) for an irreversible (cannot be resuscitated) one in an attempt to comply with the law. This substitution is not valid. We should recall the 1981 President's Commission's rationale for using 'irreversible' for both the neurological and cardiorespiratory criteria for diagnosing death. 'Since the evidence reviewed by the Commission indicates that brain criteria, properly applied, diagnose death as reliably as cardiopulmonary criteria, the Commission sees no reason not to use the same standards of cessation for both. The requirement of "irreversible cessation of functions" should apply to both cardiopulmonary and brain-based determinations.'[21] The commission was quite clear that irreversible has only one meaning, not two.

This is not a trivial matter. The physician–patient relationship is not equal. Physicians inherently hold power over a vulnerable patient. Physicians abuse this power when they give a different meaning for irreversible without approval of the public's representatives.

Conversations at the bedside without the DDR would not reflect absolute truth, a situation that is not unusual in clinical medicine. But abandoning the DDR would promote the truth. There are limits to the physician's ability to prognosticate death following terminal extubation. But these limits could be expanded using accepted scientific methods.

Suppression of self-interest and courage to support the good

The current discourse between organ procurement organizations and the public is tainted with self-interest. Organ procurement organizations downplay concerns over the determination of death while promoting altruistic gifting. Consider a pamphlet entitled *Religious Views on Organ and Tissue Donation* from Illinois' organ procurement organization.[22] It lists 35 organizations' and religions' views on organ donation. None are in opposition. The US Department of Health and Human Services prepared a similar document for faith leaders, urging them to promote organ donation within their congregations.[23] But both pamphlets excluded information about the religious and cultural controversies over neurological definitions of death and the timing of circulatory death when donating organs. This is a self-interested tactic. A full and open dialogue on current organ donation practices and controversies would be a stern test of the virtues of suppression of self-interest and the courage to support the good. Such a dialogue has yet to take place.

Compassion

The DDR may affect compassionate care for patients in irreversible apneic comas. Some anesthesiologists have expressed concern that patients diagnosed as brain dead sometimes respond to the surgeon's incision with hypertension and tachycardia without general anesthesia.[24] But DCD-required death watches certainly compromise compassion. The DDR insists that patients become apneic and pulseless before they can donate their organs and so must endure air hunger, anxiety and discomfort. Terminal sedation requires titrated doses of narcotics and sedatives. Inherent in this practice is some amount of pain and discomfort. If not, to what ends are physicians titrating? Once discomfort, pain and anxiety become evident, physicians and nurses do their best to minimize them. But this practice is less compassionate than assuring comfort with general anesthesia for organ retrieval and avoiding the pain and discomfort of an orchestrated death.

What is equally disturbing, and still unanswered, is what a DCD donor might experience when the surgeon removes his or her organs after only a few minutes of pulselessness. Even advocates of DCD acknowledge that this issue has not been studied adequately when they recommend that additional research is needed in 'the chronology of brain destruction after complete cessation of circulation.'[25] How can one be certain that all neurological function has ceased after a few minutes of absent circulation? In fact, we know that the primate brain, including the human, is not irreversibly damaged after this duration of pulselessness.[26] Peter Safar, MD, wrote over 25 years ago: 'The concept of the 5 minute limit of reversible cardiac arrest in patients is obsolete'.[27] Dr Safar's work has not been forgotten. The current practice of therapeutic hypothermia for neurological preservation after cardiac arrest acknowledges that the short period of cardiac arrest used in DCD protocols is insufficient to cause irreversible neurological injury.[28] Is it prudent to perform organ retrieval in these patients without general anesthesia?

The pressure to increase the pool of donor organs has wrestled with prudence, intellectual honesty and compassion that demand the answer to the question of possible donor experience after brief cardiac arrest before instituting DCD. These virtues have been compromised.

Practical wisdom

The DDR was an unexamined choice, not conceived by thoughtful analysis of alternatives or the result of wisdom obtained from the bedside. It was erected as a pillar for organ donation when transplantation was in its fragile infancy and physicians were concerned about what to do with patients on ventilators with irreversible illnesses and learning how to approach the ethics of organ donation.

This rule may have been the most pragmatic solution to the problems confronting transplantation in the 1960s. But now, even advocates of the DDR admit that the framers of our current system did not understand the implications of what they were doing and have forced physicians into imprudent practices at the bedside when declaring death. Robert Veatch, while advising that the DDR be maintained, nevertheless states:

> I readily concede that, if we could turn the clock back by thirty-five years, it might be better to adopt a different strategy. When we began to consider the legal and moral status of humans with dead brains, we chose to classify them as dead, thus conveying our conviction that it should be legal and ethical, with proper consent, to remove organs that are normally considered necessary to preserve life. In doing so without really understanding what we were doing, we adopted a new and radically different meaning of the word *dead*.[29]

Pellegrino also advocates maintaining the DDR but acknowledges that 'In place of a *prudent* [italics Chaten's] waiting period, we must declare a donor to be dead as soon as possible, by one or the other of two standards, both of which are subject to increasing uncertainty about their validity.'[30]

Conclusions

Why does the DDR perform so much better in the conference room than at the bedside? It insists that doctors should not cause death and demands respect for patients. Any rule based on those foundations should promote virtuous practice at the bedside. The problem is that the rule rests upon a contradiction. The DDR would be a sound pillar for organ transplantation if vital organs could be successfully transplanted after the traditional untimed cardiorespiratory determination of death. But these organs must be alive when they are transplanted. The DDR requires both simultaneous life and death within the same body and thus restricts vital organ transplantation to a biological state that is fundamentally contradictory. It is not possible to be alive and dead at the same time. As a work-around, physicians and philosophers have chosen to redefine death so that many parts of a human are still alive and yet the human in whom those living parts reside is actually dead. The apparent ethical power of the rule does not survive the walk from the conference room to the bedside because it does not fit the activity for which it has been constructed. The resulting work-around has compromised fidelity, honesty, suppression of self-interest, courage to promote the good, compassionate care and prudence. Any norm that leads physicians to less virtuous behavior loses ethical power. This is the case with the DDR. It should be retired.

One can argue that this would lead to even less virtuous behavior by physicians. After all, how virtuous would the practice of organ transplantation be if surgeons caused the death of the donor through the act of organ retrieval? But proponents of this argument must situate their concerns within the present ethics of living donor organ transplantation. As Kleinman and Lowy noted, 'living organ transplantation should be recognized as an ethical compromise to the principle of non-maleficence (doing no harm), given the risks healthy donors are allowed to assume. Nowhere else in medicine is a part of a healthy person removed without the procedure being of direct physical benefit to that individual'[31]

Society accepts that it is ethical for physicians to harm living donors to benefit the recipients with the donor's voluntary and informed consent. Every living donor is harmed and some die through the surgeon's actions. When considering the degree of harm that transplant surgeons inflict on living donors and the degree of harm donors would incur at the end of life without the DDR, it is hard to make the case that surgeons would harm dying organ donors more than current healthy living donors. Rejecting the DDR would change the system of organ procurement to one that relies almost entirely on living donors. This would allow the transplant community to practice under a unified ethical framework that assesses the balance between the good for recipients and the harm to donors, regardless of whether they are healthy or dying.

Others may argue that abandonment of the DDR would diminish trust in physicians and the transplantation system because of the fear that patients would become vulnerable to being killed for their organs. Embedded in this fear is the issue of the physician's intention. Perceptions about intention directly relate to the patient's trust in the character and virtue of their physician. Trust is at the core of both the doctor–patient relationship and the public's acceptance of organ transplantation. Theorists on trust have identified several physician attributes that promote trust: fidelity, competence, honesty and confidentiality.[32] Unfortunately, fidelity and honesty have been two of the virtues most compromised by the DDR. This has obvious implications for public trust in current organ donation practice. The best way to gain the public trust for organ transplantation is to promote *trustworthiness* in the physicians at the bedside of dying patients. Our current system does not.

At the same time, advocates of vital organ donation without the DDR must place clear boundaries on this practice. It should be restricted to the same patients currently eligible to donate organs at the end of life: patients diagnosed with irreversible apneic coma and patients who are removed from mechanical ventilation expected to die soon thereafter. The slippery slope concern over this system is valid but no more slippery than our current system.

The DDR has been described as 'the ethical linchpin of a voluntary system of organ donation, and helps maintain public trust in the organ procurement system.'[33] But the practice of organ transplantation with this supposed linchpin has led to constant erosion in many virtues integral to the excellent practice of medicine. If this rule is truly a linchpin for the public acceptance of organ donation, we must recognize and accept the tremendous cost it imposes on the physician–patient relationship of potential organ donors. Before accepting this cost, it would be prudent to promote an open public discourse about whether the DDR is vital to the public's trust. The public might embrace the idea that it is ethically acceptable and preferable for dying patients to donate vital organs on the last day of their lives rather than on the first day of their deaths.

Competing interests: None.

Provenance and peer review: Not commissioned; externally peer reviewed.

Notes

1. Veatch RM. Abandon the dead donor rule or change the definition of death? *Kennedy Inst Ethics J* 2004; 14:261–76.

2. President's Council on Bioethics: Controversies in the Determination of Death: A White Paper by the President's Council on Bioethics. Washington, DC, 2008. http://bioethics.georgetown.edu/pcbe/reports/death/index.html (accessed 19 Nov 2012).

3. Collins M. Reevaluating the dead donor rule. *J Med Philos* 2010; 35:154–79.

4. Rodriguez-Arias D, Smith MJ, Lazar NM. Donation after circulatory death: burying the dead donor rule. *Am J Bioeth* 2011; 11:36–43.

5. Joffe AR, Carcillo J, Anton N, et al. Donation after cardiocirculatory death: a call for a moratorium pending full public disclosure and fully informed consent. *Philos Ethics Humanit Med* 2011; 6:17.

6. Miller FG, Truog RD. *Death, dying, and organ transplantation: reconstructing medical ethics at the end of life.* Cary, NC: Oxford University Press, 2011.

7. Cribb A. Translational ethics? The theory-practice gap in medical ethics. *J Med Ethics* 2010; 36:207–10.

8. Pellegrino ED. Professionalism, profession and the virtues of the good physician. *Mt Sinai J Med* 2002; 69:378–84.

9. Pellegrino ED. The internal morality of clinical medicine: a paradigm for the ethics of the helping and healing professions. *J Med Philos* 2001; 26:559–79.

10. Robertson JA. The dead donor rule. *Hastings Cent Rep* 1999; 29:6–14.

11. President's Commission for the Study of Ethical Problems in Medicine and Biomedical and Behavioral Research. *Defining death: medical, legal and ethical issues in the determination of death.* Washington, DC: U.S. Government Printing Office, 1981.

12. Keenan JF. Dualism in medicine, christian theology, and aging. *J Religion Health* 1996; 35:33–45.

13. Jay CL, Lyuksemburg V, Ladner DP, et al. Ischemic cholangiopathy after controlled donation after cardiac death liver transplantation: a meta-analysis. *Ann Surg* 2011; 253:259–64.

14. Mathur AK, Heimbach J, Steffick DE, et al. Donation after cardiac death liver transplantation: predictors of outcome. *Am J Transplant* 2010; 10:2512–19.

15. Khushf G. A matter of respect: a defense of the dead donor rule and of a "Whole-Brain" criterion for determination of death. *J Med Philos* 2010; 35: 330–64.

16. Heubel F, Biller-Andorno N. The contribution of Kantian moral theory to contemporary medical ethics: a critical analysis. *Med Health Care Philos* 2005; 8:5–18.

17. Wingate D. Definition of death. *BMJ* 1968; 2:363.

18. Boucek MM, Mashburn C, Dunn SM, et al. Pediatric heart transplantation after declaration of cardiocirculatory death. *N Engl J Med* 2008; 359:709–14.

19. Pellegrino ED. Toward a virtue-based normative ethics for the health professions. *Kennedy Ins Ethics J* 1995; 5:253–77.

20. National Conference of Commissioners on Uniform State Laws: The Uniform Determination of Death Act. http://pntb.org/wordpress/wp-content/uploads/Uniform-Determination-of-Death-1980_5c.pdf (accessed 19 Nov 2012).

21. President's Commission for the Study of Ethical Problems in Medicine and Biomedical and Behavioral Research. *Defining death: medical, legal and ethical issues in the determination of death.* Washington, DC: US Government Printing Office, 1981.

22. Gift of Hope Organ and Tissue Network: *Religious Views on Organ and Tissue Donation.* Itaska, IL.

23. United States Department of Health and Human Services Health Resources and Services Administration: Sharing the Gift of Life: A Resource Guide for Faith Leaders on Organ and Tissue Donation and National Donor Sabbath. August 2010. http://www.organdonor.gov/materialsresources/donorsabbathmaterials.html (accessed 18 Mar 2013).

24. Young PJ, Matta BF. Anesthesia for organ donation in the brainstem dead-why bother? *Anesthesia* 2000; 55: 105–6.

25. Bernat JL, Capron AM, Bleck TP, et al. The circulatory-respiratory determination of death in organ donation. *Crit Care Med* 2010; 38:963–70.

26. Wolin LR, Massopust LC, Taslitz N. Tolerance to arrest of cerebral circulation in the rhesus monkey. *Exp Neurol* 1971; 30:103–15.

27. Safar P. Cerebral resuscitation after cardiac arrest: a review. *Circulation* 1986; 74:138–53.

28. Testori C, Sterz F, Holzer M, et al. The beneficial effect of mild therapeutic hypothermia depends on

the time of complete circulatory standstill in patients with cardiac arrest. *Resuscitation* 2012;83:596–601.

29. Veatch RM. The dead donor rule: true by definition. *Am J Bioeth* 2003; 3:10–11.

30. Pellegrino ED. Personal Statement of Edmund Pellegrino, M.D.: Controversies in the Determination of Death. http://bioethics.georgetown.edu/pcbe/reports/death/pellegrino_statement.html (accessed 3 Feb 2012).

31. Kleinman I, Lowy FH. Ethical considerations in living organ donation and a new approach: an advance-directive organ registry. *Arch Intern Med* 1992; 152: 1484–8.

32. Hall MA, Dugan E, Zheng B, et al. Trust in physicians and medical institutions: what is it, can it be measured, and does it matter? *Milbank Q* 2001; 79:613–39.

33. Robertson JA. The dead donor rule. *Hastings Cent Rep* 1999; 29:6–14.

Chapter 5

Brain Death without Definitions

Winston Chiong

Until recently, "brain death" was widely regarded as one of the crowning conceptual achievements of bioethics. After all, less than four decades after the whole-brain criterion of death was first proposed, it has come to supplant the traditional, cardiopulmonary criterion of death throughout much of the world. Not only doctors but also lawmakers and religious authorities have embraced the view that we die when our brains irreversibly cease to function, not, as earlier times had it, when our hearts and lungs irreversibly cease to function. This revolution in our thinking about human death has had profound practical implications. It has opened the way to vital organ donation and unilateral withdrawal of treatment from patients with beating hearts but no hope of recovering brain function.

In recent years, however, the whole-brain criterion of death has come under increasing criticism, and a growing consensus has developed among bioethicists and philosophers that brain death is actually incoherent. While the proponents of brain death have typically defended it on the grounds that the brain is necessary for the integrated functioning of the organism as a whole, recent findings appear to contradict this claim.[1] Furthermore, extensive study of the "brain dead" has shown that even

after the standard battery of diagnostic tests for brain death has been fulfilled (including documentation of coma, the absence of brainstem reflexes, and the absence of respiratory effort), many brain functions persist—including such presumably integrative functions as hormone secretion and thermoregulation.[2]

These apparent inconsistencies have led even one of brain death's most prominent defenders to admit that "Brain death was accepted before it was conceptually sound."[3] I will argue in this paper that, while the whole-brain criterion of death is roughly correct, the conceptual framework that its advocates have appealed to is deeply philosophically flawed. In their arguments in support of the whole-brain criterion, the advocates of brain death have appealed to a misguided philosophical model of what is required for the justification of a criterion of death, which their opponents have adopted and turned against them. This model depends on some claims about language that, while initially plausible, have been seriously undermined by Ludwig Wittgenstein, Saul Kripke, and Hilary Putnam, whose arguments most philosophers of language regard as decisive. Drawing upon their insights, and also upon promising recent work in the philosophy of biology, I propose a new model for our understanding of life and death, which I argue provides a more secure justification for the whole-brain criterion.

The Challenge to the Whole-Brain Criterion

According to the whole-brain criterion of death, a person dies when the whole brain irreversibly ceases to function. Coma, absence of respiratory effort, and absence of brainstem reflexes are the standard tests for the loss of whole-brain function. The two main alternatives to the whole-brain criterion are the higher-brain criterion and the traditional cardiopulmonary criterion. Advocates of the higher-brain criterion claim that it is not the irreversible loss of the functioning of the whole brain, but only of the neocortex—the part of the brain responsible for consciousness, memory, personality, and perception—that is necessary and sufficient for death. This criterion would only require permanent unconsciousness for the declaration of death, dismissing lower-brain functions such as respiratory drive and brainstem reflexes as irrelevant. Advocates of the cardiopulmonary criterion, on the other hand, claim that the irreversible loss of circulatory functioning and the irreversible loss of respiratory functioning together are necessary and sufficient for death. As the cardiopulmonary criterion is usually interpreted, it does not matter whether these functions are carried out spontaneously or via external measures (such as a ventilator or chest compressions). Thus, according to the cardiopulmonary criterion, a patient without brain function and therefore without respiratory drive can be kept alive on a ventilator in the absence of spontaneous breathing, while the whole-brain and higher-brain criteria would class such a patient as dead.

Given the abstract character of debates over the nature of death, how can we hope to make any progress in deciding between these criteria? In an influential early series of articles in support of the whole-brain criterion, James Bernat, Charles Culver, and Bernard Gert offered a framework for resolving these disputes, which I call the *definitions-criteria-tests* model. Bernat set out this framework as follows:

> This analysis of brain death should be conducted in three sequential phases: (1) the philosophical task of making explicit the *definition* of death that is implicit in our traditional conception of death; (2) the combined philosophical and medical task of identifying the *criterion* of death—that generally determinable standard that shows that the definition is satisfied by being both necessary and sufficient conditions for death; and (3) the medical task of devising a set of bedside *tests* to show that the criterion of death has been fulfilled. Thus, the optimal sequence of argument must proceed from the intangible and conceptual to the tangible and measurable.[4]

On this model, the primary philosophical problem is to arrive at the correct "definition" of death—presumably as a result of something like a conceptual analysis of our ordinary notion of death. Such a definition, intended to cover all literal biological uses of our English word "death," is supposed to be general and devoid of specific reference to human physiology; for instance, *the permanent cessation of the integrated functioning of the organism as a whole*, or *the departure of the animating or vital principle*. Once we have the proper definition, we may then proceed to a more practical level, arriving at a species-specific "criterion" of death that gives necessary and sufficient conditions for satisfying the definition of death in human beings.[5] Finally, with this criterion in hand, we can devise clinical "tests" that indicate when the criterion has been satisfied.

Bernat and other proponents of the whole-brain criterion have appealed to a definition of death as the permanent cessation of the integrated functioning of the organism as a whole, by which they mean "that set of vital functions of integration, control, and behavior that are greater than the sum of the parts of the organism, and that operate in response to demands from the organism's internal and external milieu to support its life and to maintain its health."[6] With this definition in hand, they have gone on to make the empirical claim that the destruction of the whole brain is necessary and sufficient for satisfying this definition in human beings—because the brain is the "master organ" or "critical system" that integrates the activities of the other organs into a cohesive whole.[7]

However, the empirical claim that the loss of whole-brain function is necessary and sufficient for the cessation of integrated functioning has since been cast into doubt, prompting a revival of interest in the cardiopulmonary criterion. Given advances in critical care, it is now possible to maintain bodies for long periods after they meet clinical tests for brain death, during which they exhibit numerous forms of integration and control that are "greater than the sum of the parts of the organism" and demonstrate functional responsiveness to their physiological milieu. Alan Shewmon has published a report identifying 175 cases in which the bodies of patients reliably diagnosed as fulfilling the whole-brain criterion were maintained for at least one week (and in rare cases years), sometimes with little aggressive intensive care besides mechanical ventilation.[8] These bodies exhibit a "litany of non-brain-mediated somatically integrative functions," including

- homeostasis of a limitless variety of physiological parameters and chemical substances; assimilation of nutrients;
- elimination, detoxification, and recycling of cellular wastes;
- energy balance;
- maintenance of body temperature (albeit subnormal);
- wound healing;
- fighting of infections and foreign bodies;
- development of a febrile response to infection (albeit rarely);
- cardiovascular and hormonal stress responses to incision for organ retrieval;
- successful gestation of a fetus (as in thirteen pregnant women of the prolonged survivors);
- sexual maturation (in two prolonged-surviving children); and
- proportional growth (in three children).[9]

Some defenders of the whole-brain criterion have responded by attempting to narrow the sense of "integrated functioning" so that it refers not to these functions, but only to functions that are in fact carried out by the brain. For instance, Bernat has proposed a defense of the whole-brain criterion that appeals to "critical functions," by which he means functions that are necessary for the continued health and life of the organism.[10] But since it is unclear whether only brain functions satisfy this standard, or why this standard should be preferred to the broader reading of "integrated functioning," this move has struck many critics as ad hoc.

On these grounds, advocates of the cardiopulmonary criterion have argued that the whole-brain criterion is not sufficient for the permanent cessation of integrated functioning. Instead, Shewmon's cases suggest that the irreversible loss of circulatory and respiratory functioning is necessary and sufficient for satisfying this definition of death. Thus, if the definitions-criteria-tests model is right, and if the correct definition of death is the permanent cessation of integrated functioning, then it seems that the traditional cardiopulmonary criterion is the proper criterion for human death.

Intuitive Grounds for Doubt

Ultimately, however, it is not the whole-brain criterion but the definitions-criteria-tests model that must be given up. At the level of definitions, there neither is nor need be any general feature that defines death, and at the level of criteria, there are no necessary and sufficient conditions for an organism's being dead.

Although a definition of death as "the permanent cessation of integrated functioning" would favor the cardiopulmonary criterion, there are strong intuitive grounds to reject this conclusion: the cardiopulmonary criterion gives no intrinsic consideration to consciousness as a characteristic of biological life, but on a commonsense view an organism's being conscious, in itself, counts very strongly in favor of its being alive. Consider the following example.

In many cases of sudden cardiac arrest, the victim remains conscious for several seconds after blood stops flowing to the brain. This would also be true of someone who suffered an *irreversible* cardiac arrest while simultaneously suffering a second injury that irreversibly stopped respiration. On any ordinary understanding of life, this double victim

would clearly remain alive as long as he remains conscious; if he managed to mouth a few words or flail around before lapsing into unconsciousness, we would have little inclination to say that these words and actions were produced by a dead organism (a sort of animated corpse?); we would say instead that they were produced by an organism in the process of dying. Yet on the cardiopulmonary criterion he is dead when he suffers the irreversible loss of circulation and respiration, regardless of whether he briefly retains consciousness.

We should note that this is not only a counterexample to the cardiopulmonary criterion, but also to a definition of death as the permanent loss of integrated functioning. Quite plausibly, an organism that can no longer breathe or circulate blood is no longer functioning in an integrated way. If this is right, then in this case the permanent loss of integrated functioning does not amount to death. Furthermore, this counterexample does not rely upon special assumptions about human consciousness, self-consciousness, or personhood. If mice also retain consciousness for several seconds after sudden cardiac arrest, we would be just as inclined to judge that they remain alive so long as they are conscious.

This suggests that something's being conscious is, in itself, a strong indicator that it is a living organism. Some might then suggest abandoning Bernat's proposed definition of death as the loss of integrated functioning in favor of a definition of death as the permanent loss of consciousness. Such a definition would favor the higher-brain over the whole-brain criterion: the destruction of the whole brain is not necessary for the permanent loss of consciousness, as the destruction of the neocortex is sufficient. However, there are counterexamples to this criterion and definition even more serious than the counterexamples to the cardiopulmonary criterion raised earlier. Brain injuries that destroy the neocortex while sparing the brainstem produce persistent vegetative states (PVS). Those in PVS are not conscious, but often show other classic signs of biological life—including spontaneous breathing and sleep/wake cycles (when "awake" they are not conscious, but are generally more active), and in virtue of brainstem reflexes they may cough when their throats are irritated, blink when their corneas are touched, and swallow food that is placed in their mouths. I think it intuitively clear that an organism that breathes spontaneously, has circadian rhythms, and exhibits these complex (though nonconscious) responses to stimuli is not dead on any ordinary understanding of life and death—strongly suggesting that the irreversible loss of consciousness also does not amount to death.

Against the Definitions-Criteria-Tests Model

These cases ground strong intuitive objections to the cardiopulmonary and higher-brain criteria, and also to the definitions that would most naturally be taken to justify them. They also undermine an idea implicit in the definitions-criteria-tests model: that there is some special characteristic common to all living or to all dead things, in virtue of which they are alive or dead. In the sudden cardiac arrest case, what seems to guide our judgment about whether the victim is alive or dead is the presence of consciousness. But in the PVS case, our judgments about life and death seem to track different characteristics entirely—most notably, the presence of spontaneous respiration, irrespective of the presence of consciousness. Taken together, these cases suggest that the irreversible loss of consciousness *and* the

irreversible loss of spontaneous respiration are each individually necessary for death—neither is sufficient on its own. This finding echoes claims made by defenders of the brainstem criterion of death, which is closely related to the whole-brain criterion and has been adopted in the United Kingdom. (The brainstem criterion can be thought of as the anatomical converse of the higher-brain criterion, with the rationale that while neocortical function is necessary for consciousness, brainstem activation is also required for consciousness as well as for the nonconsciously mediated behavior observed in PVS.) As Christopher Pallis and D.H. Harley write, "We consider human death to be a state in which there is irreversible loss of the capacity for consciousness combined with irreversible loss of the capacity to breathe spontaneously (and hence to maintain a spontaneous heartbeat). Alone, neither would be sufficient."[11]

Critics of the brainstem criterion have claimed that this rationale for a criterion of death does not satisfy the definitions-criteria-tests model because the definition offered is not theoretically unified. For instance, Shewmon has complained that "apneic coma as a *concept of death* is completely idiosyncratic, pulled out of philosophical thin air."[12] Similarly, Baruch Brody argues that "Neither a purely respiratory criterion nor a combined respiratory/consciousness criterion lends itself to a justifying definition. The former criterion involves only one of the traditional vital 'bodily fluids,' and it is hard to see why one is to be preferred to the other. The latter criterion comes from two very different definitions, and it is hard to see why the two criteria should be combined."[13] Shewmon and Brody thus insist that a criterion for death appeal to a nonidiosyncratic, unified "justifying definition." But what underlies this demand for a unified definition of death—particularly when this demand seems to conflict with our best intuitions about cases?

This requires a bit of reconstruction, but I think the best available rationale for this demand, and indeed for the entire definitions-criteria-tests model, relies upon a natural but flawed picture of rigorous theoretical investigation. The picture goes something like this: if we're going to investigate some phenomenon X (such as death), we must begin with a definition of the term "X" that serves both metaphysical and semantic purposes. Metaphysically, the definition of "X" is supposed to give us a unified account of *what it is* for something to be X (rather than, say, Y or Z) and thus an account of the truth-conditions of the claim that one or another particular thing is X. Otherwise, we wouldn't think that such a definition would help us to find the characteristic or characteristics that all Xs have in common that is necessary and sufficient for being X. Semantically, the definition of "X" is supposed to explain how, when we use the term "X," we succeed in referring to things that are X rather than things that are not X—the idea being that there is some implicit concept or mental content associated with the term "X" that picks out the common characteristic that is definitive of Xs. Otherwise, we wouldn't expect conceptual investigation of our traditional understanding of X to be of much use in revealing the nature of X.

This *descriptivist* picture of how terms like "death" work was similarly dominant within analytic philosophy of language and philosophy of science until the 1970s. One early challenge to this picture concerns the metaphysical role that these definitions are supposed to play. When theorists present "definitions" of death like *the permanent cessation of the integrated functioning of the organism* or *the irreversible loss of consciousness*, they are attempting to tell us what is common to all dead things in virtue of which they are dead—we might say they are attempting to state the *essence* of death. However, as Wittgenstein famously argued, in natural languages we find many terms for which there is no essential characteristic that determines whether the term applies in a given case. Consider his refusal to offer a unified definition of a "language-game":

> Instead of producing something common to all that we call language, I am saying that these phenomena have no one thing in common which makes us use the same word for all,—but that they are *related* to one another in many different ways. And it is because of this relationship, or these relationships, that we call them all "language". I will try to explain this.
>
> Consider for example the proceedings that we call "games". I mean board-games, card-games, ballgames, Olympic games, and so on. What is common to them all?—Don't say: "There *must* be something common, or they would not be called 'games'"—but *look and see* whether there is anything common to all.—For if you look at them you will not see something that is common to all, but similarities, relationships, and a whole series of them at that. To repeat: don't think, but look!—Look for example at board-games, with their multifarious relationships. Now pass to card-games; here you find many correspondences with the first group, but many common features drop out, and others appear. When we pass next to ballgames, much that is common is retained, but much is lost.[14]

These points are directed against philosophers who would demand a unified definition of what it is for something to be a game, and can be extended to bioethicists who, appealing to the definitions-criteria-tests model, demand a unified definition of death or life. The terms we use don't always require any such shared, essential characteristic to do their work.

Still more serious objections to this style of descriptivism were later presented by Saul Kripke and Hilary Putnam, who attacked the semantic role that such definitions had been thought to play. On the descriptivist model, the reference of terms like "life" and "death" is fixed by our implicit mental association of these terms with definitions that specify essential features of their referents. In other words: on this view, what enables me to use the word "death" to make claims about dead things is my grasp of some description that tells me what it *means* for something to be dead. Here Kripke argued that the mental contents associated with certain terms, particularly proper names and natural kinds, may be merely contingent or even entirely mistaken. To cite Kripke's most famous example: it could be that all of the descriptions that we use to identify Gödel are in fact not true of Gödel but instead of some more obscure mathematician; but even if this were so, in using the term "Gödel" we would still be talking about Gödel rather than his colleague.[15]

Putnam extended Kripke's suggestion that the reference of terms does not depend solely on the mental contents of the speaker, but also on contingent causal connections between the speaker and the world, the nature of which may even be inaccessible to the speaker.[16] On this view, philosophical analysis of the mental contents or concepts associated with a term may be quite irrelevant, in itself, to discovering necessary and sufficient conditions for the term's application. Instead, Putnam suggested that these mental contents or concepts might

merely provide "operational definitions" rather than essential ones: ways of picking out the referents of our terms that appeal to contingent rather than necessary and sufficient characteristics of their referents. So an English speaker before the advent of chemistry, who would have been ignorant of the fact that what *makes* something water is having the chemical composition H2O, could still refer to water by conceiving of it under some contingent description— as the primary constituent of the lakes and rivers of the actual world, for example, or as the primary constituent of some paradigmatic sample of water. Furthermore, an analysis of this speaker's "definition" of water wouldn't, in itself, get us very far in trying to find out what makes something water (that is, being H2O): this is a matter for empirical rather than conceptual investigation.

Similarly, armchair theoretical investigation of our ordinary concepts of death is unlikely to help us decide among possible criteria of death. Linguistic terms can be successfully used to refer even when the mental contents associated with them only contingently pick out their referents, and sometimes when these contents do not even truly apply to their referents. For instance, even if there is no such thing as an immaterial soul, someone whose concept of death is *the departure of the immaterial soul from the physical body* might nonetheless succeed in referring to the dead rather than the living—perhaps by deferring to authorities in her community, or by having false beliefs about the relationship of the soul to the physiological features that actually are involved in death, or by deferring to authorities with such beliefs.

A further advantage of this approach to the semantics of "life" and "death" is that it allows that people might have different concepts or mental contents associated with the terms "life" and "death" and yet still be talking about the same things. It's quite plausible to me that people in different cultures and times, and often in the same culture and at the same time, have different concepts of life and death. But we still want to be able to say that (for example) a vitalist and a materialist are actually disagreeing about the nature of life, not merely talking about two different things.

Taken together, I believe that the arguments of Wittgenstein, Kripke, and Putnam together show the definitions-criteria-tests model, and the associated demand for a unified justifying "definition," to be deeply philosophically flawed. The right way to argue for a given criterion of death is not to argue that it fits some singular "definition" of life or death that results from any conceptual analysis of these terms. Metaphysically, it may be that there is no shared characteristic common to all dead things in virtue of which they are dead; and semantically, the concepts or mental contents that we associate with death may merely be operational definitions that appeal to accidental features rather than to necessary and sufficient conditions for death. We ought, therefore, to seek some alternative theoretical model that can make sense of our best intuitive responses to cases —such as the cardiac arrest and PVS cases.

Life and Death as Cluster Kinds

When we give up the idea that criteria for death must be backed by a unified definition of death, we can abandon the claim that there need be any single characteristic, or even any conjunction of characteristics, that is both necessary and sufficient for an organism to be alive or dead. Indeed, cases like the cardiac arrest and PVS cases lead me to suspect that no single characteristic works this way; instead,

the property of being alive (like the property of being a language or a game) involves a cluster of characteristics—none of which is in itself necessary and sufficient for an organism to be alive, but all of which contribute to an organism's being alive and tend to reinforce one another in paradigm cases. To list some important examples:

1. consciousness;
2. what might be called, at the risk of circularity, spontaneous vital functions, which may vary from species to species (where "vital" means those functions that are necessary for the persistence of the other functions of the organism and "spontaneous" means that these functions are regulated and maintained by activities that are internal rather than external to the organism[17]);
3. behavior—that is, functional responsiveness to environmental stimuli, regardless of the presence of consciousness;
4. integrated and coordinated functioning of multiple subsystems— a certain degree of organizational complexity and coherence;
5. the ability to resist decay and putrefaction;
6. the capacity to reproduce; and
7. the capacity to grow via the assimilation of nutrients.

No doubt this list is incomplete, but I take it as a start. None of these characteristics appears necessary for life: the cardiac arrest victim might only exhibit the first feature, while those in PVS lack it. But at the same time, at least in paradigm cases of living things, these characteristics are related: they tend to be mutually supporting and reinforcing. For instance, in higher animals (we suspect), consciousness contributes to an organism's functional responsiveness to its environment, which helps it to respond to situations in ways that support its spontaneous vital functions and the coordination of its subsystems, which in turn support the structures necessary for consciousness and behavior.

In this proposal I appeal to Richard Boyd's influential recent work in the philosophy of biology, and more specifically to the distinction between natural kinds (or "real kinds") and nominal kinds. Natural kinds involve categories that occur in nature and independently of human interests (such as "water" or "tigers"), while nominal kinds involve categories that we take to be useful or otherwise answer to human interests ("chair" or "salad fork"). Traditionally, realists about natural kinds have held that the members of natural kinds, unlike those of nominal kinds, are unified in virtue of having in common some intrinsic characteristic or set of characteristics that is necessary and sufficient for membership.[18]

If this traditional understanding of natural kinds is correct, then the following objection could be raised to the cluster theory of life and death that I have proposed: "Languages and games are human inventions, but life and death are not human inventions. It's acceptable that languages and games don't involve shared, necessary, and sufficient membership conditions because there's no *objective*, mind-and-language-independent fact of the matter whether something is a language or game anyway. However, life and death are matters of biological fact, independent of human purposes and intentions, and therefore there must be shared, necessary, and sufficient conditions for something's being alive or dead."

However, this traditional conception of natural kinds has also been recently undermined. It turns out that almost none of the categories investigated in biology, nor in most of the other special sciences—such as psychology, meteorology, astronomy, economics, or linguistics— involve shared intrinsic characteristics that are necessary and sufficient for membership. The most-discussed controversy is over species. Michael Ghiselin and David Hull have argued on evolutionary grounds that species do not involve this sort of necessary and sufficient membership condition—for instance, there needn't be any special characteristic that tigers all have in common that makes it the case that they're all tigers—and therefore are not categories or *kinds*, but in fact are massively spatiotemporally extended *individuals* composed of numerous organisms.[19] But this proposal faces serious objections of its own, and it is difficult to see how it might be generalized to other categories in the special sciences that are also taken to be natural kinds but are not spatiotemporally continuous in the way that species may be.

In a recent series of papers, Richard Boyd has proposed an alternative understanding of natural kinds that does not involve necessary and sufficient membership conditions, but instead appeals to what he calls "homeostatic property clusters."[20] These are Wittgensteinian families of properties that tend to be nonaccidentally co-instantiated, in that something's possessing some of the properties in the cluster makes it more likely that it will also possess the other properties in the cluster. Boyd has argued that a number of biological categories (not only biological species, but also the higher taxa) involve homeostatic property clusters, as do many of the categories studied in economics and geology.

This proposal shows that cluster kinds can be natural kinds: that categories can occur in nature prior to our classificatory schemes without any intrinsic characteristic that all members of the category have in common. Thus, against Ghiselin and Hull's presuppositions, two animals might both belong to the natural kind "tiger" even though there is no special characteristic that both possess that all nontigers lack—because some of the characteristics that they do possess have the natural higher-order property of being members of a homeostatic property cluster. Another such natural kind, I think, is "living organism." Even though there is no single special characteristic that a recent victim of cardiac arrest and a PVS patient possess and that all nonliving things lack, both of them might belong to the natural kind "living organism" because some of the characteristics that they do possess (for the cardiac arrest victim, consciousness, and for the PVS patient, the capacity for spontaneous respiration, integrated functioning, and so on) have the higher-order property of being members of a homeostatic property cluster. At least in humans and higher animals, these characteristics are coinstantiated in the vast majority of cases and function to sustain one another.

The Indeterminacy of Life and Death

While the properties in a Wittgensteinian cluster tend to be coinstantiated, they are not always coinstantiated. In some cases, an individual will possess some but not all of the properties in the cluster. When some property is central to the cluster—as I've argued consciousness is—then possessing only this one property may be sufficient for membership in the natural kind. However, merely possessing one or several properties that are peripheral to the cluster may not be sufficient for membership. Consider organizational complexity and behavior: some robots are organizationally

complex and functionally responsive, though intuitively not alive. In between the clear cases of membership and exclusion from the natural kind will be borderline cases, in which it is indeterminate whether something is a member of the kind.[21]

Intuitively, viruses strike me as a borderline case: there seems to be no determinate answer to the question of whether viruses are alive. Of the various characteristics I have identified as relevant to life, viruses exhibit only the capacity for reproduction.

While consciousness may be determinately sufficient for something to be alive, I take it to be indeterminate whether reproductive capacity is by itself sufficient, which is why the question of whether viruses are alive admits no determinate answer.

It is also very plausible to think that, in the course of dying, many people pass through a borderline state in between being determinately alive and determinately dead: think of a comatose patient in multisystem organ failure, losing one bodily function or capacity after another. Before the advent of critical care and mechanical ventilation, this progression might have advanced so quickly as to escape notice—but now we often face patients in whom this process may be arrested indefinitely. How should we deal with these indeterminate cases?

One response might be to refuse to treat such people as either alive or dead, perhaps devising some third category for the indeterminate cases. But this approach faces serious practical and theoretical problems. One practical problem is that there is as yet no moral or legal consensus on how to treat those who are "neither alive nor dead," which would likely be troubling and confusing for their families. A theoretical problem is that this approach would only succeed in pushing off the basic problem to a higher level. This approach would not account for the phenomenon of higher-order indeterminacy. Just as there are borderline cases between determinate life and death, there are also borderline cases between determinately determinate life and the determinately indeterminate cases. So even on this approach, at some point a discontinuous boundary must be introduced. A different approach, commonly applied to indeterminacy elsewhere, is to sharpen an originally indeterminate distinction by introducing an artificially defined cutoff that can be used to sort the borderline cases determinately into different categories.[22] Consider adulthood, which also often admits of borderline cases. When for legal or social purposes it is important to make a dichotomous distinction between adults and children, we may do so by introducing a cutoff at eighteen years. This cutoff is not entirely "arbitrary"—it clearly fits better with the original category than a cutoff at six years or thirty—but it is no more consistent with the original category than many other cutoffs, such as a cutoff at seventeen-and-a-half years. So some ways of sharpening an indeterminate distinction are admissible, while others are not: a cutoff at seventeen-and-a-half years is admissible, a cutoff at six or thirty is not. For a cutoff to be admissible it must agree with the original distinction in the determinate cases, and a seven-year-old is very definitely not an adult.

We may then look upon competing criteria for death not as attempts to state necessary and sufficient conditions for death, but instead as proposals for sharpening the distinction between life and death. Presumably there is no uniquely admissible cutoff; however, some proposals can be ruled out as inadmissible,

while some admissible cutoffs may be preferred to others on practical grounds (how easily and reliably they can be clinically determined, for example, and their degree of fit with longstanding cultural traditions).

A proposed sharpening is inadmissible if it disagrees with the original distinction in the determinate cases. Recall that something might lack some of the properties in a cluster and yet nonetheless belong determinately to the relevant kind: for instance, mules cannot reproduce, but healthy mules are nonetheless determinately alive. Similarly, I have claimed that recent, still-conscious victims of cardiac arrest and people in PVS are determinately alive. Thus, the cardiopulmonary and higher-brain criteria are not admissible cutoffs: adopting one of these would be tantamount to revising, rather than sharpening, the boundaries of life and death.

A similar case could be made against the whole-brain criterion if it made some determinately living individual count as determinately dead—or some determinately dead individual count as determinately alive. To my knowledge, the best potential counterexamples are the cases of "chronic brain death" documented by Shewmon, in which individuals have retained numerous integrative functions over long periods when maintained on mechanical ventilation. Clearly these cases undermine the traditional rationale for the whole-brain criterion, which defines death in terms of integrated functioning. But since I've argued that demands for such analytic definitions are misguided, the relevant question for our present purposes is whether these intuitively are determinate cases of life, determinate cases of death, or borderline cases in between.

Shewmon's original reaction to these cases—which I suspect he would now dis-claim—was that these individuals are determinately alive.[23] I would claim, however, that these are borderline cases, in contrast with those in PVS, whom I regard as determinately living. Think, after all, of the many significant functions that those in PVS exhibit and that Shewmon's patients lack, such as spontaneous breathing, sleep-wake cycles, and complicated functional responses to stimuli such as protective coughing, protective blinking, and swallowing. By contrast, I think that Shewmon's cases of "chronic brain death" are so dependent on the external provision of such paradigmatically vital functions as breathing that they cannot be considered clear, determinate cases of life. And if there are no better potential counterexamples, then adopting the whole-brain criterion is an admissible way of sharpening the boundary between life and death.

This defense of the whole-brain criterion as an admissible sharpening of death, rather than as a necessary and sufficient condition for death, is much more modest than the defenses that others have offered for this criterion. As such, it avoids another serious objection raised against the whole-brain criterion. Critics have noted that, as this criterion is usually employed, it does not literally require the irreversible loss of all brain functions. This is to say that, even after the clinical tests for brain death have been met, other untested functions often persist—for instance, hormone secretion and thermoregulation.[24] Yet few advocates of brain death have proposed that we should adopt a more extensive clinical examination for determining brain death, which would test for *all* brain functions that could persist—in part because such testing might prove both difficult and costly and might thereby delay organ procurement or the process of grieving. But on what principled ground can one maintain,

for example, that although brainstem reflexes are relevant to the determination of death, neurohormonal regulation is not?

Treating the whole-brain criterion as an admissible cutoff helps to defuse this objection. On the view I've proposed, there are many admissible cutoffs—including some that require the loss of neurohormonal regulation, and others that do not (such as the whole-brain and brainstem criteria). Choosing between these is like choosing between cutoffs for legal adulthood at seventeen-and-a-half, eighteen, and eighteen-and-a-half years—all agree with one another (and the original distinction) in the originally determinate cases, though they disagree about the borderline cases. The choice between them must then be settled on practical rather than purely biological grounds—for instance, by how easily and reliably they can be clinically confirmed. (A major consideration favoring the cardiopulmonary criterion in earlier times was that the relevant tests could be reliably performed by any doctor with a stethoscope.)

A Nonrelativistic Pluralism

The account of life and death presented here is pluralistic, in that it admits numerous ways of sharpening the indeterminate boundary between life and death. If the whole-brain criterion is to be preferred to these other potential cutoffs, this must be on practical grounds rather than on biological or metaphysical grounds. Yet while this position is pluralistic, it is not relativistic: many other proposed sharpenings of this distinction are objectively inadmissible—as I have argued in the case of the cardiopulmonary and higher-brain criteria. Ultimately, these proposals must answer to a mind-and-language-independent standard: agreement with the original boundary between life and death in determinate cases. Thus, any proposal that would treat conscious people as dead would be ruled out, while any proposal that would treat spontaneously breathing people as dead would most likely also be ruled out.

On such a pluralistic view, the adoption of different criteria for death in different societies is unproblematic in itself, so long as these different criteria all represent admissible cutoffs. If the brainstem and whole-brain criteria are both admissible ways of sharpening the distinction between life and death, then we need not be troubled by the fact that the brainstem criterion is accepted in the United Kingdom, while the whole-brain criterion is accepted in the United States. Note, by contrast, that if we held to Bernat's claim that criteria must give necessary and sufficient conditions for being dead, then we would have to regard at least one of these different criteria as objectively wrong.

Must a uniform standard be imposed in all contexts within a given society? I believe there is a default presumption in favor of simplicity and universality; however, the account of life and death presented here is compatible with a limited degree of context-dependence. For instance, some states have adopted "conscience clauses" to accommodate the convictions of people whose cultural or religious traditions do not accord with the whole-brain criterion, such as Orthodox Jews, Japanese, and some Native Americans. In essence, such clauses allow individuals (or their families) considerable discretion in choosing which standard of death will be applied to them. If the different candidate criteria for death made available by such a conscience clause are all admissible ways of sharpening the original distinction between life and death, then such a statute need not be inconsistent with the account of life and death defended here. Whether such

conscience clauses make sense as a matter of policy is thus not a matter to be settled solely by attending to the nature of life and death, but also to various practical considerations at stake in balancing the social benefit of unanimity against due respect for the adherents of admissible minority views.

An even more controversial example of context-dependence can be seen in the efforts of some organ procurement agencies to expand the pool of potential organ donors by applying different criteria for death in different circumstances. These efforts make use of the fact that the Uniform Determination of Death Act proposed by the President's Commission in 1981 calls for the declaration of death given *either* the irreversible loss of cardiopulmonary function or the irreversible loss of whole-brain function (although the commission's report suggests that cardiopulmonary arrest was recognized only as an indicator of the loss of brain function).[25] Thus, some organ procurement organizations employ two different protocols for vital organ donation: one for donors declared dead on the basis of neurological testing, and another for donors who are declared dead after a two-to-five minute interval following cardiopulmonary arrest ("non-heart-beating donors," or NHBDs). These NHBD protocols are used to facilitate organ procurement from people with neurological injuries that impair only some crucial brain functions—for instance, in conscious people who can no longer breathe spontaneously and wish to be organ donors. In these cases, mechanical ventilation is withdrawn in accordance with the patient's wishes to discontinue life-sustaining treatment, thereby inducing a hypoxic cardiac arrest; following a two-to-five minute interval (depending on the site), the organs are removed quickly to minimize ischemic injury.

Most NHBDs in whom mechanical ventilation is withdrawn in this way would not meet the whole-brain criterion of death—while five minutes of cerebral ischemia likely would result in the permanent destruction of cortical structures required for consciousness, some brainstem structures could survive for many more minutes. (Nancy Cruzan was estimated to have suffered twelve to fourteen minutes of cerebral ischemia, which left her persistently vegetative rather than brain-dead.) However, such a protocol might represent a different admissible cutoff between life and death—recall that the protocol is implemented in people who have already lost the capacity for spontaneous respiration, and then lose integrated functioning and the capacity for consciousness following the withdrawal of mechanical ventilation. If so, then applying the whole-brain criterion to one group of potential donors while applying the NHBD protocol to another group of potential donors would represent another instance of a context-dependent application of different admissible cutoffs for the boundary between life and death.

What remains potentially troubling about this practice, of course, is the idea of tailoring our standards of death in different circumstances to meet the purpose of facilitating organ procurement. Depending on how these disjunctive policies are implemented and applied, they could easily invite confusion and mistrust about organ transplantation among patients; there is also a danger that the ventilator-dependent may be subtly coerced into assenting to withdrawals of treatment that they would not otherwise have chosen for themselves. In general, I suspect that the potential benefits of such policies as a means of meeting the demand for organs have been overstated. Instead, their advocates might do well to emphasize the potential that these policies present for enhancing the autonomy of the terminally ill and ventilator-dependent in determining the character and circumstances of their deaths. On such a view, NHBD protocols might have more in common with "conscience clauses" than is generally recognized.

Acknowledgments

I would like to thank William Ruddick, Derek Parfit, John Richardson, Wade Smith, James Bernat, and Alan Shewmon for many valuable conversations about the material in this paper. I would also like to thank the editors and reviewers for their input and suggestions for improvement.

Notes

1. D.A. Shewmon, "Chronic 'Brain Death': Meta-analysis and Conceptual Consequences," *Neurology* 51 (1998): 1538–45.

2. A. Halevy and B. Brody, "Brain Death: Reconciling Definitions, Criteria, and Tests," *Annals of Internal Medicine* 119 (1993): 519–25; and R.D. Truog, "Is It Time to Abandon Brain Death?" *Hastings Center Report* 27, no. 1 (1997): 29–37.

3. J.L. Bernat, quoted in G. Greenberg, "As Good As Dead," *The New Yorker*, August 13, 2001.

4. J.L. Bernat, "How Much of the Brain Must Die in Brain Death?" *Journal of Clinical Ethics* 3 (1992): 21–28, at 21–22. See similar passages in J.L. Bernat, C.M. Culver, and B. Gert, "On the Definition and Criterion of Death," *Annals of Internal Medicine* 94 (1981): 389–94, at 389, and "Defining Death in Theory and in Practice," *Hastings Center Report* 12, no. 1 (1982): 5–9, at 5–6. Culver and Gert have changed their views about the definition of death in ways that resemble the definition offered by defenders of the brainstem criterion of death, but they remain committed to this model. See B. Gert, C.M. Culver, and K.D. Clouser, *Bioethics: A Return to Fundamentals* (Oxford, U.K.: Oxford University Press, 1997), ch. 11.

5. I interpret Bernat's claim that criteria are meant to give "necessary and sufficient" conditions for death as a claim about nomological, rather than metaphysical, necessity and sufficiency. After all, the whole-brain criterion, the cardiopulmonary criterion, and the higher-brain criterion must be intended as criteria for death in a given actual species (that is, *Homo sapiens*)—they could not seriously be proposed as criteria for death in plants or microorganisms, or in possible species with unknown physiologies.

6. J.L. Bernat, "A Defense of the Whole-Brain Concept of Death," *Hastings Center Report* 28, no. 2 (1998): 14–23, at 17.

7. See J.L. Bernat, "The Biophilosophical Basis of Whole-Brain Death," *Social Philosophy and Policy* 19 (2002): 324–42.

8. Shewmon, "Chronic 'Brain Death.'"

9. D.A. Shewmon, "'Brainstem Death,' 'Brain Death' and Death; A Critical Re-Evaluation of the Purported Equivalence," *Issues in Law and Medicine* 14 (1998): 125– 45, at 139–40.

10. J.L. Bernat, "Refinements in the Criterion of Death," in *The Definition of Death: Contemporary Controversies*, ed. S.J. Youngner, R.M. Arnold, and R. Schapiro (Baltimore, Md.: Johns Hopkins University Press, 1999), 83–92.

11. C. Pallis and D.H. Harley, *ABC of Brainstem Death* (London, U.K.: BMJ Publishing Group, 1993), 28. See also Gert, Culver and Clouser, *Bioethics*.

12. Shewmon, "'Brainstem Death,' 'Brain Death' and Death," 132.

13. B. Brody, "How Much of the Brain Must Be Dead?" in *The Definition of Death:Contemporary Controversies*, 71–82, at 78.

14. L. Wittgenstein, *Philosophical Investigations*, third ed., tr. G.E.M. Anscombe (New York: MacMillan, 1958), secs. 65–66.

15. S. Kripke, *Naming and Necessity* (Cambridge, Mass.: Harvard University Press, 1972).

16. H. Putnam, "Meaning and Reference," *Journal of Philosophy* 70 (1973): 699–711.

17. I take the terms "spontaneous," "internal," and "external," as used here, to admit of borderline cases—see the discussion of indeterminacy in the next section.

18. "Intrinsic characteristics" is a term of art for properties that are nondisjunctive and nonrelational. Much traditional thinking about natural kinds is put in terms of intrinsic characteristics—see Robert A. Wilson's discussion of the role of "intrinsic properties" in "traditional scientific realism" in "Promiscuous Realism," *British Journal for the Philosophy of Science* 47 (1996): 303–16, at 304–5. See also a related discussion of the reality of cluster concepts as "class terms" in D.L. Hull, "A Matter of Individuality," *Philosophy of Science* 45 (1978): 335–60, at 355.

19. See Hull, "A Matter of Individuality."

20. R. Boyd, "Homeostasis, Species, and Higher Taxa," in *Species: New Interdisciplinary Essays*, ed. R.A. Wilson (Cambridge, Mass.: MIT Press, 1999), 141–85, at 143–44. See also "What Realism Implies and What it Does Not," *Dialectica* 43 (1989): 5–29; and "Realism, Anti-Foundationalism and the Enthusiasm for Natural Kinds," *Philosophical Studies* 61 (1991): 127–48.

21. Boyd: "Moreover, there will be many cases of extensional indeterminacy, which are not resolvable even given all the relevant facts and all the true theories. There will be things that display some but not all of the properties in [the cluster] such that no rational considerations dictate whether or not they are to be classed under [the natural kind term], assuming that a dichotomous choice is to be made." "Homeostasis, Species, and Higher Taxa," p. 144.

22. In the philosophical literature on indeterminacy, this sort of sharpening is called "precisification." Let me note here that, while the notion of precisification is usually associated with supervaluationist approaches to indeterminacy, I don't think that this sort of practical application of precisification commits one to supervaluationism. For instance, an epistemicist who thinks there is a discontinuous but unknowable boundary at which adulthood begins can still admit the option of precisifying adulthood by introducing a cutoff at age eighteen for the purposes of epistemically challenged creatures like ourselves.

23. For his original reaction to these cases see his comments about "T.K." in "'Brainstem Death,' 'Brain Death,' and Death," 136. In recent articles he has expressed doubts about his earlier views, on grounds similar to those presented in this paper: see D.A. Shewmon and E.S. Shewmon, "The Semiotics of Death and its Medical Implications," in *Brain Death and Disorders of Consciousness*, ed. C. Machado and D.A. Shewmon (New York: Kluwer Academic, 2004), 89–114.

24. See again Halevy and Brody, "Brain Death," and Truog, "Is It Time to Abandon Brain Death?"

25. President's Commission for the Study of Ethical Problems in Medicine and Biomedical and Behavioral Research, *Defining Death: Medical, Legal and Ethical Issues in the Determination of Death*, (Washington, D.C.: U.S. Government Printing Office, 1981). This sort of disjunctive legal standard is also employed in many states that did not adopt the Uniform Determination of Death Act.

Chapter 6

Accepting Brain Death

David C. Magnus, Benjamin S. Wilfond, and
Arthur L. Caplan

Two cases in which patients have been determined to be dead according to neurologic criteria ("brain death") have recently garnered national headlines. In Oakland, California, Jahi McMath's death was determined by means of multiple independent neurologic examinations, including one ordered by a court. Her family refused to accept that she had died and went to court to prevent physicians at Children's Hospital and Research Center in Oakland from discontinuing ventilator support. Per a court-supervised agreement, the body was given to the family 3 weeks after the initial determination. The family's attorney stated that ventilatory support was continued and nutritional support added at an undisclosed location.

In Fort Worth, Texas, Marlise Muñoz's body was maintained on mechanical ventilation for 8 weeks after the medical and legal criteria for death were met, in an attempt to "rescue" her fetus. Muñoz was 14 weeks pregnant when she died from pulmonary embolism. Her family asserted that continuing ventilatory support was contrary to what the patient would have wanted, but John Peter Smith Hospital cited a state law requiring that support not be terminated if a patient is pregnant. A judge ultimately ordered that the hospital follow the medically and legally indicated steps of declaring the patient dead and removing ventilatory support.

The McMath family's attorney claimed that their constitutional rights were violated and their religious beliefs (both about when death occurs and about prognosticating a possibility of recovery) were not respected. In making this argument, proponents of allowing family members to determine death threaten to undermine decades of law, medicine, and ethics.

The current U.S. approach to determining death was developed in response to the emergence of technologies that made the traditional standard of cardiopulmonary death problematic. In 1968, an ad hoc committee at Harvard Medical School published an influential article arguing for extending the concept of death to patients in an "irreversible coma."[1] The emerging neurologic criteria for death defined it in terms of loss of the functional activity of the brain stem and cerebral cortex. Although clinical criteria were developed in the 1960s, it took more than a decade for consensus over a rationale for the definition to emerge. In 1981, the President's Commission for the Study of Ethical Problems in Medicine and Biomedical and Behavioral Research provided a philosophical definition of brain death in terms of the loss of the critical functions of the organism as a whole.[2]

Shortly thereafter, the National Conference of Commissioners on Uniform State Laws produced the Uniform Determination of Death Act, which has been adopted in 45 states and recognized in the rest through judicial opinion.[3] In response to pressure from a vocal religious minority, New York and New Jersey added religious exceptions that affect the timing of the declaration of death. Even in these states, however, the vast majority of the time, the standard medical criteria for death are followed. Over the past several decades, brain death has become well entrenched as a legal and medical definition of death. It is clearly defined by the neurologic community (see box), standards for diagnosis are in place, and it is established in law.

It has become the primary basis of organ-procurement policy for transplantation. Ironically, the other standard for defining death, irreversible cessation of circulation, lacks consensus about diagnosis.

The concept of brain death has periodically come under criticism.[4] The primary objections focus on inadequacies in the philosophical rationale for the concept that the unifying functioning of the body has been lost with loss of brain functioning, combined with a concern that biologically, there is still a sense that the body is alive, often long after brain death occurs. Wound healing can continue to occur, most organs continue to function for some period, hormonal and body-temperature regulation may be maintained. It has been reported that a child's growth can continue. And as the Muñoz case demonstrates, a pregnancy can be maintained even after the pregnant woman has met the neurologic criteria for death.

Even many of the most vocal critics of brain death agree that there is no obligation to continue providing mechanical support after brain death. Although they do not consider brain death to be death, many of them agree that the person has ceased to exist and has no interests at stake in the discontinuation of ventilator support. Although some physicians accommodate a family's grief by allowing a brief delay either before completing brain-death examinations or before discontinuing mechanical support after a brain-death determination, these actions are for the family, not the patient. In addition, many believe that it is appropriate to procure organs after such declarations.

Unfortunately, these views raise severe difficulties for public policy. In a society tolerant of individual values and views, family views are appropriately given great weight in deciding exactly when to discontinue mechanical support. If brain death were not defined as death, it would be more difficult to justify routine decisions to discontinue mechanical support in this context. Families often need time to accept death, and that can be particularly complicated in cases of brain death. For the family's benefit, a short-term accommodation can be ethically justified. But these psychological realities do not undermine the important social construction of death when the brain has ceased all meaningful activity.

Rejecting brain death by shifting toward a more fluid and variable standard might undermine support for cadaveric organ donation. The "dead-donor rule," a fundamental concept of transplant ethics, requires that patients not be killed by the removal of vital organs necessary for life. Some critics of brain death seek to abandon the dead-donor rule. Whatever one thinks of the arguments for that as a philosophical position, it is far out of touch with currently accepted medical and legal standards and public opinion.[5]

We believe that there is no good reason to

Determination of Brain Death*

1. Absence of neurologic function with a known irreversible cause of coma
2. Correction of conditions affecting evaluation of brain death (performed before neurologic evaluation):
   - hypotension
   - hypothermia
   - metabolic disturbances
3. Discontinuation of medications affecting the neurologic examination (performed before neurologic evaluation):
   - sedatives
   - neuromuscular blockers
   - anticonvulsants
4. Timing of neurologic evaluation should be more than 24 to 48 hours after cardiopulmonary resuscitation or other severe acute brain injury
5. Duration of observation (pediatric cases):
   - 24 hours for neonates (37 weeks of gestation to 30 days after birth for term infants)
   - 12 hours for infants and children (>30 days to 18 years of age)
6. Clinical evaluation:
   - absence of pupillary response to a bright light
   - absence of movement of bulbar musculature
   - absence of gag, cough, sucking, and rooting reflexes shown by examining the cough response to tracheal suctioning
   - absence of corneal reflexes demonstrated by touching the cornea; no eyelid movement should be seen
   - absence of oculovestibular reflexes shown by irrigating each ear with ice water; movement of the eyes should be absent during 1 minute of observation
7. Apnea testing:
   - Pretest: confirmation of complete absence of spontaneous respiratory effort — preoxygenate with 100% oxygen, maintain core temperature above 35°C, normalize pH, blood pressure, and arterial blood gas (partial pressure of carbon dioxide [$PaCO_2$])
   - Test: demonstration of increase in arterial $PaCO_2$ of at least 20 mm Hg above baseline and of a total $PaCO_2$ of at least 60 mm Hg, with no observed respiration
   - Ancillary study: indication to perform if there is a medical contraindication to the apnea test, hemodynamic instability, desaturation to less than 85%, or the inability to reach a $PaCO_2$ of at least 60 mm Hg
   - Evidence of any respiratory effort is inconsistent with brain death, and the apnea test should be terminated
8. Ancillary studies:
   - electroencephalography
   - radionuclide cerebral blood flow
   - spinal cord reflexes if abnormal movements present

* Derived from the American Academy of Neurology.

take such a drastic step. Dying is a process. Parts of the body die, and then other parts do. Eventually, gradually, all the cells die. Where in that process should the line between life and death be drawn? Given the brain's importance in determining who we are and its crucial role in driving the activity of bodily organs and systems, it is not surprising that loss of cortical and brain-stem function should be equated with death. Seen in this light, the decision reached by the medical and particularly the neurology community to articulate and promulgate the concept of brain death as the right place to draw the line between life and death is extremely reasonable. There are clear medical criteria that can be reliably and reproducibly utilized to determine that death has occurred. If professional standards are followed properly, there are no false positives. Brain-dead patients are clearly past the point of any possibility of recovery. Although one could conceivably draw the line somewhere else, such as loss of cognitive functioning, the reliability and social consensus that has emerged around brain death as death is reflected in the broad legal agreement under which brain death is recognized in every state.

Medical and legal acceptance that the irreversible loss of brain functioning is death enables families to grieve the loss of their loved ones knowing that they were absolutely beyond recovery, as distinct from patients in a coma or a vegetative state. It errs on the side of certainty when organ procurement is requested. The determination of death is a highly significant social boundary. It determines who is recognized as a person with constitutional rights, who deserves legal entitlements and benefits, and when last wills and testaments become effective. Sound public policy requires bright

lines backed up by agreed-on criteria, protocols, and tests when the issue is the determination of death. The law and ethics have long recognized that deferring to medical expertise regarding the diagnosis of brain death is the most reasonable way to manage the process of dying. Nothing in these two cases ought to change that stance.

Disclosure forms provided by the authors are available with the full text of this article at NEJM.org.

From the Center for Biomedical Ethics, Stanford University, Palo Alto, CA (D.C.M.); the Treuman Katz Center for Pediatric Ethics, Seattle Children's Hospital, Seattle (B.S.W.); and the Division of Medical Ethics, New York University, New York (A.L.C.).

Notes

1. A definition of irreversible coma: report of the Ad Hoc Committee of the Harvard Medical School to Examine the Definition of Brain Death. JAMA 1968; 205:337–40.

2. President's Commission for the Study of Ethical Problems in Medicine and Biomedical and Behavioral Research. Defining death: a report on the medical, legal and ethical issues in the determination of death. Washington, DC: Government Printing Office, 1981.

3. National Conference of Commissioners on Uniform State Laws. Uniform Determination of Death Act, 1981(http://www.uniformlaws.org/shared/docs/determination%20of%20death/udda80.pdf).

4. Truog RD, Miller FG, Halpern SD. The dead-donor rule and the future of organ donation. N Engl J Med 2013;369:1287–9.

5. Bernat JL. Life or death for the dead-donor rule? N Engl J Med 2013; 369:1289–91.

Chapter 7

Address to the International Congress on Transplants

Karol Wojtyła (Pope John Paul II)

Distinguished Ladies and Gentlemen:

1. I am happy to greet all of you at this International Congress, which has brought you together for a reflection on the complex and delicate theme of transplants. I thank Professor Raffaello Cortesini and Professor Oscar Salvatierra for their kind words, and I extend a special greeting to the Italian authorities present. To all of you I express my gratitude for your kind invitation to take part in this meeting and I very much appreciate the serious consideration you are giving to the moral teaching of the Church. With respect for science and being attentive above all to the law of God, the Church has no other aim but the integral good of the human person.

Transplants are a great step forward in science's service of man, and not a few people today owe their lives to an organ transplant. Increasingly, the technique of transplants has proven to be a valid means of attaining the primary goal of all medicine: the service of human life. That is why in the encyclical letter *Evangelium Vitae* I suggested that one way of nurturing a genuine culture of life "is the donation of organs, performed in an ethically acceptable manner, with a view to offering a chance of health and even of life itself to the sick who sometimes have no other hope."[1]

2. As with all human advancement, this particular field of medical science, for all the hope of health and life it offers to many, also presents certain critical issues that need to be examined in the light of a discerning anthropological and ethical reflection. In this area of medical science too the fundamental criterion must be the defense and promotion of the integral good of the human person, in keeping with that unique dignity which is ours by virtue of our humanity.

Consequently, it is evident that every medical procedure performed on the human person is subject to limits: not just the limits of what it is technically possible, but also limits determined by respect for human nature itself, understood in its fullness: "what is technically possible is not for that reason alone morally admissible."[2]

3. It must first be emphasized, as I observed on another occasion, that every organ transplant has its source in a decision of great ethical value: "the decision to offer without reward a part of one's own body for the health and well-being of another person."[3] Here precisely lies the nobility of the gesture, a gesture which is a genuine act of love. It is not just a matter of giving away something that belongs to us but of giving something of ourselves, for "by virtue of its substantial union

with a spiritual soul, the human body cannot be considered as a mere complex of tissues, organs and functions . . . rather it is a constitutive part of the person who manifests and expresses himself through it."[4] Accordingly, any procedure which tends to commercialize human organs or to consider them as items of exchange or trade must be considered morally unacceptable, because to use the body as an "object" is to violate the dignity of the human person. This first point has an immediate consequence of great ethical import: the need for informed consent. The human "authenticity" of such a decisive gesture requires that individuals be properly informed about the processes involved, in order to be in a position to consent or decline in a free and conscientious manner. The consent of relatives has its own ethical validity in the absence of a decision on the part of the donor. Naturally, an analogous consent should be given by the recipients of donated organs.

4. Acknowledgment of the unique dignity of the human person has a further underlying consequence: vital organs which occur singly in the body can be removed only after death, that is from the body of someone who is certainly dead.

This requirement is self-evident, since to act otherwise would mean intentionally to cause the death of the donor in disposing of his organs. This gives rise to one of the most debated issues in contemporary bioethics, as well as to serious concerns in the minds of ordinary people. I refer to the problem of ascertaining the fact of death. When can a person be considered dead with complete certainty? In this regard, it is helpful to recall that the death of the person is a single event, consisting in the total disintegration of that unitary and integrated whole that is the personal self. It results from the separation of the life principle

(or soul) from the corporal reality of the person. The death of the person, understood in this primary sense, is an event which no scientific technique or empirical method can identify directly.

Yet human experience shows that once death occurs certain biological signs inevitably follow, which medicine has learned to recognize with increasing precision. In this sense, the "criteria" for ascertaining death used by medicine today should not be understood as the technical-scientific determination of the exact moment of a person's death, but as a scientifically secure means of identifying the biological signs that a person has indeed died.

5. It is a well-known fact that for some time certain scientific approaches to ascertaining death have shifted the emphasis from the traditional cardio-respiratory signs to the so-called "neurological" criterion. Specifically, this consists in establishing, according to clearly determined parameters commonly held by the international scientific community, the complete and irreversible cessation of all brain activity (in the cerebrum, cerebellum and brain stem). This is then considered the sign that the individual organism has lost its integrative capacity. With regard to the parameters used today for ascertaining death—whether the "encephalic" signs or the more traditional cardio-respiratory signs—the Church does not make technical decisions. She limits herself to the Gospel duty of comparing the data offered by medical science with the Christian understanding of the unity of the person, bringing out the similarities and the possible conflicts capable of endangering respect for human dignity.

Here it can be said that the criterion adopted in more recent times for ascertaining the fact of death, namely, the complete and irreversible cessation of all brain activity, if rigorously applied, does not seem to conflict with the essential elements of a sound anthropology. Therefore a health-worker professionally responsible for ascertaining death can use these criteria in each individual case as the basis for arriving at that degree of assurance in ethical judgment which moral teaching describes as "moral certainty." This moral certainty is considered the necessary and sufficient basis for an ethically correct course of action. Only where such certainty exists, and where informed consent has already been given by the donor or the donor's legitimate representatives, is it morally right to initiate the technical procedures required for the removal of organs for transplant.

6. Another question of great ethical significance is that of the allocation of donated organs through waiting-lists and the assignment of priorities. Despite efforts to promote the practice of organ-donation, the resources available in many countries are currently insufficient to meet medical needs. Hence there is a need to compile waiting-lists for transplants on the basis of clear and properly reasoned criteria. From the moral standpoint, an obvious principle of justice requires that the criteria for assigning donated organs should in no way be "discriminatory" (i.e., based on age, sex, race, religion, social standing, etc.) or "utilitarian" (i.e., based on work capacity, social usefulness, etc.). Instead, in determining who should have precedence in receiving an organ, judgments should be made on the basis of immunological and clinical factors. Any other criterion would prove wholly arbitrary and subjective, and would fail to recognize the intrinsic value of each human person as such, a value that is independent of any external circumstances.

7. A final issue concerns a possible alternative solution to the problem of finding human organs for transplantation, something still very much in the experimental stage, namely xenotransplants, that is, organ transplants from other animal species. It is not my intention to explore in detail the problems connected with this form of intervention. I would merely recall that already in 1956 Pope Pius XII raised the question of their legitimacy. He did so when commenting on the scientific possibility, then being presaged, of transplanting animal corneas to humans. His response is still enlightening for us today: in principle, he stated, for a xenotransplant to be licit, the transplanted organ must not impair the integrity of the psychological or genetic identity of the person receiving it; and there must also be a proven biological possibility that the transplant will be successful and will not expose the recipient to inordinate risk.[5]

8. In concluding, I express the hope that, thanks to the work of so many generous and highly-trained people, scientific and technological research in the field of transplants will continue to progress, and extend to experimentation with new therapies which can replace organ transplants, as some recent developments in prosthetics seem to promise. In any event, methods that fail to respect the dignity and value of the person must always be avoided. I am thinking in particular of attempts at human cloning with a view to obtaining organs for transplants: these techniques, insofar as they involve the manipulation and destruction of human embryos, are not morally acceptable, even when their proposed goal is good in itself. Science itself points to other forms of therapeutic intervention which would not involve cloning or the use of embryonic cells, but rather would make use of stem cells taken from adults. This is the direction that research must follow if it wishes to respect the dignity of each and

every human being, even at the embryonic stage. In addressing these varied issues, the contribution of philosophers and theologians is important. Their careful and competent reflection on the ethical problems associated with transplant therapy can help to clarify the criteria for assessing what kinds of transplants are morally acceptable and under what conditions, especially with regard to the protection of each individual's personal identity.

I am confident that social, political and educational leaders will renew their commitment to fostering a genuine culture of generosity and solidarity. There is a need to instill in people's hearts, especially in the hearts of the young, a genuine and deep appreciation of the need for brotherly love, a love that can find expression in the decision to become an organ donor. May the Lord sustain each one of you in your work, and guide you in the service of authentic human progress. I accompany this wish with my blessing.

Notes

1. No. 86.

2. Congregation for the Doctrine of the Faith, *Donum vitae*, introduction., no. 4.

3. "Address to the Participants in a Congress on Organ Transplants," June 20, 1991, no. 3.

4. *Donum vitae*, introduction, no. 3.

5. Cf. "Address to the Italian Association of Cornea Donors and to Clinical Oculists and Legal Medical Practitioners," May 14, 1956.

Chapter 8

Brain Death

Can It Be Resuscitated?

D. Alan Shewmon

Introduction

Why is a patient with a destroyed brain considered dead rather than moribund and irreversibly comatose? The world has been grappling with this question for the past four decades with little success. The recently released white paper of the President's Council on Bioethics is in many respects a refreshing, thoughtful, and comprehensive reexamination of this complex topic.[1] It offers a very helpful analysis of the major positions on the determination of death, and it proffers a creative new solution of its own. Unfortunately, the new solution does not put the problem to rest, but the humility with which the council discusses its own position and the honesty with which it confronts the consequences of being wrong alone make this report a very commendable document.

Historical Backdrop

What is refreshing about the white paper emerges best when it is put in historical perspective. In 1968, the Harvard Committee catalyzed a monumental socio-medico-legal revolution: the reformulation of death in terms of brain function.[2] The only rationale given by the committee for why the irre-

versible cessation of all brain functions should be equated with death was legal utility: it would free up beds in intensive care units and facilitate organ transplantation.

The Harvard report ushered in a brief era of wild transplantation.[3] In a domino effect beginning in 1970, state after state revised its statutory definition of death, despite the absence not just of official diagnostic criteria for irreversible cessation of all brain functions, but also of any generally accepted philosophical rationale for why irreversible non-function of the brain should constitute death. By 1978, over thirty different diagnostic criteria had been published, none of them validated; neither had any consensus on the conceptual basis emerged.[4]

The next milestone in the history of "brain death" was the 1981 President's Commission.[5] Its comprehensive report included a proposed Uniform Determination of Death Act (UDDA), which served as the model for the remaining twenty-three states that had not yet revised their death statutes to include a brain-based criterion. Its medical consultants proposed a set of diagnostic criteria that instantly became the standard for the United States. And most importantly, it articulated a then plausible rationale for equating irreversible cessation of all brain function with death—namely, the loss of integrative unity of the organism. It argued that the brain is the body's central integrator, without which the body necessarily and imminently literally "dis-integrates" and succumbs to asystole despite all technological interventions. The President's Commission also maintained that "brain death" and ordinary death are physiologically identical states, only in the former case the equivalence is "masked" by artificial ventilation and circulatory support. That same year, James Bernat, Charles Culver, and Bernard Gert published an influential paper promoting even more forcefully the integrative unity rationale, which quickly became the mainstream conceptual justification for brain death in the United States and many other countries.[6]

Over the next two decades, however, new clinical data made it increasingly clear that patients with total brain failure were not physiologically identical to non-heart-beating corpses, and they did not necessarily "dis-integrate" despite all technological support. Moreover, the rare longer-surviving ones exhibited holistic properties such as homeostasis, proportional growth (of a child), teleological repair, and general ability to survive outside a hospital setting with relatively little support (ventilator, tube feedings, and nursing care much less than many sick patients in intensive care units require, who are nevertheless clearly living organisms). Such properties are difficult to reconcile with the mainstream assumption that these bodies were nothing but bags of partially interacting subsystems.

The mainstream rationale also made little headway into the minds of people at large. Even now, reporters refer to "brain-dead" patients as being "kept alive" by machines or as "dying" when the ventilator is turned off. Much of the public and a surprising proportion of the medical profession still consider "brain-dead" patients "as good as dead" or "better off dead," but not yet really dead. Moreover, many who do regard them as dead do so on the grounds of loss of personhood (by virtue of permanent unconsciousness) from a biologically still living human organism grounds that would also categorize patients in a permanent vegetative state as dead.[7]

Medical organizations have been strangely silent on their own rationale for equating "brain death" with death, limiting their official statements to purely diagnostic considerations.[8] The same can be said about various highly respected neurologists, apart from Bernat, who have authored books and chapters on brain death. But every now and then a Freudian slip reveals that the author's unstated rationale is not the mainstream one. In their popular textbook Principles of Neurology, for example, Allan Ropper and Robert Brown wrote: "In exceptional cases [of brain death], however, the provision of adequate fluid, vasopressor, and respiratory support allows preservation of the somatic organism in a comatose state for longer periods."[9] Regarding a series of seventy-three brain-dead patients, Fred Plum wrote that "half experienced asystole by the third day but the bodies of 2 lived on until the 10th and 16th day."[10] And the late Dr. Ronald Cranford wrote, regarding patients in permanent vegetative state, "that permanently unconscious patients have characteristics of both the living and the dead. It would be tempting to call them dead and then retrospectively apply the principles of death, as society has done with brain death."[11]

Philosophers and bioethicists have become increasingly unconvinced by the organismic unity rationale, many preferring instead some variation of the personhood rationale.[12] In this they are joined by certain prominent neurologists, such as Plum and Calixto Machado, as well as by many rank-and-file neurologists.[13] Some experts have opined that "brain death" is not death after all, but that it doesn't matter anyway for ethical organ harvesting.[14]

Thus, the much-touted international "consensus" on a neurological standard of death is only skin deep.[15] The widespread superficial agreement that "brain death" is death conceals a widespread disagreement over the reason why, and even much schizophrenic tacit belief to the contrary. "Brain death as death" began as a utilitarian legislative decree and has remained a conclusion in search of a justification ever since: a conclusion clung to at all costs for the sake of the transplantation enterprise that quickly came to depend on it.

The White Paper

Against this backdrop, the President's Council's white paper stands out as a beacon and a breath of fresh air in a number of respects. The council articulately and concisely summarizes the issues and the various positions that have been advanced over the years. The superb chapter on terminology discards the question-begging and ambiguous term "brain death," replacing it with the philosophically neutral and physiologically clearer term "total brain failure." The council upholds the Kantian prohibition against using human beings merely as means to an end and not also as ends in themselves (p. 72), thereby excluding any relaxation of the "dead donor rule" and warning of the ethical dangers inherent in relying on non-heart-beating donors.[16] Also, its cautionary attitude regarding patients diagnosed as being in a persistent vegetative state—whether they truly lack all subjective awareness, as is commonly assumed—is noteworthy and should be widely heeded (pp. A2–4A).

Regarding the various proposed rationales for equating total brain failure with death, the council explicitly rejects the 1968 Harvard Committee's social construct approach (pp. 49–50). It also follows most other commentators in rejecting the "higher-brain-death" position (according to which death occurs when the higher brain functions that are purportedly responsible for personhood are lost) (pp. 50–52). More remarkable, however, is the council's studied rejection of the mainstream rationale of organismic integrative unity. "If being alive as a biological organism requires being a whole that is more than the mere sum of its parts, then it would be difficult to deny that the body of a patient with total brain failure can still be alive, at least in some cases" (p. 57).

In effect, the council rejects all previously advanced rationales for a neurological standard of death. In the face of this unsettling conclusion, it sees only two possible options. Position one is simply to conclude that "there is no sound biological justification for today's neurological standard." Position two is to posit a completely novel rationale, "a more compelling account of wholeness that would support the intuition that after total brain failure the body is no longer an organismic whole and hence no longer alive" (p. 60). A majority of the council came down in favor of position two.

Death remains a condition of the organism as a whole and does not, therefore, merely signal the irreversible loss of so-called higher mental functions. But reliance on the concept of "integration" is abandoned and with it the false assumption that the brain is the "integrator" of vital functions. Determining whether an organism remains a whole depends on recognizing the persistence or cessation of the fundamental vital work of a living organism—the work of self-preservation, achieved through the organism's need-driven commerce with the surrounding world. When there is good reason to believe that an injury has irreversibly destroyed an organism's ability to perform its fundamental vital work, then the conclusion that the organism as a whole has died is warranted. . . . Thus, on this account, total brain failure can continue to serve as a criterion for declaring death—not because it necessarily indicates complete loss of integrated somatic functioning, but because it is a sign that this organism can no longer engage in the essential work that defines living things, (pp. 60, 64–65)

The council singles out two forms of environmental commerce as conceptually important: breathing and consciousness. According to position two, at least one of these is necessary for a higher organism to be a living whole; conversely, the irreversible loss of both suffices to constitute cessation of the organism as a whole—that is, death (p. 64). The council thereby aligns itself in many respects with the "brainstem death" notion of the United Kingdom and Canada, although with a purportedly more robust philosophical justification (pp. 65–67).

The council is to be commended for its creativity in developing the first new rationale for the neurological standard of death in many years. Although the majority of council members found position two "more compelling" than the integrative unity rationale, it remains to be seen how many others will find it so after thorough public debate. A minority of members disagreed with position two, including chairman Ed Pellegrino. (At least one member, Floyd Bloom, disagreed with position two in the opposite direction, opining in essence that irreversible unconsciousness alone suffices for death on the basis of loss of human personhood—the "higher brain-death" standard.)

The Problems with Position Two

Alas, this commentator is yet another who fails to be convinced by position two, for multiple reasons. First and foremost, the concept of "wholeness" is never defined. If it is to be understood as a necessary characteristic of life, it certainly cannot be read as meaning "entire" or "complete." I'm sure the council would agree; otherwise, amputees would not qualify as living organisms. On numerous occasions, the council employs the phrase "organism as a whole" to describe the kind of wholeness that is relevant. But by what contortion of semantics can an admittedly integrated unity that is more than the sum of its parts not be a "whole"? And what lexicon defines "wholeness" exclusively in terms of externally directed "work"?

Furthermore, why is it simply assumed, without argument, that the only kind of "fundamental vital work of a living organism" is "the work of self-preservation, achieved through the organism's need-driven commerce with the surrounding world"? Why should immanent work on a holistic level such as self-development (for instance, of an embryo) and self-maintenance (for instance, internal homeostasis, orderly turnover of cells and tissue components, or teleological repair) not also count as legitimate examples of "fundamental vital work of a living organism"? Perhaps only because of a tacit a priori determination to save the neurological standard at all intellectual costs?

The council seems to backtrack on its rejection of internal integration when it states about some cases of total brain failure that "globally coordinated work continues to be performed by multiple systems, all directed toward the sustained functioning of the body as a whole. If being alive as a biological organism requires being a whole that is more than the mere sum of its parts, then it would be difficult to deny that the body of a patient with total brain failure can still be alive, at least in some cases" (p. 57, emphasis added). So it may be a "whole" after all. But then a few pages later: "If these kinds of integration were sufficient to identify the presence of a living Organism as a whole, total brain failure could not serve as a criterion for organismic death, and the neurological standard enshrined in law would not be philosophically well-grounded" (p. 60). Given that the white paper then presents what it considers to be its "more compelling" philosophical grounds for preserving the neurological standard, the council in this section is in effect claiming that the body of a patient with total brain failure is not a "whole" after all. There can be no logical flow when a pivotal term such as "whole" is never defined, is often juxtaposed against what is ordinarily taken as a synonym ("unity"), and keeps changing implicit meaning.

But suppose we grant, just for the sake of argument, that it is possible for a unity not to be a whole, and that holistic, self-preserving, immanent dynamisms are not fundamental, vital works of a living organism. Position two still faces serious challenges. One problem is that it conflates physical necessity for staying alive (in the wild) with logical necessity for being alive (ontologically). Breathing, eating, drinking, seeking sustenance, and avoiding predators are (physically) necessary for self-preservation in the wild, but not in a hospital. The cessation of any or all of them in the wild will inextricably lead to death, but that cessation is not already death per se. External assistance for an organism with such disabilities will forestall death, not "mask" it (p. 61).

The council also conflates "sufficiency of sign X to prove life" with "sufficiency of irreversible-lack-of-X to prove death." (For simplicity, let "life" and "death" refer to the organism as a whole, and let "lack" mean "irreversible lack.") The white paper frequently alludes to self-preserving commerce with the environment as a fundamental and characteristic sign of organismic wholeness and life, which is undeniably true but utterly irrelevant to the search for a reliable sign of death (pp 62–64). The key logical equivalences are these: the claim "X is sufficient to prove life" is equivalent to the claim "lack-of-X is necessary to prove death," and "lack-of-X is sufficient to prove death" is equivalent to "X is necessary to prove life." Of all the potential candidate-signs X, the council reviews the traditional three: conscious awareness, breathing, and circulation. Let us call them A, B, and C. The council asserts several points regarding their respective sufficiency or necessity as signs of life or death:

1. The lack of any one of them alone is insufficient to prove death.
2. Presence of A or B alone (but not C alone) suffices to prove life.
3. In combination, the absence of both B and C (and as a physical consequence, also A) is sufficient to prove death (this is equivalent to the first arm of the bifurcated UDDA, the traditional cardiopulmonary criterion).
4. The absence of both A and B is also a sufficient sign of death (this is equivalent to the second arm of the UDDA, the neurological standard).

When individual signs are combined into a composite criterion for life or death, the logic of sufficiency and necessity quickly becomes complicated. In fact, the possibilities that must be considered increase exponentially with each independent factor: sign A, B, or C; presence or absence; sufficiency or necessity; proving life or death.

The white paper blurs these critical distinctions, forsaking logical rigor. The logical counterpart of "either A or B suffices to prove life" is "lack of both A and B is necessary to prove death." But what position two asserts is: "lack of both A and B is both necessary and sufficient to prove death." That may be true, but it does not logically follow from the painstakingly established premise that the presence of A or B is sufficient to prove life. To establish that lack of both A and B is sufficient to prove death, the council would have had to demonstrate that, of the myriad possible candidate signs, A and B are the only two that are individually sufficient to prove life. (If some other sign were also sufficient, its presence, despite the joint absence of A and B, would prove life; hence the joint absence of A and B would be insufficient to prove death.[17]) Yet the council makes no attempt at such an argument, perhaps because the claim would hardly be plausible.

This brings us to another serious problem with position two. What exactly characterizes signs A and B, whose joint absence purportedly suffices to prove death? The very notion of "self-preserving commerce with the environment" needs clarification if it is to serve as the cornerstone of position two. The white paper seems ambivalent and at times inconsistent regarding what it considers key: is it the actual exchange of substances with the environment (or adaptive sensorimotor interaction, in the case of consciousness), or rather the inner drive to exchange substances (or to adaptively interact). The discussion of "vital functions" in chapter three (preceding the presentation of position two) repeatedly emphasizes that it is the actual exchange of gases across the alveolar membrane that is the "vital work" and environmental "commerce" that counts with regard to respiration (pp. 22–25). Regarding the inner drive to breathe, mediated by the brainstem, the council states that, "For the purposes of our inquiry, the crucial fact about the mechanics of breathing is this: When the brainstem's respiratory centers are incapacitated, the organism will not make or display any respiratory effort. . . . If the death of the organism is to be prevented some external 'driver' of the breathing process—a mechanical ventilator—must be used" (pp. 26–27).[18]

Taken together, such passages indicate that the critical respiratory "commerce," as understood by the council, is the actual exchange of gases between organism and environment and not the inner drive to breathe per se. Something analogous could be said about a comatose or totally paralyzed patient's self-preserving sensorimotor interaction with the environment. Paraphrasing the emphasized quoted sentence just above, "If the death of the organism is to be prevented, some external 'sensorimotor interactor'—a caregiver—must be used." Other passages from the white paper also reinforce the idea that the "fundamental vital work" at issue is the actual self-preserving "commerce" with the environment, and not a purely internal drive towards it (pp. 60–61).

On the other hand, still other passages seem to indicate just the opposite. For example: "[A]rtificial, non-spontaneous breathing produced by a machine . . . is not driven by felt need, and the exchange of gases that it effects is neither an achievement of the organism nor a sign of its genuine vitality" (p. 63, emphasis in original). A footnote of the white paper and the personal statement of Gilbert Meilaender supporting position two also emphasize that the inner drive to self-preserving commerce with the environment is what counts for organismic wholeness, not the actual commerce itself.[19]

The inner drive to breathe, mediated by the medullary respiratory centers, is of course absent in patients with total brain failure. But it can also be absent in conscious patients with lower brainstem lesions, and during sleep in patients with Ondine's curse (in whom the lack of drive is arguably also "irreversible," insofar as the person will die during sleep, at least without ventilatory assistance). So even the inner drive to breathe is not a necessary feature of organismic wholeness. Neither is inner consciousness, as acknowledged repeatedly in the white paper. The council fails to offer any reasoned argument why the combined absence of these two inner drives, neither of which alone suffices as an indicator of organismic death, together should suffice. Moreover—and very importantly—if primacy is to be given to inner drive over actual "commerce," then position two comes perilously close to conceding that purely internal properties, apart from any self-preserving exchange with the environment, can be relevant for organismic wholeness after all.

There are also counterexamples that undermine the logic of position two. For example, a human fetus has neither breathing (since the rhythmic contraction of the respiratory muscles moving amniotic fluid in and out of the lungs is not "breathing" in the life-preserving sense of position two), nor a drive to breathe, nor conscious self-preserving interaction with the (maternal) environment, yet it is unquestionably alive and a "whole" organism. And this is true not only (not even primarily) because eventually, after birth, it will breathe and consciously interact, but because of its manifestly holistic properties while still in utero.

For the fetus with an undeveloped brain, the placenta is analogous to the ventilator and feeding tube for a brain-damaged patient who depends on them for survival.

Finally, there is a logical disconnect between apneic coma being the conceptual essence of the neurological standard of death and the requirement of total brain failure. The council explains that, given the pathophysiological vicious cycle of brain swelling and herniation, the only way to guarantee the irreversibility of both coma and apnea is to require that herniation has run its full course—that is, that there is total brain failure (pp. 66–67). (In this respect, position two differs significantly from the British notion of "brainstem death.") Using totality as a surrogate for irreversibility assumes that all cases of irreversible apneic coma are the endpoint of the classical rostral-caudal sequence of brain destruction caused by transtentorial herniation. But if the medullary respiratory centers were always and necessarily the last thing to go, then it would be superfluous, in a case of known herniation, to require examination of all cranial nerve reflexes; demonstration of apnea alone would suffice to establish totality. Yet all published diagnostic criteria require explicit demonstration of absence of each and every cranial nerve reflex, in addition to an apnea test (notwithstanding that the apnea test is typically the last item performed in the sequence of tests). The experts responsible for these criteria would not have needed to formulate them that way if it were pathophysiologically impossible for herniation to-the-point-of-apnea to be incomplete, sparing some brainstem functions (at least for a while) despite reaching the medullary respiratory centers.

Moreover, rostro-caudal herniation is not the only pathophysiological pathway to irreversible apneic coma. Primary brainstem lesions, such as infarcts, hemorrhages, and tumors, can be patchy, yet if strategically placed, can result in destruction of the medullary respiratory centers and critical portions of the reticular activating system, causing both irreversible apnea and coma, while mostly sparing other brainstem structures and the cerebral hemispheres. If irreversible apneic coma is the reason why total brain failure is death, then such cases of partial brain failure should equally qualify as dead.

In short, it seems doubtful that, even with a lot more work, position two could be made compelling enough to save the neurological standard.

Implications

These objections aside, the council's white paper is both remarkable and courageous. It is remarkable for its reasoned assessment and rejection of all previously proposed justifications for a neurological standard of death. Although the council does not say it in so many words, it implies that over the past forty years, prior to the introduction of its own novel "commerce with the environment" rationale, all statutory death laws, all diagnostic criteria for "brain death," and all transplantations from heart-beating donors have, in retrospect, been based on an invalid conceptual framework and incorrect empirical "facts" about bodies with total brain failure.

The council is courageous for its explicit readiness to accept the full ethical consequences if its proposed "commerce" rationale turns out not to hold any more conceptual water than its forerunners: "If indeed it is the case that there is no solid scientific or philosophical rationale for the current 'whole brain standard,' then the only ethical course is to stop procuring organs from heart-beating indi-

viduals" (p. 12, emphasis in original). This and similar statements are truly audacious in light of the council's humility about its own conceptual innovation: regarding patients in total brain failure, for example, the council admits that "there is still reason to wonder if our knowledge of their condition is adequate for labeling them as dead" (p. 54).

The final sections of the paper, on the implications for policy and practice and on non-heart-beating organ donation, are also thoughtful and morally cautious. One point deserves greater elaboration, however. This is that although the council reaffirms the traditional requirement of consent for organ donation (p. 10), not once does it pair the term "consent" with "informed." Yet this curious omission is actually typical for the literature on organ donation. "Informed" has never been a characteristic of the consent process for organ donation. With the council's white paper, it is high time to confront this elephant in the room. Just as cigarette ads are required to contain a footnote warning of health risks, ads promoting organ donation should contain a footnote along these lines: "Warning: It remains controversial whether you will actually be dead at the time of removal of your organs. This depends on the conceptual validity of 'position two' in the analysis of the determination of death conducted by the President's Council on Bioethics. You should study it carefully and decide for yourself before signing an organ donor card."

Similarly, in conversations with families of patients in total brain failure, representatives of organ procurement organizations should frankly disclose the existence of ongoing controversies over whether their loved one is dead or in a deep, irreversible coma. Of course such information is never given, neither to the public nor to individuals, because it would likely decrease the number of donated organs. But perhaps the time has come for patient dignity and autonomy to take precedence over utility for the good of others, by reforming the consent process in this area to come up to the high standard of all other consents in health care—that is, by allowing the decision-maker to be truly informed.

Author Affliation

D. Alan Shewmon is professor of neurology and pediatrics at the David Geffen School of Medicine at the University of California Los Angeles, and chief of neurology at Olive View-UCLA Medical Center, Sylmar, California. He has a special interest in philosophical-neurological interface issues such as brain death and the vegetative state and is strongly critical of equating brain death with death.

Notes

1. President's Council on Bioethics, Controversies in the Determination of Death (Washington, D.C.: President's Council on Bioethics, 2008).

2. H.K. Beecher et al., "A Definition of Irreversible Coma," Journal of the American Medical Association 205 (1968): 337–40.

3. MA. DeVita, J.V. Snyder, and A. Grenvik, "History of Organ Donation by Patients with Cardiac Death," Kennedy Institute of Ethics Journal 3 (1993): 113–29.

4. PM. Black, "Brain Death (Second of Two Parts)," New England Journal of Medicine 299 (1978): 393–401, at 395–96.

5. President's Commission for the Study of Ethical Problems in Medicine and Biomedical and Behavioral Research, Defining Death: Medical Legal and Ethical Issues in the Determination of Death (Washington, D.C.: U.S. Government Printing Office, 1981).

6. J.L. Bernat, C.M. Culver, and B. Gert, "On the Definition and Criterion of Death," Annals of Internal Medicine 94 (1981): 389–94.

7. S.J. Youngner et al., "'Brain Death' and Organ Retrieval: A Cross-Sectional Survey of Knowledge and Concepts among Health Professionals," Journal of the American Medical Association 261 (1989): 2205–2210; LA. Siminoff, C. Burant, and SJ. Youngner, "Death and Organ Procurement: Public Beliefs and Attitudes," Kennedy Institute of Ethics Journal 14 (2004): 217–34.

8. American Academy of Neurology, Quality Standards Subcommittee, "Practice Parameters for Determining Brain Death in Adults (Summary Statement)," Neurology 45 (1995): 1012–14; E.F. Wijdicks, "Determining Brain Death in Adults," Neurology 45 (1995): 1003–1011.

9. AH. Ropper and RH. Brown, Adams and Victor's Principles of Neurology (New York: McGraw-Hill, 2005), 962, emphasis added.

10. F. Plum, "Clinical Standards and Technological Confirmatory Tests in Diagnosing Brain Death," in The Definition of Death: Contemporary Controversies, ed. S.J. Youngner, R.M. Arnold, and R. Schapiro (Baltimore, Md.: Johns Hopkins University Press, 1999), 34–65, at 53, emphasis added.

11. R.E. Cranford and D.R Smith, "Consciousness: The Most Critical Moral (Constitutional) Standard for Human Personhood," American Journal of Law and Medicine 13 (1987): 233–48, at 243, emphasis added.

12. For criticisms of organismic unity, see Journal of Medicine and Philosophy 26, no. 5 (2001), entire issue. On the personhood rationale, see J.P. Lizza, Persons, Humanity, and the Definition of Death (Baltimore, Md.: Johns Hopkins University Press, 2006); R.M. Veatch, "The Impending Collapse of the Whole-Brain Definition of Death," Hastings Center Report 23, no. 4 (1993): 18–24; R.M. Veatch, "The Death of Whole-Brain Death: The Plague of the Disaggregators, Somaticists, and Mentalists," Journal of Medicine and Philosophy 30 (2005): 353–78; M.B. Green and D. Wilder, "Brain Death and Personal Identity," Philosophy and Public Affairs 9 (1980): 105–33; RM. Zaner, ed., Death: Beyond Whole-Brain Criteria (Dordrecht,

the Netherlands: Kluwer Academic Publishers, 1988); RJ. Devettete, "Neocortical Death and Human Death," Law, Medicine and Health Care 18 (1990): 96–104.

13. F. Plum and J.B. Posner, The Diagnosis of Stupor and Coma (Philadelphia, Penn.: FA Davis Company, 1983), at 325; C. Machado, "A New Definition of Death Based on the Basic Mechanisms of Consciousness Generation in Human Beings," in Brain Death. Proceedings of the Second International Conference on Brain Death, ed. C. Machado (Amsterdam, the Netherlands: Elsevier, 1995), 57–66.

14. S.J. Youngner and R.M. Arnold, "Philosophical Debates about the Definition of Death: Who Cares?" Journal of Medicine and Philosophy 26 (2001): 527–37; RD. Truog and W.M. Robinson, "Role of Brain Death and the Dead-Donor Rule in the Ethics of Organ Transplantation," Critical Care Medicine 31 (2003): 2391–96; N. Fost, "Reconsidering the Dead Donor Rule: Is It Important That Organ Donors Be Dead?" Kennedy Institute of Ethics Journal 14 (2004): 249–60; F.G. Miller and R.D. Truog, "Rethinking the Ethics of Vital Organ Donations," Hastings Center Report 38, no. 6 (2008): 38–46.

15. E.F.M. Wijdicks, "Brain Death Worldwide: Accepted Fact but No Global Consensus in Diagnostic Criteria," Neurology 58 (2002): 20–25.

16. All parenthetical references are to the white paper; President's Council on Bioethics, "Controversies in the Determination of Death: A White Paper by the President's Council on Bioethics" (Washington, D.C.: President's Council on Bioethics, 2009); http://www.bioethics. gov/reports/death/index.html.

17. The council acknowledges this reasoning when it explains that breathing is not a necessary sign of life: "Even if the animal has lost that capacity, other vital capacities might still be present" (p. 64). But it fails to use the same logic as applied jointly to breathing and consciousness.

18. Emphasis added. Curiously, this statement is contradicted later in the white paper by another claim: "This drive [to breathe] is the organism's own impulse, exercised on its own behalf, and indispensable to its continued existence" (p. 62). The claim that the drive to breathe is indispensable is patently false.

19. The footnote states: "Shewmon fails to convey the essential character of breathing. . . . [He] misses the critical element: the drive exhibited by the whole organism to bring in air, a drive that is fundamental to the constant, vital working of the whole organism" (p. 63, emphasis in original).

Chapter 9

The Boundaries of Organ Donation after Circulatory Death

James L. Bernat

Organ donation after circulatory (or cardiac) death has become an accepted medical practice over the past 15 years.[1] Programs permitting such donations satisfy two needs: they provide organs in addition to those procured after brain death, and they fulfill the wish of family members that relatives with severe brain injuries serve as organ donors after cessation of life-sustaining therapy and subsequent death. The proliferation of protocols for donation after circulatory death has been spurred by the publication of three reports by the Institute of Medicine (IOM), support by the Department of Health and Human Services, and the establishment of criteria for such donation by the Joint Commission, which accredits U.S. hospitals. A 2005 national conference on the topic identified areas of consensus in an effort to standardize practice.[2]

Now that donation after circulatory death has become mainstream, researchers have begun to design innovative protocols that aim to improve the function of transplants and expand the donor pool. These protocols test the conceptual limits of donation after circulatory death—by permitting invasive intervention in living organ donors or by altering the tests required to determine death. In this issue of the *Journal*, Boucek et al. (pages 709–714) report their success with a research protocol for the donation of infant hearts after circulatory death, in which they shortened the duration of asystole required for the determination of death to less than that in prevailing standards of practice. To determine whether such protocols should be incorporated into standards of practice, we must analyze them within the context of accepted principles of organ transplantation from deceased donors (see table) and test them against the conceptual basis for death determination.

The decision of a patient (or a surrogate) to have life-sustaining therapy withheld should precede and remain independent of the decision to donate organs. The strict separation of these two decisions ensures that society's need or a physician's request for organs does not drive the decision to withdraw treatment—a possibility that may be even more of a concern when the patient and potential organ donor is a child.[3] In most cases, the inherent conflict may be mitigated (but not eliminated) by having a representative from the local organ-procurement organization, rather than physicians in the intensive care unit (ICU), speak to families about donation.

The physician team determining death must be strictly separated from the procurement team to prevent organ-procurement considerations from influencing the death determination. This separation of roles is even more critical in donation after circulatory

Principles Governing Organ Transplantation Involving Deceased Donors.		
Principle	**Donation after Brain Death**	**Donation after Cardiac Death**
Respect the dead donor rule	Yes	Yes
Determine death using accepted tests and procedures	Yes, using brain-death tests	Yes, using circulatory-death tests
Separate death-determination team from organ-procurement team	Yes	Yes
Separate decision to refuse life-sustaining therapy from decision to donate	Not applicable	Yes
Obtain surrogate consent for withdrawal of life-sustaining therapy	No	Yes
Obtain surrogate consent for organ donation	Yes	Yes
Provide palliative care during dying	No	Yes
Provide end-of-life family support	Yes	Yes
Properly design and scrupulously follow protocol; document findings	Yes	Yes

death than in donation after brain death, because the former requires the withdrawal of life-sustaining therapy, which should be done by the donor's ICU physician. The recent allegations against Dr. Hootan Roozrokh in San Luis Obispo, California, demonstrates the serious problems that may result from the conflict created when a transplantation surgeon manages the terminal care of a potential organ donor.

The process of withdrawing life-sustaining therapy and providing appropriate palliative care for a dying patient should be the same, irrespective of the patient's donor status. The situation becomes complicated, however, when a protocol permits intervention in the living donor through the administration of intravenous heparin or vasodilators, not to benefit the donor patient but only to improve the function of transplantable organs. Protocols instituting extracorporeal membrane oxygenation (ECMO) in the donor after the declaration of death permit much more invasive intervention, including the insertion

of arterial catheters before death. Advocates assert that surrogate consent sufficiently justifies these interventions, because they are minimally harmful to the patient and they benefit the organ recipient. Opponents argue that respect for the dying patient is being compromised.

The dead donor rule states that the donor must be dead before vital organs are procured. Death statutes require the irreversible cessation of circulation and respiration or the irreversible cessation of brain functions; the former constitutes an adequate criterion for death because, in the absence of cardiopulmonary resuscitation (CPR) or autoresuscitation, it inevitably leads to the fulfillment of the brain criterion.[4]

What duration of asystole proves irreversibility? The IOM has recommended that after the withdrawal of life-sustaining therapy, physicians wait 5 minutes after the onset of asystole to be certain that a heart rhythm sufficient to generate a pulse does not resume spontaneously. In such circumstances, autoresuscitation has never been reported after 65 seconds of asystole. Physicians can confidently declare the donor dead after 5 minutes of asystole and apnea, because without autoresuscitation or CPR, the cessation of circulatory and respiratory functions is permanent (will not return), and it inevitably and rapidly becomes irreversible (cannot return).[4]

In their investigational protocol, Boucek et al. shortened the interval of required asystole to 75 seconds on the grounds that 60 seconds was the longest reported duration of asystole that had been followed by autoresuscitation and that the sooner death can be declared after asystole, the less damage from warm ischemia will occur in the organs. What minimum duration of asystole ensures that autoresuscitation will not occur is an empirical question that can be answered conclusively only after observing many hundreds of patients. The recommended duration of asystole required for donation after circulatory death should be determined by scientific and public policy considerations. The IOM and the Canadian Council for Donation and Transplantation purposely chose a conservative duration of 5 minutes, which has been adopted by most donation programs, but a few protocols use as short a span as 2 minutes. In 2005, participants in a national conference on donation after circulatory death agreed with the recommendation by the Society of Critical Care Medicine to wait at least 2 minutes and at most 5 minutes.[2]

An unanswered question is whether cardiac transplantation from a donor declared dead according to a circulatory criterion retroactively negates the determination of death. Does the fact that a donor's heart is restarted in another patient prove that circulatory cessation was not irreversible? Or should the requirement of irreversibility be restricted to circulation within the donor?

Another unconventional protocol used by several hospitals for donation after circulatory death involves providing ECMO to the donor immediately after death is declared. If ECMO adequately provided circulation and oxygenation to the donor's entire body, it would retroactively negate the death determination by preventing the loss of circulation and respiration from becoming permanent or irreversible, potentially "reanimating" the heart and preventing the progression to brain destruction on which the circulatory criterion of death is predicated.

A University of Michigan ECMO protocol for procuring abdominal organs apparently avoids this problem.[5] During ECMO, an intraaortic occlusion balloon blocks all blood flow above the diaphragm so that only the abdominal organs are perfused with oxygenated blood. The thoracic organs and brain are isolated from this perfusion circuit and are destroyed by ischemic infarction. If blood flow above the diaphragm is successfully blocked, this protocol does not negate the previous determination of death. Ex vivo ECMO, in which the procured organ is temporarily perfused and preserved after removal from the donor's body, is another technique that is under investigation.

These investigational protocols test the permissible societal boundaries of donation after circulatory death. To what extent should society permit manipulation of an organ donor or alteration of the determination of human death for the good of organ recipients? A consensus-driven oversight process should determine whether investigational protocols reflect appropriate medical treatment and whether their translation into accepted clinical practice is sound public policy. Leaders of the critical care, neurology, and transplantation communities need to jointly draft practice guidelines for organ donation after circulatory death that establish acceptable boundaries of practice. These boundaries should be based on scientific data and accepted principles and should be demarcated conservatively to maintain public confidence in the integrity of the transplantation enterprise. I predict that when prudent boundaries are created, they will exclude whole-body ECMO of the donor and death determinations at 75 seconds of asystole.

No potential conflict of interest relevant to this article was reported.

Dr. Bernat is a professor of neurology and medicine at Dartmouth Medical School, Hanover, NH.

Notes

1. Steinbrook R. Organ donation after cardiac death. N Engl J Med 2007; 357:209–13.

2. Bernat JL, D'Alessandro AM, Port FK, et al. Report of a national conference on donation after cardiac death. Am J Transplant 2006; 6: 281–91.

3. Mandell MS, Zamudio S, Seem D, et al. National evaluation of healthcare provider attitudes toward organ donation after cardiac death. Crit Care Med 2006; 34:2952–58.

4. Bernat JL. Are organ donors after cardiac death really dead? J Clin Ethics 2006;17: 122–32.

5. Magliocca JF, Magee JC, Rowe SA, et al. Extracorporeal support for organ donation after cardiac death effectively expands the donor pool. J Trauma 2005; 58:1095–102.

Chapter 10

AN EXCERPT FROM

Should We Allow Organ Donation Euthanasia?

Alternatives for Maximizing the Number and Quality of Organs for Transplantation

Dominic Wilkinson and Julian Savulescu

Conclusions

In this paper we have argued that one of the ethical principles that should influence, and in the past *has* influenced transplantation policy is the need to maximize the number and quality of organs for transplantation. There is a substantial shortfall in organs for transplant. We could overcome this in a range of ways. Future developments in xenotransplantation, stem cell-based therapies, or neo-organs might make the use of organs from deceased donors unnecessary. However, such solutions are some time off, and in the meantime thousands of patients per year die for want of a transplanted organ.

The most promising immediate source of organs for transplantation is the large number of patients who die in intensive care units in hospitals following diagnosis of brain death, or decisions to withdraw Life Support Treatment (LST) on the basis of poor prognosis, the group that we have referred to as Life Support Withdrawal (LSW) donors. At present the majority of such organs are buried or burned with the patient.

We have suggested a set of options for increasing the number of organs that could be made available from LSW donors. Simple measures should be adopted, including

improved efficiency of approaching families for consent or a switch to an opt-out consent system; however, they may not be enough to resolve the organ shortfall. Organ Conscription would have the greatest potential to increase the numbers of organs available for transplantation, though it would come at the cost of patient and family autonomy. If Organ Conscription is not acceptable, the alternative that would have the greatest potential in terms of organ numbers would be Organ Donation Euthanasia.

Proposal for allowing Organ Donation Euthanasia (ODE)

Definition

Removal of organs from a patient under general anesthesia. Death follows removal of the heart.

Eligibility criteria:

1. The patient is dependent on life support in intensive care
2. Withdrawal of life support is planned on the basis of poor prognosis
3. Death is predicted to occur within a short period after withdrawal of life support
4. Prognosis has been independently confirmed

5. The patient has consented specifically for Organ Donation Euthanasia

Arguments in favor of Organ Donation Euthanasia

1. It would promote patient autonomy
2. It would provide patients with the greatest chance of being able to donate their organs after death
3. It would be a Pareto improvement over current practice for treatment withdrawal and increase the number and quality of organs available for transplantation.
4. Suffering or discomfort for the patient would be less likely than with withdrawal of life support

Arguments against Organ Donation Euthanasia

1. It may lead to a fall in organ donation rates due to community non-acceptance
2. It could lead to the killing of patients who would not otherwise have died

Organ Donation Euthanasia would conflict with the dead donor rules, and the injunction against physician killing. Yet it would not (if appropriate safeguards were provided) lead to the death of any patients who would otherwise live. The justification for this is not limited to utilitarian considerations. It is a Pareto improvement on current practice for withdrawal of LST and organ donation, and may be Pareto optimal. ODE would apply to patients who are going to die—and soon. It is already accepted that it is permissible to withdraw life support from these patients. It would prevent those individuals from suffering as a consequence of withdrawal of life support. And it would save the lives of up to 9 other individuals. Many potential LSW donors, even

if they would have wanted to donate their organs, and their families consent, are currently unable to donate. Their organs die with them.

The most acceptable way to introduce Organ-Donation Euthanasia would be to make it available as an option for prospective organ donors. It must be noted, though, that if ODE were made available in this way, it would have (at least in the short term) only a small impact upon the organ shortfall since only a few individuals would be likely to embrace it. This would undermine to some degree the case in terms of organ supply for ODE. But if we can save even one life, that is something of great moral importance. Many lives could be saved even if only a small percentage of people opted for ODE. And there is also a strong autonomy-based argument for allowing individuals who wish to donate their organs to opt in to ODE (in the circumstance that they are severely ill in intensive care and going to have life support withdrawn.) We should allow people to make advance directives indicating that they would like to be eligible for this alternative. We should encourage and support such altruistic desires.

To some degree at least, there is a conflict between the need to supply organs to the largest number of individuals able to benefit from them, and our beliefs about how we ought to care for those who are dying or dead. We have outlined seven alternatives that may increase the supply of organs. These alternatives clash with one or more of the traditionally accepted ethical principles that govern transplantation, though they potentially promote other ethical values including those of autonomy and beneficence. Whichever transplantation policy is adopted, we should ensure that decisions about withdrawal of life-sustaining treatment are separated from decisions about organ donation, and that organ donation procedures carry minimal risks of causing suffering to organ donors. But continuing current transplantation practice comes at a cost, in terms of a significant number of patients who die or continue to suffer organ failure for want of an available organ. We should think seriously about whether it is time to embrace an alternative strategy.

Chapter 11

The Ethics of Non-Heart-Beating Donation

How New Technology Can Change the Ethical Landscape

Kristin Zeiler, Elisabeth Furberg, Gunnar Tufveson, and Staffen Welin

Abstract

The global shortage of organs for transplantation and the development of new and better medical technologies for organ preservation have resulted in a renewed interest in non-heart-beating donation (NHBD). This article discusses ethical questions related to controlled and uncontrolled NHBD. It argues that certain preparative measures, such as giving anticoagulants, should be acceptable before patients are dead, but when they have passed a point where further curative treatment is futile, they are in the process of dying and they are unconscious. Furthermore, the article discusses consequences of technological developments based on improvement of a chest compression apparatus used today to make mechanical heart resuscitation. Such technological development can be used to transform cases of non-controlled NHBD to controlled NHBD. In our view, this is a step forward since the ethical difficulties related to controlled NHBD are easier to solve than those related to non-controlled NHBD. However, such technological developments also evoke other ethical questions.

Non-heart-beating donation (hereafter referred to as NHBD) was common in the 1970s. At that time, NHBD was the only way that the donation of vital organs could be performed according to "the dead donor rule" since organ donation was only acceptable after irreversible cardiac arrest. The acceptance of the whole-brain-death definition, that is, death defined as "the irreversible cessation of all functions of the entire brain, including the brain stem," (1) changed this and it made transplantation of vital organs from brain-dead donors possible.

During the 1980s and 1990s, the number of heart-beating, brain-dead donors increased and NHBD gradually became less common. The development of new and better medical technologies for organ preservation and the global shortage of organs for transplantation have resulted, however, in a renewed interest in NHBD.

At present, there are protocols for both non-controlled and controlled NHBD (2–7). Non-controlled NHBD protocols are applied when resuscitation efforts fail after cardiac arrest. This situation usually occurs in the hospital, and most often in the emergency room. Controlled NHBD typically involves a patient who is on a ventilator. There is no hope of recovery, but the patient has brain activity. Furthermore, the heart as well as other organs still function. If further treatment is deemed futile, the medical team stops the artificial ventilation. After cardiac arrest has occurred and death has been declared, organs can be removed if the patient wanted to donate and if there are no medical contraindications against NHBD. The required time span between cardiac arrest and the declaration of death varies between countries and NHBD/transplantation programmes (compare for example (2–7)).

We consider NHBD to be an interesting way to increase the number of organs available for transplantation. However, it evokes a number of ethically difficult questions, some of which we will discuss in this paper.

- How long should one wait after cardiac arrest before declaring death and removing organs, if the donor wanted to donate when alive?
- For whose sake are preparations made? Donation, we will argue, is done for the benefit of recipients and out of respect for the donor's autonomy.

One well-known controversy concerns whether preparative measures, such as giving anticoagulants, are acceptable before the patient is dead, in the interest of the recipients-to-be as well as for the donor-to-be. We will argue that such treatment is acceptable when a still living patient has reached a point where further curative treatment is futile, the patient is in the process of dying and she or he is deeply unconscious. We will call this point the point of no return and we will argue that this is the ethically important point. When the patient has passed beyond this point, nothing can be done to stop the process of dying and restore health. In practice, the existence of such a point has been accepted in all countries where it is deemed acceptable to abort treatment because it is futile.

- Another ethical question concerns how and when informed consent should be obtained.

Obtaining informed consent before one starts organ donation preparatory treatment is more complicated in the non-controlled NHBD case than in the controlled case. Below, we will argue that whereas explicit consent should be obtained before one starts organ donation preparatory treatments in controlled NHBD, and whereas it is an advantage to get an explicit consent for these treatments also in the early phase of the non-controlled NHBD, it should not be necessary when the person has passed the point of no return. Our reasons for holding this view are both practical and ethical.

Finally, even if these ethical questions were to be resolved, there are still problems—particularly in the case of non-controlled NHBD—related to the change from life-saving efforts to preparatory measures for organ donation. This paper discusses how NHBD can be done in an ethically acceptable way. It discusses the three ethical questions presented above. We will also discuss the consequences of a possible technological development based on improvement of a chest compression apparatus used today to perform mechanical heart resuscitation. Such technological development can be used to transform cases of non-controlled NHBD into cases of controlled NHBD. In our view, this is a step forward since the ethical difficulties related to controlled NHBD are easier to solve than those related to non-controlled NHBD. Most of the ethical and psychological difficulties with NHBD are associated with the non-controlled case, where one starts with a life-saving treatment and then changes to preparatory measures for organ donation.

On the Relation between Ethics and Law

In most countries, transplantation laws regulate the medical practice of organ donation. In our view, the ideal situation is that the relevant laws harmonise with ethics. However, it is not difficult to imagine scenarios in which laws and ethics do not harmonise. In such cases we suggest that the law should be changed. However, medical professionals should follow the existing laws—but they may argue and work for a change of the law.

The Ethics of Present-Day NHBD

First ethical question: time span between cardiac arrest and declaration of death

When the British Transplant Society refers to brain-related death criteria, it states that it is a key requirement that a certain interval has elapsed without circulation, long enough to ensure that profound hypoxic injury to the brain has occurred—so that the capacity for consciousness and the capacity to breathe are irreversibly lost (8). An interval of five minutes "hands-off" is recommended,[1] provided that the patient has normal core body temperature.[2]

This time span is disputed and NHBD protocols differ on what time is required without circulation. According to the Maastricht protocol, a ten-minute hands-off period is required to ensure that irreversible brain death has occurred (2–4). Other protocols state that it is mandatory to observe a no-touch interval of five minutes (5–9). Still others, such as the University of Pittsburgh Medical Center policy, argue that death could be declared only two minutes after loss of cardiopulmonary function (7, 10–12).

How long the waiting time needs to be should depend on what exact death criteria is being used.[3] However, for the present discussion, the important issue is not the exact minutes for the hands-off time. It is more important to consider when someone has passed the point of no return. For this reason, we will allow ourselves not to enter the discussion of exactly how long this hands-off time should be.[4]

Second ethical question: for whose sake is treatment done?

In order to discuss patients' medical treatment a distinction can be made between:

- treatment *before the point of no return*, i.e., the point when (a) there is no curative treatment nor hope of spontaneous improvement, (b) the patient is in the process of dying and life cannot be prolonged more than marginally even with intensive care, and (c) the patient is deeply unconscious,
- treatment when the patient has passed this point, which we will call *treatment after the point of no return*,
- measures undertaken *after the patient is dead*.

We need also to distinguish between treatment for the health of the person and treatment for the sake of respecting the will of the person.

Clearly, *after death* nothing can be done for the sake of the patient's health. After the declaration of death, organ donation can take place if the patient has given her or his consent during life. If interventions are performed on the deceased after the declaration of death these are performed in the interest of the recipients-to-be. They are *also*, in our view, performed for the sake of respecting the will of the person *if* she or he wanted to become a donor.

What, then, about treatment *before the point of no return*? Before this point, the patient should *only* be treated for her/his own sake. This general rule, which obviously applies to the whole health care system, is important in order to maintain people's trust that medical treatment is given to patients in order to improve their situation and that no efforts are spared as long as the patient has not passed the point of no return.[5]

After the point of no return, we will argue, it is ethically acceptable to start preparatory measures aiming at organ donation—for example, to give a large amount of heparin. In this stage, the patient is in the process of dying and is deeply unconscious. By definition, nothing curative can be done for the patient at this time though the patient is still alive. Since nothing curative can be done for the patient, s/he is in the process of dying and is deeply unconscious, we suggest that treatment may be initiated whose primary goal is good consequences for a future organ recipient.

Let us give an example from the Swedish situation. According to the Swedish transplantation act, (13) the known will of the deceased person should always be respected. However, if the will of the deceased person is *not* known, which is often the case, presumed consent applies (and relatives have the right to say no to donation).

Organ donation is allowed when the patient has been declared dead and up to 24 hours after the declaration of death. Furthermore, when death has been declared, medical treatment for the sake of enabling a later organ donation *is* allowed even if the will of the deceased person is not yet known (14). It should be noted that in Sweden, the medical staff are advised not to discuss the patient's organ donation wishes, with her or his family members, before the declaration of death. Whereas it is possible to register one's view on donation in a national Donation Registry, medical professionals are *not allowed* to look into this Register for Organ Donation Advance Directives before the patient has been declared dead.

Consider now the following case: a patient is declared dead, and no preparatory treatment is initiated prior to death in order to make organ donation possible. The patient has not registered in the Donation Registry, but relatives (after death has been declared) say that the patient wanted to donate organs. However, due to the time-factor, and since donation preparatory measures were not performed earlier on, donation is no longer possible.

In cases of this sort, the will of the deceased who did want to donate cannot be respected. We believe that those who want to donate should be given this possibility, since donation is a beneficent and possibly life-saving act. In accordance with the Swedish law, we hold that it is important that steps can be taken to enable donation when death is declared even if the will of the patient is yet unknown. However, in accordance with our ethical view—but in contrast to the Swedish law—we suggest that donation preparatory measures should be allowed *also* before death but after the point of no return, provided that it is not known that the patient did not want to donate organs and, in the case of controlled NHBD, provided that relations have given their informed consent.

It should be noted that this implies not that a human being is treated as a means only; she or he is treated as a means but also as an end. She or he is given heparin in the interest of others, *and* in order to ensure the possibility of respecting her/his will.[6]

We suggest that the will of those who did not want to donate is not harmed, even if they are given heparin *while information is being sought about what they wanted*: if they did not want to donate organs, such donation will not take place. If it is known beforehand that the patient did not want to donate organs, no preparatory measures aiming at organ donation should take place.[7]

Third ethical question: how and when should informed consent be obtained?

Informed consent for donation needs to be distinguished from informed consent for preparatory treatments in order to enable a possible organ donation. The third ethical question in need of being addressed is whether, and if so what kind of, informed consent for preparatory treatment is necessary in cases of NHBD.

It is commonly assumed that medical treatment should require informed consent in some form. There are also exceptions to be noted, such as when the patient is unconscious and in need of emergency treatment. In these cases, medical professionals act paternalistically, on the basis of what is assumed to be for the best of the patient, and consent is presumed. (However, also in these circumstances, relatives should be contacted expeditiously.)

It should be noted that many ethicists argue that one must put emphasis on the informed part of the informed consent. Although there are various ideas about how this part of the informed consent should be understood, many ethicists agree that the person who makes the decision (if not the patient, then perhaps some relative) needs to go through some process of deliberation (15). In the case of controlled NHBD, informed consent for preparatory treatments can in principle always be obtained (at least from the patients relatives) since there is more time. One may simply wait to stop ventilation and other treatment that is not palliative until informed consent

from relatives has been obtained, or from the consent registrar, if such exist in the particular country. However, in most cases of non-controlled NHBD there is no time for such a deliberative process, provided that there is no answer to be found in a registry or in a written advance directive. The need for a very hasty decision, and the lack of time needed to make an informed one, therefore renders it problematic to *require* informed consent for preparatory treatments in the acute phase of non-controlled NHBD when the person has reached the point of no return. It is practically complicated, as well as ethically questionable, to urge relatives to make such a hasty decision.

We conclude that whereas informed consent for preparatory treatments should be required in cases of controlled NHBD, it should not be required in the acute phase of non-controlled NHBD when the person has reached the point of no return. Obviously, regarding valid informed consent, it would be advantageous if non-controlled NHBD could be transformed into controlled NHBD—as this would ease the problem of obtaining informed consent.

Controlled NHBD is less problematic than non-controlled NHBD since decisions do not need to be made in such haste. We believe that a change from a non-controlled to controlled NHBD situation would be positive and that it will be possible—given some technological development.

A Future Scenario

Consider the following future scenario in which a pneumatic chest compression/decompression apparatus will be used. Such apparatuses, for example LUCAS (Joliffe AB, Lund, Sweden), are already approved for use in mobile emergency units (16). Our scenario is based on the possibility of further improving the present technology. Assume that a person outside the hospital suffers a myocardial infarction that leads to cardiac arrest. The ambulance arrives within a few minutes and resuscitation efforts by means of a highly effective pneumatic chest compression/decompression apparatus start immediately. This is aimed at saving the patient's life. Assume also that the patient can be intubated and ventilated immediately.

Even if resuscitation fails (the heart does not regain its function), pneumatic chest compression/decompression and ventilation may be continued until arrival to the emergency room. After arrival, the blood is still flowing to the brain and the patient is still alive. (We assume that the patient has not developed a total brain infarction though there has been severe brain damage.) When the patient is still attached to a heart compressor in the hospital (she or he has no spontaneous heart activity), relatives can be contacted in order to find out the patients' will. If the patient is *beyond the point of no return*, the compressor is withdrawn and, after relevant medical examination, death is declared. Organ donation may proceed, if the patient so wanted when alive. If the wish of the patient is not known, the relatives' consent should be sought.

This is a future controlled NHBD scenario, different from the controlled NHBD scenarios of today. Still, it resembles the present-day NHBD scenario in important ways. Resuscitation efforts start as soon as the ambulance arrives, the highly effective pneumatic chest compression/decompression apparatus making sure that heart as well as other organs function when the ambulance arrives at the hospital, and (we assume) during the next couple of hours. Relatives are contacted. If the patient wanted to donate, and if there are no

medical contraindications against NHBD, the medical staff stops the artificial ventilation, after consent from the relatives, and waits until cardiac arrest occurs.

In discussions of future scenarios, it is difficult to assess how many organs can be retrieved. It is also difficult, for obvious reasons, to assess the quality of these organs. However, non-controlled NHBD that result in transplantations of kidneys, livers and pancreas do occur today (16, 17). Furthermore, there are reasons to believe that the future scenario can become reality. The pneumatic chest compression/decompression apparatus LUCAS has been used in cases of non-controlled NHBD. Steen and colleagues in Lund, Sweden, transplanted a lung in such a case, where the lung was reconditioned *ex vivo* (18, 19). The transplantation was possible thanks to the usage of LUCAS.[8]

We may expect better results, the more similar to the present day controlled donation after cardiac death that the future scenario will become.[9]

The future scenario would do away with the special ethical and psychological problems surrounding non-controlled NHBD, such as the problem of informed consent in a very urgent situation and the change from life-saving efforts to organ donation preparation. It is an example of a scenario where some feasible technical advance may solve some ethical problems. However, the use of such future technology may also result in a new category of patients who survive a cardiac arrest and who live supported by the artificial heart compressor until their hearts either regain their activity or are replaced or supported by a medical device.

Ethical Issues Raised in the Future Scenario

Suppose the new chest compression technology is so effective that the scenario may occur. However, the use of chest compression technologies and artificial ventilation may not always restore the patient's health, nor may the patient die. In some cases the heart may regain its activity but only after there has been severe brain damage and the patient may end up in a vegetative state needing continuous life-supporting treatment. Here, the personal suffering of the patients and relatives, and the will of the patients need to be taken into account.

Another issue raised by new methods in transplantation and in particular the use of non-optimal organs (which may be the case at least in the early stages of our future scenario) is who should receive these "marginal" organs and what kind of informed consent is needed. However, this is a general problem in any expansion of what counts as acceptable organs for transplantation and not special to our scenario.

Concluding Remarks

Although some of the ethical problems outlined in this paper remain, this transformation of uncontrolled NHBD candidates into controlled NHBD candidates would give the medical staff the time needed to find out if consent for organ donation can be obtained, either through an advance directive of some sort or by giving the proxy enough time for reflection and a truly informed decision. The possible development of chest compression technologies may help to ease the ethical problems surrounding present-day NHBD.

However, the new advances in technology suggest that there will be a grey area between resuscitation efforts and measures that are undertaken in the interest of future transplant recipients. It is hard to define when resuscitation efforts including a heart compressor, such as LUCAS, stop being a tool for rescuing the patient's life and turn into a means for maintaining function, at least partly, of the organs in a possible organ donor.

Usually, attempts at resuscitation are made in the case of patients with cardiac arrest. We suggest that these attempts continue either until the patient recovers or reaches the point of no return. This may seem problematic, since the longer cardio-pulmonary resuscitation continues, the more severe mechanical damage to myocardium and lungs occurs. However, the actual Swedish scenario described above, which resembles our future scenario, did result in a lung transplant.

In the best possible scenario, the patient will survive with minimal or no brain damage. In another scenario, the patient would be a candidate for controlled NHBD, if she or he so wanted when alive.

Competing interests: None.

Notes

1. It should also be noted that a brain-stem concept of death is used in the United Kingdom.

2. During hypothermia, the human brain is able to withstand much longer periods of circulation arrest. See for example Litasova et al. (20).

3. Since most (but not all) countries have accepted the whole-brain death definition as the legally valid definition, we will allow ourselves not to discuss death definitions in this article. Furthermore, we will argue as if the whole-brain death definition was the legally accepted version. See (21) for a death declaration law that accepts not only the whole-brain death definition as legal, but also the traditional heart-lung death.

4. If one holds the view that all the functions of the entire brain, including the brain stem, should be irreversibly lost, this may result in a longer necessary timespan than if one holds the view that it is the irreversible loss of higher brain functions that matters. A higher-brain-death definition implies that death is defined as the irreversible loss of higher cognitive functions.

5. Obviously, if the patient is conscious, the rules of informed consent apply.

6. In a recent EU opinion poll, a majority of the Swedish population (74%) stated that they would like to donate their own organs after death (22).

7. One more ethical argument can support our view of the acceptability of organ-preserving treatment after the point of no return. The doctrine of double effect can be applied to this specific scenario. Even though giving a large amount of heparin could cause further haemorrhage in patients with brain injuries and thereby hasten death, this act meets the requirements of the double effect principle. The act is performed for the sake of something good: to ensure fulfilment of the patients' wishes. The intention is not to hasten the patient's death. Furthermore, the risk of death due to heparin is not a means to achieve organ viability. And, the patient is already in the process of dying.

8. However, it should also be noted that this lung was first rejected as non-acceptable by the Scandinavian transplant centres; later it was accepted for transplantation.

9. Of course, it could be argued that this is an expensive way of obtaining organs for donation and that living organ donation, as one example, is much less expensive. This, however, presumes that there are living organ donors that want to donate organs. This is not always the case.

References

1. Ott BB. Defining and redefining death. In: Caplan AL, Coelho DH, eds. *The ethics of organ transplantation.* New York: Prometheus Books, 1998:18.

2. Brook NR, Waller J, Richardson, AC, *et al.* A report on the activity and clinical outcomes of renal non-heart-beating donor transplantation in the United Kingdom. *Clin Transplant* 2004; 8:627–33.

3. Booster MH, Wijnen RMH, Ming Y, *et al.* In situ perfusion of kidneys from non-heart-beating donors: the Maastricht Protocol. *Transplant Proc* 1993; 25: 1503.

4. Daemen JW, Kootstra G, Wijnen RM, Yin M, Heineman E. Non-heart-beating donors: the Maastricht experience. *Clin Transplant* 1994; 8:303.

5. US Institute of Medicine. *Non-heart-beating organ transplantation: medical and ethical issues in procurement.* Washington DC: National Academy Press, 1997.

6. Feest TG, Riad HN, Collins CH, *et al.* Protocol for increasing organ donation after cerebrovascular death in a district general hospital. *Lancet* 1990; 335: 1133–35.

7. University of Pittsburgh Medical Centre. UMPC Policy for the management of terminally ill patients who may become organ donors after death. *Kennedy Inst Ethics J* 1993; 3:217–30.

8. British Transplant Society. *Guidelines relating to solid organ transplants from non-heart-beating donors.* London: British Transplant Society, 2004.

9. Bos MA. Ethical and legal issues in non-heart-beating organ donation. *Transplant Proc* 2005; 37: 574–76.

10. Younger SJ, Arnold RM, DeVita MA. When is "dead"? *Hastings Cent Rep* 1999; 29:14–21.

11. Zawistowski CA, DeVita MA. Non-heartbeating organ donation: a review. *J Intensive Care Med* 2003; 18:189–197.

12. DeVita MA. The death watch: certifying death using cardiac criteria. *Prog Transplant* 2001; 11: 1158–66.

13. The Swedish Transplantation Act [Lagen om transplantation]. *SFS* 1995:831.

14. The Swedish law on criteria for the assessment of death [Lag (1987:269) om kriterier för bestämmande av människans död]. *SFS* 1987:269.

15. Beauchamp T, Childress J. *Principles of biomedical ethics.* Oxford: Oxford University Press, 2001.

16. Foley DP, Fernandez LA, Leversen G, et al. Donation after cardiac death. The University of Wisconsin experience with liver transplantation. *Ann Surg* 2005; 242:724–31.

17. Fernandez LA, Di Carlo A, Odorico JS, *et al.* Simultaneous pancreas-kidney transplantation form donation after cardiac death. Successful long-term outcomes. *Ann Surg* 2005; 242:716–23.

18. Jolife. *Certificate for LUCAS*, 2003. Available at http://www.jolife.com (accessed 13 May 2008).

19. Steen S, Ingemansson R, Eriksson L, et al. First human transplantation of a non-acceptable donor lung after reconditioning ex vivo. *Ann Thorac Surg* 2007: 832:191–5.

20. Litasova EE, Beliaev AM, Lomivorotov VN, *et al.* [A procedure for compensating for the blood loss in heart operations under hypothermia without perfusion]. *Vestnik Khirurgii Imeni i—i—Grekova* 1992; 149:280–84.

21. New Jersey Statutes. Annotated. *Declaration of death*. 26:6A–5. St Louis, Mo: West Publishing, 1991: 232–35.

22. Zoki no Ishoku nikansuru Horitsu [The Japanese Law concerning organ transplantation], July 16th, 1997, Law no. 104 of 1997.

23. European Opinion Research Group, European Commission. Europeans and Organ donation. Special Eurobarometer 272D, 2007. Available at http://ec.eu ropa.eu/public_opinion/archives/ebs/ebs_272d_en.pdf (accessed 13 May 2008).

Part II

The Use of Anencephalic Infants as Organ Donors

James J. McCartney

At first glance, the use of anencephalics as organ donors appears to be a dated issue, because while this controversy seemed very important in the 1980s, public policy ultimately maintained an approach that was not in favor of using the organs of these damaged infants. However, the first chapter by Alex Capron shows that the issues raised by the use of anencephalic organs are very germane to the controversies discussed in part I of this book. Capron points out that there is no principled reason for considering anencephalics to be dead under the standards of the Uniform Determination of Death Act. To accept anencephalics as donors would, in fact, raise questions about the necessity of the dead donor rule in general and would not just be confined to anencephalics. In this context, Capron supports the dead donor rule and describes the far-reaching implications and possibilities that could come about if it were abandoned. We believe that, should the dead donor rule be abandoned as advocated by some authors in the previous part, the issue of anencephalic donors would again be raised and reconsidered anew. Capron holds that adding anencephalics to the category of dead persons would be a radical change, both in the social and medical understanding of what it means to be dead and in the social practices surrounding death. He argues that anencephalic infants may be dying, but they are still alive and breathing. He also presents arguments based on "personhood," "misdiagnosis," and the "slippery slope" to defend his contention that anencephalics ought not be used as organ donors.

The chapter by Zaner that we have chosen emphasizes first that empathy toward parents who have an anencephalic child should move us to allow them to donate their child's organs, since, by this donation, they would be able to bring about at least some good from this tragic event. Then Zaner goes on to consider Capron's article in detail and argues point by point against the positions Capron holds. Zaner very clearly supports anencephalic organ donation (and probably some of its broader implications) based on empathy for the parents and rational argument and persuasion.

Caplan's chapter presents cautious support for using anencephalics as donors. He first argues that public trust in the health care professions is weak already and that therefore anencephalic donation must provide appropriate safeguards and protections. This is so that the public will not see this only as utilitarian opportunism but rather as respecting the wishes of the parents of anencephalics to bring solace out of tragedy. He also discusses the moral status of the fetus and shows that allowing anencephalic donation would probably result in significant opposition from those who respect and want to protect all fetal life, and who also would want to extend protection to the anencephalic as well. Nonetheless, he argues that from his ethical perspective, donation of organs by the parents of anencephalics could be justified, but he acknowledges the public policy challenges this position would engender.

The final chapter included in part II is a relatively recent Position Statement of the Canadian Paediatric Society (CPS). This statement presents current information for clinicians supporting the previous CPS position that did not support the use of anencephalic infants as organ donors in the clinical setting. The statement holds that infants with anencephaly require the same respect for life given to all human beings and that organ donation may only be considered if the anencephalic infant has satisfied the criteria for brain death or somatic death as applied to other human beings. Finally, the statement presents several ethical reasons for opposing organ donation from living anencephalic infants.

Chapter 12

Anencephalic Donors

Separate the Dead from the Dying

Alexander Morgan Capron

In biomedical ethics, some cases involving individuals present true dilemmas: choosing between two evils (shorter life or longer suffering). Others are perplexing in another way: choosing between two goods (one person's privacy or another's well-being). When biomedical ethics moves to the realm of law and public policy, we face even more complex challenges. Consider, for example, several recent bills that aim to facilitate organ transplantation in infants by allowing organs to be taken from other babies who are born with most of their brains missing. These proposals aim to do good, but they create the possibility of doing great harm.

The Need and the Technology

In the past few years, medical interest in pediatric organ transplantation has rapidly expanded. Extensive press coverage of developments in immunosuppression and refinement of surgical techniques—particularly cardiac replacement in newborns—has created hope for some parents whose children have otherwise fatal heart, kidney, and liver problems.

Before these transplant procedures move from experimental to therapeutic, they must improve technically. Yet an inadequate supply of usable cadaver organs poses an even more formidable impediment. Cadaver organs for transplantation in older patients come primarily from the victims of accidents, especially automobile and motorcycle collisions. Relatively few newborns and very young children die under these or other circumstances that would make them suitable organ donors. Present methods of identifying possible donors and receiving permission to harvest their organs provide only a small fraction of the estimated 400 to 500 infant hearts and kidneys and 500 to 1,000 infant livers that are needed in the U.S. each year.

The supply is likely to increase somewhat as transplant techniques are perfected for newborns and infants. And some refinements now underway in the methods for obtaining organs generally—such as the development of a national computerized registry and more intensive local organ procurement efforts—may partially ameliorate the shortage. The chance to make "the gift of life" to another infant may in time become a source of solace commonly offered to the parents of dead infants as it is to relatives of older accident victims.

The present (and perhaps long-range) inadequacy of organ supply for infants has led to proposals that the law be altered to allow organs to be taken from another group of babies—those born with a fatal neurologic condition called anencephaly, the absence of all or most of the cerebral hemispheres. According to Godfrey Oakley of the Centers for Disease Control, approximately 2,000 to 3,000 such babies are born every year. The initiative comes from surgeons who are developing the techniques for infant transplants, but parents of anencephalic infants have also publicly supported the idea, as they search for some meaning and comfort in the face of the death of their newborn.

The legislation takes two forms. The first, illustrated by a proposal made but subsequently withdrawn in the California Senate, is to modify the statutory standards for determining human death set forth in the Uniform Determination of Death Act (UDDA) or similar state laws so that they will encompass anencephalic babies. The second, illustrated by New Jersey Assembly Bill No. 3367, is to permit parents of an anencephalic child to donate its organs even though the child does not meet the requirement set forth in the Uniform Anatomical Gift Act (UAGA) that organs may be removed only after a physician not involved in the transplant procedure determines that the organ donor has died.

Both these attempts are well meaning but in my view misguided. They would create very substantial problems, as well as undermine the very goal they seek.

Amending the Determination of Death Act

For many years, death was "defined" by the law through judicial decisions which, following accepted medical and popular opinion, held that death occurs when all bodily functions, specifically heartbeat and breathing, cease.

With the development of technology to sustain circulation and respiration, medical and popular views diverged. Physicians knew that other functions besides heart and lung activity had to be measured when artificial ventilation and drugs might be causing observable cardiopulmonary activity. By the late 1960s, medical studies had verified that tests detecting the complete absence of brain functions provide an accurate alternative way to establish the same physiologic state of death as the heart and lung measurements that are done on persons not on artificial life supports.

Thus, although people frequently speak of new "definitions" of death, what was actually involved was merely an updating of the means for determining death. Beginning with Kansas in 1970, many states gave legal recognition to two standards for determining that death has occurred: the traditional one of irreversible cessation of circulatory and respiratory functions, and the new one—irreversible cessation of all functions of the entire brain, including the brain stem—which is relevant when respirators and other treatments render the traditional standard unreliable.

By the late 1970s, when Congress wrote the mandate for the President's Commission for the Study of Ethical Problems in Medicine and Biomedical and Behavioral Research, a consensus existed among public officials, as well as legal, medical, and ethical commentators, on the need for simple and uniform legislation recognizing the new (brain) standard for determining death alongside the old (heart and lungs). From the joint efforts of the National Conference of Commissioners on Uniform State Laws, the American Medical Association, the American Bar Association, and the President's Commission, the UDDA emerged in 1982. It has been adopted in sixteen states legislatively, and in two others through explicit judicial recognition; statutes with provisions similar to the UDDA have been enacted in twenty other states, and the highest courts in an additional four states have accepted neurological determinations of death, without explicitly recognizing the UDDN's formulation of the appropriate language to achieve this end.

In February 1986 California Senator Milton Marks introduced Senate Bill 2018. He was apparently moved by an article in the San Francisco *Chronicle* that recounted the frustration of a couple who were unable to donate the organs of their anencephalic baby for transplantation to an infant patient at the University of California Medical Center. As originally proposed, the bill would have amended the UDDA by adding the statement that "an individual born with the condition of anencephaly is dead." Sen. Marks subsequently modified his bill and proposed that a state health advisory board make recommendations about the care of infants with life-threatening conditions, including the "feasibility and necessity" of infant organ transplants, the donation of organs from infants born with anencephaly, and any "necessary changes" in the UAGA or the UDDA.

Adding anencephalics to the category of dead persons would be a radical change, both in the social and medical understanding of what it means to be dead and in the social practices surrounding death. Anencephalic infants may be dying, but they are still alive and breathing.

Calling them "dead" will not change physiologic reality or otherwise cause them to resemble those (cold and nonrespiring) bodies that are considered appropriate for post-mortem examinations and burial. The amendment of the UDDA to include anencephalics is therefore unwise, for several reasons.

To begin with, the UDDA provides that determinations of death "must be made in accordance with accepted medical standards." In the case of anencephalics, this provision creates enormous difficulty because physicians do not consider anencephalic infants as dead, but as dying. Their perception is borne out by statistics. One study of liveborn infants with anencephaly, conducted over a thirty year period, found an equal distribution among males and females. Significantly more males survived the first day of life, but none lived longer than seven days, while female survival was comparable to male after the first day. One female (1.1 percent) survived 14 days:

> The results of this study show that over 40 percent of anencephalic infants can be expected to survive longer than 24 hours (51% males; 34% females), and of these, 35 percent will still be alive on the third day and 5 percent on the seventh day.[1]

For most of the infants in this study, anencephaly was the only neural tube defect, and most of these had no anomalies in other organ systems. Among those infants who also had spina bifida or encephalocele (a protrusion of the brain substance through an opening in the skull), one third had defects in another major organ system.

The UDDA's requirement that determinations of death accord with "accepted medical standards" might be read in another way were anencephaly added to the statute. This would hold that the requirement is met if accepted medical standards for determining anencephaly are applied. Although the diagnosis is usually made accurately by neurologists, authors of the thirty-year study just mentioned found that in "conducting this study, it became obvious that it is important to verify the diagnosis of anencephaly." They describe several cases of long survival:

> One infant initially coded as anenceph-
> aly, who survived over 4 months, had
> hydranencephaly rather than anencephaly,
> and another who lived for 12 days actually
> had amniotic band syndrome mimicking
> anencephaly.

Misdiagnosis by itself would not appear to be a great enough risk to preclude the use of anencephaly as a category to trigger further action (such as declaration of "death"). But the observed relationship to—or even overlapping with—other congenital neurological defects underlines the problems that the proposal would create. For example, hydranencephalics have normal brain development early in gestation; as a result of some event (such as an in utero infection) their cerebral hemispheres are destroyed and replaced with fluid. Like anencephalics, hydranencephalics survive depending upon the extent to which their brain stems are able to regulate vegetative functioning, but they usually survive somewhat longer because their skulls are intact and thus their brains are not open to infection.

To further complicate the picture, other neurological conditions, such as certain types of microcephaly, are also inconsistent with long-term survival. Microcephaly—literally, a small head—covers a spectrum of problems, including cases in which the hemispheres fail to form. Whatever their clinical differences from anencephalic babies, hydranencephalic and some microcephalic infants are *conceptually* indistinguishable if the characteristic separating anencephalics from normal children is their lethal neurological condition.

Because of the existence of these other diagnostic categories, decision makers will be pressured to expand the "definition" to sweep in other similarly situated "dead" neonates. Indeed, Dr. Alan Shewmon, a pediatric neurologist at UCLA, has pointed out that babies—such as hydranencephalics—who typically live a little longer than anencephalics are actually likely to be more attractive sources of organs because of the extra time for development. At present, the regional organ procurement association for California does not accept organs from infants younger than two months of age because of physiologic difficulties (such as the tendency of vessels to clot).

More important, these other diagnostic categories serve as a reminder that the proposals involve a variety of infants who are going to die in a relatively short time. Distinguishing those who will die within a day or two from those (including some microcephalics and hydranencephalics as well as the remaining anencephalics) who will die over the following two weeks is inevitably imprecise. The distinctions rest on clinical judgment, not moral principle.

What the Law Now Provides

Amending the UDDA would also open the door to other changes that the proponents of this particular amendment are unlikely to favor. Perhaps those who have proposed the change do not think it involves a major break with existing law because they are confused about what the law now provides.

Part of that confusion can be traced to the use of the term "brain death" to describe the newer standard for determining death. This terminology is misleading because it wrongly suggests that organs rather than organisms die, and because it implies that there are several kinds of death, when in fact death is a unitary concept that can be determined by several standards, each appropriate under particular circumstances.

"Defining" anencephalics as dead would place these patients into the same category as patients who lack the capacity to breathe on their own, which has always been taken as a basic sign of life. Perhaps the proponents of this change do not see this as a major alteration because they think the law already lumps together some people who are "more dead" (those whose hearts have stopped) with others who are merely "brain dead." But all persons found to meet the standards of the UDDA are equally dead; it is merely the means of measuring the absence of the integrated functioning of heart, lungs, and brain that differs between those who are and those who are not being treated by methods that can induce breathing and heartbeat.

Defining anencephalics as dead so that they may be used as organ donors could, ironically, actually decrease organ donation. Imagine the effect of the law on the process of seeking organ donations from the relatives of a deceased person. At present, when that situation arises, the person seeking permission can explain that the patient is dead; despite the heaving chest and other appearances of life. If the physicians were to cease the mechanical interventions, it would immediately be apparent that the body is in the same state that we have always recognized as dead. The next-of-kin are told that they do not face a difficult decision over whether to let the patient die; instead they face the reality that their loved one is now a corpse—albeit a corpse with artificially generated heartbeat and breathing—whose organs are still being maintained in a way that would make them useful for transplants. (Remember that only a fraction of persons declared dead on the basis of absence of brain functions are candidates for organ donation.)[2]

If anencephalic babies were also regarded as dead bodies suitable for organ donation, this certainty would be lost. For in these cases, decisions about the extent of treatment remain—indeed, some parents may even wish to try heroic or experimental means to lengthen their child's life. The message to those involved in organ transplantation—both as relatives of potential donors and as physicians, nurses, and others seeking permission for donation—is thus likely to introduce new elements of uncertainty. Is *any* particular patient—and not just an anencephalic baby—*really* dead? Or do the physicians mean only that the outlook for the patient's survival is poor, so why not allow the organs to be taken and bring about death in this (useful) fashion?

Alternatively, perhaps some who favor the anencephalic standard for death *do* mean to change the law radically. A few commentators have argued for many years that the statutes on death should move beyond new means for measuring the traditional state of death and should instead declare that persons who have lost only the higher (neocortical) functions of their brains are also dead.[3] These suggestions have been uniformly rejected by legislators across the country—as well as by most medical, ethical, and legal writers. Yet the inclusion of anencephalics in the "definition" of death would amount to the first recognition of a "higher brain" standard—and a first step toward a broader use of this standard—because these babies, despite the massive deficit in their brains, still have some functions (principally at the brain stem level).

To state that such patients are dead would be equivalent to saying that the late Karen Quinlan was "dead" for the more than ten years that she lived after her respirator was removed. Like the anencephalic babies, Ms. Quinlan and other patients in a persistent vegetative state lack the ability to think, to communicate, and probably even to process any sensations of pain and pleasure (at least in the way that we think of these phenomena). Some people may consider such a life as unrewarding, but that does not justify loose use of language about who is "dead." Emotionally, one may be tempted to say that a person in a permanent coma is "as good as dead" because he or she cannot participate in any of the activities that give life meaning. But such a breathing, metabolizing patient does not embody what we mean by dead and is not ready for burial—or organ donation.

A statute that labels anencephalics "dead" is a bad idea because either it will treat differently another group that is identical on the relevant criteria (the permanently comatose, who are dying and lacking consciousness) or it will lead to a further revision in medical and legal standards under which the permanently comatose would also be regarded as "dead" although many of them can survive for years with nothing more than ordinary nursing care.

For many people, the prospect of being in a permanent coma is unacceptable; if that occurred, they would want to be allowed to die without further treatment. But that is a separate problem to which society is already responding in other ways. It would be highly controversial—and, indeed, would be rejected by most people—to call people who are in a coma but who still breathe on their own "dead," especially when the purpose is to allow removal of their vital organs, which would then cause their death as that term is now used. This was the nightmarish scenario that took place in the Jefferson Institute in Robin Cook's novel *Coma*.

Amending the Anatomical Gift Act

Amending the UDDA would thus open up the possibility of an ever-increasing category of persons who are defined as "dead" because their organs might be useful in a legally sanctioned "Jefferson Institute." Moreover, the change in "definition" would apply far beyond transplantation to all contexts in which death arises, from burials to probate to criminal law. Amending the Anatomical Gift Act to permit organ harvesting from anencephalics might be subject to some of the same pressures for extension to other groups of dying, unconscious patients. But at least such a change in the law would be limited to organ donation and would thus avoid the conceptual problems that arise when dying is confused with death. Certainly, the need for infant organ donors requires serious consideration of proposals such as the one introduced in October 1986 by New Jersey Assemblyman Walter Kern, Jr.

Though the idea of living people choosing to give vital organs (as a better way of dying than simply getting old or sick) has been around for quite a while,[4] it has not been accepted. Anencephalic newborns should not be the opening wedge in such a revision of the organ donor process, for several reasons.

First, if society wants to adopt a policy of sacrificing living patients for their organs, it seems very strange—and a very bad precedent —to start with the most vulnerable patients. Unconsenting, incompetent patients who have never had a chance to express their views about whether, if near death but not yet dead, they would want their bodies cut up for purposes of organ donation, are the least suitable source. Moreover, how would one distinguish anencephalics from other possible candidates for involuntary sacrifice for organ donation, such as comatose, demented, or severely retarded patients?

Second, the argument that anencephalics *are* suitable because they are not living *persons* (since they are born with such profound mental defects that they will never be able to establish meaningful human interactions) is a radical redefinition of the accepted criterion for being considered a person, namely, live birth of the product of a human conception. If an anencephalic is not a living person for purposes of organ removal, what about for purposes of homicide, which might be justified on the same utilitarian grounds as organ removal (a greater benefit to the community) or even on the grounds that the death would be better for the parents or other members of the baby's family? This concern raises the general issue of the justice of a proposal that would treat one being as a means of achieving a good for other beings (the grieving donor parents, the ailing recipient child). Certainly, one can imagine cases where there would be sufficient justification for sacrificing one child to save the life of another. For example, suppose that Siamese twins were joined by a six-chambered heart and the only chance of saving either one lay in performing an operation in which the twin with just a two-chambered heart was killed. But the agonizing process that would lead to a decision to proceed in such a rare case is very different from establishing a general rule that would be applied (inevitably, not always in such a conscientious fashion) to the thousands of anencephalic children born each year, to say nothing of other potential organ "donors" with other lethal conditions.

Third, even more than other potential involuntary organ "donors," the anencephalic opens the door to manipulation. The diagnosis of anencephaly is now often made prenatally.

The parents are usually offered the option of abortion or of normal delivery, after which the child will die. If anencephalics come to be regarded as an attractive source of transplantable organs, women who would otherwise choose abortion may be pressured by physicians or others to carry the fetus to term and then perhaps to deliver by a riskier method (cesarean section) that would optimize the usefulness of the child as a source of organs.

Finally, amending the UAGA to allow organs to be removed from anencephalic babies seems likely to undermine, rather than reinforce, the public's support for, and confidence in, organ transplantation. Indeed, if the UAGA were to be amended in such a fashion, legislators might well insist on many protections. They would want to ensure the absolute reliability of the diagnosis and prognosis, for example, and to guard against any conflicting interests on the part of those seeking organs or consenting to organ removals from anencephalics. This could lead to the misguided addition of such safeguards for organ removal from dead bodies under the existing UAGA, thus undermining public confidence ("With safeguards like this, organ donation must be a bad or risky thing!") and diminishing the number of donated organs. At the very least it would unnecessarily encumber the process of organ retrieval, increasing its costs and reducing its yield. These would be ironic results for a measure with the well-intentioned purpose of increasing the organs available for transplantation.

Medical ingenuity should be directed toward finding ways to care for dying anencephalic (and other) babies so that when they become brain-dead, they can be organ donors (with their parents' permission). Medicine should not embark on a course of sacrificing living but incompetent patients for the admitted social good of transplanting organs.

Notes

1. P. A. Baird, and A. D. Sadovnick. "Survival in Infants with Anencephaly," *Clinical Pediatrics* 23 (1984), 268–72.

2. President's Commission for the Study of Ethical Problems in Medicine and Biomedical and Behavioral Research, *Defining Death* (1981), p.23.

3. See, e.g., Robert M. Veatch, "The Whole Brain Oriented Concept of Death: An Outmoded Philosophical Formulation," *Journal of Thanatology* 3 (1975), 13.

4. Belding H. Scribner, "Ethical Problems of Using Artificial Organs to Sustain Human Life," *Transactions of American Society for Artificial Internal Organs* 10 (1964), 209, 211, stating personal preference, if ill with a fatal disease, to be able to have physician put him to sleep "and any useful organs taken prior to death."

Chapter 13

AN EXCERPT FROM

Anencephalics as Organ Donors

Richard M. Zaner

Abstract

This paper reviews objections to the proposal to allow parents of anencephalics to donate their infant's organs for transplantation and finds them unpersuasive. Instead, interpretations of 'Baby Doe' legislation, a 'higher-brain' functional conception of death, the idea of 'viability' in many abortion statutes, and the wishes of many patients, give strong support for the proposal—for organ transplantation using anencephalics.

The idea of utilizing babies born without or with only partial brains—anencephalics—as organ donors has gained momentum over the past several years. Organs and tissues suitable for transplant into infants are in short supply (for all ages of potential recipients) (Rowland, 1988). If the approximately 2,500 anencephalies born each year in the United States could become organ donors, the estimated 40 to 70 percent of babies who die while currently on transplant waiting lists could be saved (Blakeslee,1987; Gianelli, 1987).

A number of people have expressed opposition to the idea, in part because it is seen as evoking other controversial issues (the 'whole brain' definition of death, abortion, or treating donors as 'organ farms') (Warren et al., 1978), and in part because some believe the idea too risky and even immoral. Among others in support of the idea are physicians and ethicists who emphasize the therapeutic opportunity of the procedure, as well as many parents wanting to donate their anencephalic infant's organs and tissues, so as to realize what good they can from what they often see as a hopeless situation (Sahagun, 1987; Walters, 1987).

The Proposal

The recent Loma Linda case (Gianelli, 1987; Parachini, 1986; Pear, 1987), in which the heart of Baby Gabrielle was transplanted into Baby Paul Hole (Ferrell, 1987), illustrates the issue. Diagnosed late in pregnancy as anencephalic, her parents "insisted that they wanted their infant's organs used" for transplantation, "to touch others and contribute to life in some way" (Blakeslee, 1987, p. AI). Placed on supports to keep her heart and other organs viable, her body was transported to California after being declared brain dead by clinical determination of absent pulmonary reflex. In another Loma Linda case, the Winners, learning that their unborn child was anencephalic, decided to continue the pregnancy with the aim of having its organs donated for transplantation. As it was still-born, the ethical and legal issues were mooted (ABC News Nightline, 1987).

Although a number of technical problems must still be resolved to make use of these organs and tissues, the proposal is thought to have definite advantages. As the pediatric surgeon, Michael Harrison says, most important "is that use of fetal organs may need less immunosuppression than will use of mature organs" (Harrison, 1986, p. 1384), a point also emphasized by Mahowald et al. (1987, p. 10).

It nevertheless remains uncertain whether these organs can be legally or ethically retrieved for transplanting. Harrison believes that the difficulty concerns the whole-brain death statutes enacted by most states since the mid-1970s. As anencephalics are born with at least some portion of the brain stem, they are legally 'alive' (Blakeslee, 1987; Ferrell, 1987; Gianelli, 1988; Tennessee Annotated Code), and thus are obstacles to an important therapeutic opportunity. By the time the functions of the entire brain (and brain stem) have ceased, "the organs and tissues are irreparably damaged" (Harrison, 1986, p. 1384; see also Ferrell, 1987).[1]

To make the procedure allowable, Harrison argues that the whole-brain definition of death should be amended so that "failure of brain development, or brain absence, is recognized as the only exception to present brain death statutes . . ." (Harrison, 1986, p. 1385). He points out that neither the President's Commission (see President's Commission, 1981) nor the several states had ever considered 'brain absence' or 'failure of the brain to develop' in making recommendations for brain-death legislation. The primary concern in requiring safeguards regarding brain death, he alleges, was the chance of *recovery* of brain function after injury   which is irrelevant for

anencephalics. Even though anencephaly is somewhat variable, it can be diagnosed pre-natally and defined with considerable clarity. To ensure proper respect and prevent possible abuse, Harrison thinks the best approach is to define the anencephalic as a 'dying person' whose death is inevitable at or shortly after birth. This approach would "give us the chance to recognize the contribution of this doomed fetus to mankind" (Harrison, 1986, p. 1385), and allow parents to realize something positive "from a seemingly wasted pregnancy" (Harrison, 1986, p. 1384).

As fetal organs are not sufficiently mature until the third trimester of pregnancy, however, Harrison acknowledges that his proposal evokes the abortion controversy. Still, since the chance for the anencephalic to survive is nil, "termination is justifiable even in the third trimester" (Harrison, 1986, p. 1383; see also Holzgreve et al., 1987). In support of this, Harrison cites a 1984 study, by Chervenak et al., of 28 cases of fetal anencephaly (Chervenak et al., 1984), a study that concerned only the 'moral justifiability' of third-trimester abortions. Chervenak and his team contend that one can morally justify third-trimester abortions, beyond those done to preserve the life and/or health of the mother. For that, two conditions must be met:

> (1) the fetus is afflicted with a condition that is either (a) incompatible with post-natal survival for more than a few weeks or (b) characterized by the total or virtual absence of cognitive function; and
> (2) highly reliable diagnostic procedures are available for determining prenatally that the fetus fulfills either condition 1a or 1b (Chervenak et al., 1984, p. 501).

Of the 28 fetuses studied between 1978 and 1982, 18 were diagnosed as anencephalic prior to 24 weeks gestational age. Abortion was elected in each, and the ultrasound diagnosis confirmed at autopsy. In the other 10 cases, the fetuses were between 28 and 36 weeks, and each was alive at the time of diagnosis with no maternal complications requiring delivery. Termination of pregnancy was elected by all ten women, with the diagnosis confirmed by autopsy.

At present, Chervenak et al. contend that only anencephaly fulfills the required conditions. They argue that termination in such cases serves the best interests of both the pregnant woman and the fetus (assuming, of course, that it is coherent to say that anencephalics have any interests, a point to be considered later). Abortion reduces the time during which she would suffer from carrying a fetus with a hopeless prognosis, and allows the parents to initiate another pregnancy earlier than otherwise. Second, for the anencephalic, "prenatal death does not constitute a harm, nor does the prenatal termination . . . constitute an injury" (Chervenak et al., p. 502). On the other hand, allowing such pregnancies to continue does not benefit the fetus (although it surely does benefit the parents when organ donation is an option).

Chervenak et al. insist that the argument requires a high degree of diagnostic reliability (ibid.). Specifically, they argue for serial ultrasonographic imaging "from different institutions, in which there are no false-positive diagnoses"; this "would ensure that an unaffected fetus would not be mistakenly aborted" (ibid.). In addition to their study, they note that five European centers also reported using ultrasound on 102 cases, each of which was correctly diagnosed with no false-negative or false-positive results (Murken et al., 1979). In this regard, Holzgreve et al. report that courts in the Federal Republic of Germany now accept the idea that the anencephalic "has never been alive," and "termination of such pregnancies is now allowed" at any time of gestation (p.1069).[2] Although statutory acceptance of this may prove difficult in this country (Capron, 1987, p. 6; Gianelli, 1987, pp. 2, 32), Holzgreve's team and others (e.g., Beller et al., 1980; Kinnaert et al., 1981) have already done successful transplants using anencephalic fetuses aborted in the third trimester.[3]

Objections to the Proposal

Alexander Capron has perhaps been the most vocal critic. He argues that while Harrison's idea of modifying California's brain-death definition is "well-meaning," it is misguided" (Capron, 1987, p. 5): anencephalics are *dying*, not *dead*, and no amendment can change that fact. A proposal to change organ donation statutes, moreover, harbors the "possibility of doing great harm" (Capron, 1987, p. 6) by creating serious confusion about the meaning of death.

Second, there is a risk of misdiagnosis, as Capron claims has been documented in a thirty-year study (Baird et al., 1984). One infant in this study was later found to have hydranencephaly, and another amniotic band syndrome mimicking anencephaly (Baird et al., p. 270). Capron also notes that anencephaly is frequently presented with other congenital anomalies (e.g., certain types of microcephaly). Although these other conditions cannot always be easily distinguished from anencephaly, he contends that there is a seductive slippery slope here. We may easily "be pressured to expand the 'definition' to sweep in other similarly situated 'dead' neonates" (Capron, 1987, p. 7). Rothenberg and Shewmon agree: transplanting Gabrielle's heart into Baby Paul "raises profound legal, scientific and ethical questions that should not be avoided simply because we wish the best for Baby Paul and other babies in his situation" (Rothenberg et al., 1987, p. 11).

Capron is worried, third, that altering the definition of death would seriously confuse matters (Rothenberg et al., 1987, p. 11). On the other hand, the idea behind amending the whole-brain definition of death seems to him little more than an attempt to change the definition, and define it as the irreversible loss of only higher, neocortical, brain functions, which Capron rejects. The permanently comatose patient is not dead, however unfortunate, and is ready for neither burial nor organ donation (Capron, 1987, p. 8).

Nor should anencephalic newborns be "the opening wedge" in revising the organ donor process (Capron, 1987, p. 8). On the one hand, "if society wants to adopt a policy of sacrificing living patients for their organs, it seems very strange—and a very bad precedent—to start with the most vulnerable patients" (Capron, 1987, ibid.). He is also worried about distinguishing anencephalics from other unconsenting and incompetent patients: the comatose, demented, or severely retarded, of any age.

Moreover, behind the proposal is "a radical redefinition of the accepted criterion for being considered a person," that is, "live birth of the product of human conception" (Capron, 1987, p. 8; Ferrell, 1987, p. 24). This is also unacceptable because it involves treating one being simply as a means to achieve a good for another (Rothenberg et al., 1987, p. 11). Thus, although anencephaly is fatal, so long as organic functions continue such infants should be regarded as alive and treated accordingly.

Finally, the risks of coercion are increased.

If diagnosis of anencephaly is a sufficient reason for abortion (as it has been for many parents), it is likely that women would be coerced to continue their pregnancies merely to "optimize the usefulness of the child as a source of organs" (Capron, 1987, ibid.; Mahowald et al., 1987, p. 13).[4]

Convinced that the proposal will more likely undermine than encourage the public's support for organ transplantation, Capron concludes that we would do better to learn to care for dying anencephalic babies, so that "when they become brain-dead, they can be organ donors . . . Medicine should not embark on a course of sacrificing living but incompetent patients for the admitted social good of transplanting organs" (Capron, 1987, p. 9).

Response to the Objections

Of the main arguments against the proposal to use anencephalic organs for transplantation, one concerns the implications of being a 'person.' To keep an anencephalic infant alive (or presumably to continue a pregnancy with a fetus with anencephaly) for organ donation is illicit, as it reduces that 'person' to being a mere means, and is a "radical redefinition" of what it means to be a person (Capron, 1987, p. 8).

A second argument concerns possible misdiagnosis: what is diagnosed as anencephaly may be another anomaly or a combination of anomalies. A mistake could be significant: if the diagnosis is incorrect, transplant surgeons might retrieve organs from a baby whose conditions may not be lethal—or, perhaps, who could survive longer than an anencephalic (Capron, 1987, pp. 7–8).

Third, there is a version of the 'slippery slope': there will inevitably be pressures to expand the range of potential candidates for organ transplants, to the point that wholly unacceptable consequences will follow.

(1) *The 'Person' Argument.* On the other side of the argument from Capron, Harrison seems to agree that a key issue is 'personhood,' although it is for him mainly political or legal (Harrison, 1986, p. 1384). Since society cannot reach 'consensus about personhood' (Harrison, 1986, p. 1385), the way to avoid violating their rights is to say that brain absence has the 'same medico-legal implications as brain death' (ibid.).

Capron is more direct. He argues that "the accepted criterion for being considered a person" is "live birth of the product of a human conception" (Capron, 1987, p. 8). So long as "basic bodily functions" continue to be present in anencephalics, they are alive and must be treated as persons. Rothenberg and Shewmon obviously agree, as we saw.

Such a view ignores different and legitimate senses of the term, 'person,' and, as Engelhardt emphasizes, it ignores the "many ways in which rights are accorded to humans" (Engelhardt, 1986, p. 119). The primary distinction, he argues, is between moral agents who have both rights and duties, and human beings as "bearers of rights, but not of duties" (ibid.). No infant is a moral agent in that sense, for one can neither blame nor praise them until and if they become more fully responsible for their actions. At most, one can only act on behalf of an infant, for the specific moral status it enjoys is strictly a function of the particular community into which it is born: its 'rights' are conferred by and are operative within that community.

Furthermore, there are clear differences between human beings who are capable of performing social roles and those who cannot (or can no longer) do so—permanently comatose and anencephalic individuals are prime examples of the latter. The 'rights' society may confer on the former do not at all devolve automatically on the latter. Rather, to regard anencephalics or the permanently comatose as 'persons' would be to give them a strictly derivative status (conferred, if at all, by that community). Therefore, he concludes, the strongest claims of rights "that can be advanced in favor of humans who are not persons in the strict sense depend on consequentialist, if not indeed on utilitarian, considerations" (p. 120)—that is, on grounds extraneous to their moral status in the strict sense. This does not imply that any such individuals will or should be treated capriciously. It is rather to recognize quite familiar social practices: "In dealing with competent adults, young infants, and newborn severely defective infants, we make decisions within moral practices supposing quite different senses of bearers of rights" (ibid.).

Capron's idea, then, that being a person is nothing more than 'having a biologically functioning body,' can hardly be called the 'accepted criterion,' for it flies in the face of well-recognized moral and social distinctions. Moreover, to identify 'person' with 'organic functions' is plainly wrong: even less than infants can one coherently argue that 'organic functions' are bearers of rights or duties.

Finally, where there are *no* neurological supports for personal, conscious life, there is no reason to suppose that an individual has interests of its own, in the strict sense in which the person does. This does not imply that to use anencephalic as organ donors is therefore to treat them inhumanely. Thus, while Harrison may be correct to urge that anencephalics be treated with dignity and respect, it is quite incorrect to say that this can be assured only if they are defined as 'persons.' That is as incoherent as it is to make them exceptions to the whole brain act, when they are obviously not whole-brain dead.

The culprit, it seems to me, is not the proposal to use anencephalics as organ donors, but rather the whole-brain definition of death. For in its terms, an infant with only biological conditions of human life—continued biological functioning such as spontaneous breathing, cephalic reflexes, regulation of body temperature, etc.—would qualify as an alive person. Indeed, Puccetti points out, in those terms even

> a hypothetical decapitated human body treated so as to prevent the outpouring of blood, but with brain stem left intact so that these janitorial functions are performed unaided, qualifies as a live person . . . , whereas if someone lops off the stem and substitutes a mechanical respirator in its place, the patient becomes a dead person thereby (Puccetti, 1988, p. 84).

Capron's view illicitly presumes that *personal* life is equivalent to *human biological life*. Crucial to clarifying these issues, especially regarding legislative proposals, is making a careful distinction among the *concept* (or definition) of death, the *criteria* for determining that death has occurred, and diagnostic *tests* showing whether or not the criteria have been fulfilled. Capron gives almost exclusive focus to the biological integration of essentially reflex, vegetative functions of the brain. Capron's 'human being' is a merely biological entity bereft of any distinctly personal presence. In Puccetti's terms, it is mainly the 'janitorial' functions of the central nervous system, those requiring no conscious direction whatsoever, that are given priority.

In effect, however, Capron's position evades the central issue: who, after all, has died? In effect, what is claimed as a concept of death is actually a criterion—irreversible cessation of whole-brain functions—which puts the cart before the horse. The physiological processes (even if these are said to be those of the 'wholebrain') clearly function as criteria, not as a definition. As Bartlett and Youngner emphasize, while a definition of death is a conceptual and philosophical issue, criteria "set the general physiological standards for determining whether death, as defined conceptually, has occurred. Once criteria have been determined, specific medical tests can be developed to demonstrate their fulfillment" (Bartlett et al., 1988, p. 200).

The philosophical dispute over the meaning of 'person' continues. Still, there seems little question that the irreversible destruction of higher, cerebral brain functions is quite sufficient as a criterion to determine that the 'person' is dead (Bartlett et al., 1988; Puccetti, 1988), as the physiological and neurological basis to support personal life has been lost or was never present. As new tests appear (PET-scan, cerebral blood-flow studies) and current ones enhanced, fulfilling the criterion is increasingly in reach (Puccetti, 1988).

Anencephaly, indeed, constitutes one of the clearest, most convincing instances demonstrating the need for a statutory revision of the definition of death as death of the person. In these terms, it is not that anencephalics are 'dying' and then at some later point 'dead.' Rather, they are never 'alive' in the only significant sense for morality and social policy—as persons (potential or actual moral agents), as has been recognized by courts in the Federal Republic of Germany (Holzgreve et al., 1984, p. 1069).

(2) *The Misdiagnosis Argument.* The spectre of possible misdiagnosis, on the other hand, seems unproblematic. Chervenak et al. studied 28 cases, and reported that 102 others

were studied at five European centers. In each case, the diagnosis of anencephaly by ultrasonography was confirmed at autopsy, with no misdiagnoses. In the thirty-year study by Baird and Sadovnick cited by Capron, a total of 181 cases of anencephaly were reported, in only two of which were misdiagnoses found. One turned out to be hydranencephaly, and another amniotic band syndrome. Both conditions, however, are incompatible with survival; even though the time of survival may vary (the first infant lived over four months, while the second survived only twelve days). Thus, not only is the risk of misdiagnosis quite small (2 infants of a total of 311 cases reported from the three studies), but considering the vast improvement in prenatal and neonatal diagnosis over the past decade (which Capron ignores), even this risk has been reduced.

Furthermore, even where there are other anomalies in addition to anencephaly, the fact remains that anencephalics cannot survive, whatever else may also be present. Thus, of the 181 cases in the Baird and Sadovnick study, 143 had anencephaly alone; 20 had anencephaly plus other malformations; and 18 had anencephaly plus either spina bifida (16 of 18) or encephalocele (2 of 18). As the authors emphasize, "the presence of these additional malformations is not responsible for the deaths *in utero*" or after live birth (Baird et al., 1984, p. 270). The anencephaly is lethal, whatever other malformations may be found. Even though it is important to emphasize the need for extraordinary caution when diagnosing (either *in utero* or *ex utero*), the risk potential for misdiagnosis seems nil.

(3) *The 'Slippery Slope' Argument.* Capron and others worry a great deal about slippery slopes, cunning wedges, and doors being subtly opened to subsequent disasters.[5] Allowing organ retrieval from anencephalics might

introduce the prospects of profiteering and manipulation by making fetuses into "organ farms" (Warren et al., 1978). Rothenberg and Shewmon worry: "Will those with advanced dementia or severe mental retardation also be killed as they were in Nazi Germany—except, in this case, it would be for their organs" (Rothenberg et al., 1987, p.11)?

Such purported arguments seem quite fallacious: they either deny the antecedent, affirm the consequent, or are a form of *ignorantio elenchi*. More to the point: if it is maintained merely that the initiation of a course of action (e.g. altering brain death or organ donor statutes) *might* bring about certain unhappy results, then quite obviously those results also *might not* come about. What is implied is thus not absolute prohibition but the contrary, great caution and specific justification at every stage. But then the persuasive force of appealing to possible disaster is lost. As Mahowald et al. point out, such arguments are simply not compelling: confronting a real slippery slope "requires placing wedges at the right places, in order to restrict or stop travel at those points where one is most likely to fall" (Mahowald et al., 1987, p.15). Thus, if organ retrieval from anencephalics is permitted, it is important to ensure that there are reliable checks to prevent organ donation from "living, viable individuals, and against commercialization, which would trivialize human life in its nonviable stage. These wedges are "neither new nor ineffective; they have been successfully applied to organ and tissue retrieval from cadaver donors" (Mahowald et al., 1987, ibid.; see also Maguire, 1986, p. 291).

It must be emphasized, however, that those who are seriously considered as potential organ donors in the present proposal have lethal conditions, and are clearly different from anomalies that can be treated, even if only partially. Only the former, not the latter, are under discussion, and for that very reason the slippery slope is simply irrelevant.

Notes

1. Using a ventilator to preserve organs and tissues may make it difficult to determine cessation of whole-brain functioning. It is uncertain, too, whether the case of Baby Paul would respond to Harrison's concern about brain death in fetuses. Loma Linda's current protocol requires placing the anencephalic on a ventilator, and organs removed for transplant only if whole-brain death occurs within a week; if death does not occur by then, the infant is removed and allowed to die. Statutes do not disallow such clinical determination, nor do they specify any empirical test. Some tests, such as the EEG, have not proven very effective in early infancy. Other tests, such as PET-scans and cerebral blood-flow studies, are currently under investigation, but none at this writing have been established as definitive. It might also be mentioned that neurological determination of 'brain activity' may not be equivalent to the statutory requirement of 'brain functioning;' it is unclear which of these is disclosed or measured by any of these tests.

2. Several other fetal disorders might be considered candidates for such abortions, but as of 1984 Chervenak et al. contend that none fulfill both conditions. They point out that diagnostic and clinical improvements could result in adding certain anomalies (e.g., renal agenesis). And, some formerly untreatable conditions (e.g., biliary atresia) could become treatable and thus eliminated from consideration. Some of these, e.g., those with hypoplastic left heart syndrome, could well become candidates for heart transplants, as others could become donors.

3. Such a step, however, might be problematic in some states, such as Tennessee, whose abortion statute states, in the information that must be conveyed to the pregnant woman contemplating abortion, that "if more than twenty-four (24) weeks have elapsed from the time of conception, her child may be viable" (Tennessee Annotated Code, p. 31). Even though "may be viable" clearly implies that "her child" may not be viable at that point in gestation, the phrase has been regularly interpreted as prohibiting abortion after 24 weeks unless there is a threat to the life or health of the mother. (The use of "her child" only serves to make the issue emotionally and politically loaded.)

4. It is interesting to note that one of the cases reported by Holzgreve involved continuation of pregnancy for the sake of organ donation. In this case, the two potential pediatric recipients were not appropriate candidates, and both kidneys were transplanted into a 25-year-old patient. After two minor rejection crises, the kidneys continued to function and the recipient remains well and active (Holzgreve, 1987, p. 1069). Similarly, Debrah Winner elected to continue her pregnancy with organ donation in mind (Associated Press, 1987). She explicitly denied any coercion (ABC News Nightline, 1987); whether coercion was present in Holzgreve's case cannot be determined from the report (see also Kinnaert, 1981; Murten et al., 1979).

5. Capron has elsewhere raised the question of possible conflict of interest where it is known in advance that a fetus is anencephalic and a decision by parents and physician is made to utilize its organs for transplantation. "Treatments" for the delivered baby cannot be construed as "for its benefit," but rather merely for the transplant program (ABC News Nightline, 1 987, p. 7). But surely this is unjust. The Winner case on the same program is illustrative. The couple learned in August that their fetus was anencephalic and wanted to have its organs donated for use as transplants. However, at delivery in mid-December, the infant was stillborn and, except for corneas, none of the organs were suitable for transplant. I fail to see how any conflict of interest arises here, as the question of 'interest' is quite irrelevant as regards anencephalic fetuses. Beyond that, the 'benefit' in such cases is not simply for the transplant program: it benefits other grievously afflicted infants and adults; it benefits the parents of anencephalic infants; it also benefits transplant programs and physicians, of course.

References

ABC News Nightline: 1987, 'Infant transplants and medical ethics,' *ABC News Nightline Transcripts*, Executive Producer Richard Kaplan, Show # 1713 (Dec 16), Journal Graphics, Inc., New York.

Associated Press: 1987, 'Couple wants baby to be organ donor,' *The Nashville Banner* (Dec 7), A-16.

Baird, P. A., and Sadovnick, A. D.: 1984, 'Survival in infants with anencephaly,' *Clinical Pediatrics* 23, 268–272.

Bartlett, E. T., and Youngner, S. J.: 1988, 'Human death and the destruction of the neocortex,' in R. M. Zaner (ed.), *Death: Beyond Whole-brain Criteria*, Kluwer Academic Publishers, Dordrecht, pp. 199–216.

Beller, F. K., and Quakernack, K.: 1980, 'Fragen zur Bioethik: Terminierung der Schwangerschaft im II. und III. Trimenon aus eugenischeer Indikation,' *Geburtshilfe Frauenheilkd.* 40, 142–144.

Blakeslee, S.: 1987, 'Baby without brain kept alive to give heart,' *The New York Times* (October 19), A-I, B-9.

Capron, A. M.: 1987, 'Anencephalic Donors: Separate the Dead from the Dying,' *Hastings Center Report* 17(1), 5–9.

Chervenak, F. A. et al.: 1984, 'When is termination of pregnancy during the third trimester morally justifiable?,' *New England Journal of Medicine* 310, 501–504.

Department of Health and Human Services: 'Child abuse and neglect prevention and treatment program; final rule,' *Federal Register* 50: 72, 14877–14901.

Engelhardt, H. T., Jr.: 1986, *The Foundations of Bioethics,* Oxford University Press, New York.

Ferrell, D.: 1987, 'Source of new heart ignites ethics debate,' *The Los Angeles Times* (November 11), Pt.1–3, 1–24.

Gianelli, D. M.: 1987, 'Anencephalic infant moral dilemma,' *American Medical News* (April 17), 2, 32.

Gianelli, D. M.: 1988, '1987 saw collision of law, ethics, medicine,' *American Medical News* (January 8), 12.

Harrison, M. R.: 1986, 'Organ procurement for children: the anencephalic fetus as donor,' *The Lancet,* 1383–1385.

Holzgreve, W. et al.: 1987, 'Kidney transplantation from anencephalic donors,' *The New England Journal of Medicine* 316, 1069–1070.

Kinnaert, P. et al.: 1981, Transplantation of both kidneys of an anencephalic newborn to a 23-year-old patient,' *European Urology* 7, 373–376.

Maguire, D.: 1986, 'Deciding for yourself: the objections,' in R. F. Weir (ed.), *Ethical Issues in Death and Dying,* Columbia University Press, New York, pp. 284–310.

Mahowald, M. B. et al.: 1987, 'The ethical options in transplanting fetal tissue,' *Hastings Center Report* 17: 1, 9–15.

Mahowald, M. B., Areen, J., Hoffer, B. J., Jonsen, A. R., King, P., Silver, J.,. Sladek, J. R., Jr., and Walters, L.: 1987, 'Transplantation of neural tissue from fetuses,' *Science* 235 (13 March), 1307–1308.

Murken, J. D. et al.: 1979, *Prenatal Diagnosis of Genetic Disorders*, Ferdinand Enke, Stuttgart.

Parachini, A.: 1986, 'Science, ethics clash over infant organ donations bill,' *Los Angeles Times* (December 2), I, 5.

Pear, R.: 1987, 'Use of fetal tissues assailed,' *The New York Times* (September 9), 19.

President's Commission for the Study of Ethical Problems in Medicine and Biomedical and Behavioral Research: 1981, *Defining Death*, U.S. Government Printing Office, Washington, D.C.

Puccetti, R.: 1988, 'Does anyone survive neocortical death?,' in R. M. Zaner (ed.), *Death: Beyond Whole-brain Criteria*, Kluwer Academic Publishers, Dordrecht, pp. 75–90.

Rothenberg, L. S., and Shewmon, D. A.: 1987, 'No life should be traded for another,' *The Los Angeles Times* (December 10), Pt. II, 11.

Rowland, C.: 1988, '"Critical" lack of donor hearts taking its toll,' *The Nashville Tennessean* (February 1), pp. lA, 6A.

Sahagun, L.: I 987, 'Baby to be kept alive for use as

organ donor,' *The Los Angeles Times* (December 8), Pt. I 3.

Tennessee Annotated Code, Section 39–302 (3), Supplement.

Titmuss, R.: 1971, *The Gift Relationship: From Human Blood to Social Policy*, Vintage Books, New York.

Walters, J. W.: 1987, 'Transplant of their organs can save lives,' *The Los Angeles Times* (December 10), Pt. II, 11.

Warren, M. A. et al.: 1978, 'Can the fetus be an organ farm?,' *Hastings Center Report* 8(5), 23–25.

Zaner, R. M.: 1986, 'Soundings from uncertain places: difficult pregnancies and imperiled infants,' in P. R. Dokecki and R. M. Zaner (eds.), *Ethics of Dealing With Persons With Severe Handicaps: Toward a Research Agenda*, Paul H. Brookes Publishing Company, Baltimore, 71–92.

Zaner, R. M.: 1988, *Ethics and the Clinical Encounter*, Prentice-Hall, Inc., Englewood Cliffs, NJ.

Chapter 14

Ethical Issues in the Use of Anencephalic Infants as a Source of Organs and Tissues for Transplantation

Arthur L. Caplan

Recent Interest in the Use of Anencephalics as the Source of Organs or Tissues

Interest in the use of anencephalic infants as the source of organs and tissues for the purposes of either transplantation or research has grown in recent years. In part this is as a result of recent efforts to use such infants as donors in Europe and Japan.[1] In part it is a result of the attempt by Dr Leonard Bailey and his team at Loma Linda University Medical Center to use a baboon as the source of a heart for a young infant, popularly known as Baby Fae, who was born with hypoplastic left heart syndrome.[2]

At the time the xenograft was attempted, it appeared that little effort had been made to locate a human donor. Reports appeared in the popular press quoting officials of California regional organ procurement agencies to the effect that they were not aware that a search had been undertaken to find a child who might donate a heart to Baby Fae.

Many commentators were highly critical of Dr Bailey and Loma Linda for failing to aggressively seek a human organ donor.[2] Whatever the chances of successfully performing a xenograft, there was no dispute that a human source was far preferable to a primate source when transplantation was concerned.

Subsequent to the Baby Fae experiment, the Loma Linda University team undertook five transplants using hearts from human sources for children born with the same condition as Baby Fae. Other medical centers in the United States and in other countries have also attempted transplants using infant sources for young children born with congenital organ failure. While doubts still exist about the feasibility of using animals as tissue or organ sources, the success achieved using organs from infant donors has encouraged many surgeons as to the prospects for successfully undertaking transplants in young children dying of end-stage organ failure.

However, even when aggressive attempts are made to locate them, prospective infant donors are exceedingly rare. Brain death is, fortunately, not a common occurrence in newborns or very young infants.

One source of tissues and organs from very young children are those born dead as a result of asphyxia or other birth injuries. Children who die in sudden infant death syndrome (SIDS), accidents or child abuse are other possible sources. These children may meet existing definitions of death and, therefore, qualify as potential organ donors. However, there is a great deal of dispute about the validity of current techniques that are used to determine brain death when applied to very young children.

The gap between the need for organs and tissues from young infants and the supply available from these sources is quite large. Indeed, as progress continues to be made in the field of transplantation it is quite likely that the demand for organs and tissues from infant and fetal sources will become increasingly acute in the years to come.[3]

There are a variety of conditions for which organs and tissues from newborns or young infants might be used. Heart and kidney transplants have successfully been conducted using infants as the source of these organs. Other organs and tissues may be transplantable in ways that can extend life or significantly improve the quality of life for young children born with various congenital diseases and defects.[4] There is even the possibility that tissues and organs obtained from infants might prove useful for transplantation to adults.[5] As the demand for organs and tissues from infants increases, consideration is being given to the use of alternative sources.[3] One source of tissues and organs that is not being used in the United States or Canada is anencephalic infants. While efforts to detect and prevent this condition prenatally are increasing, there are still a significant number of children born with this severe and lethal condition every year.[6]

Such infants appear to have organs and tissues that can be harvested for the purposes of transplantation or research. However, they are born with a small portion of the cerebellum present, which can manifest electrical activity. Consequently, despite the absence of a cortex and all other portions of the brain, they do not meet current definitions of brain death

and thus fail to meet existing definitions of eligibility for organ donation.[7,8] While such infants cannot survive for more than a few weeks, even with aggressive life-supporting interventions, medical centers in the United States and Canada are unwilling to accept organs or tissues from such infants for fear of legal complications.

Despite the impermissibility of using anencephalic infants as organ or tissue sources, the parents of such children sometimes initiate requests to have their children used as the source of organs or tissues. The general public is constantly reminded by the media about the plight of children who await transplants. As a result, it occurs to many parents who have been told that their child has anencephaly that organ or tissue donation might prove helpful to other children in need of transplants.

In societies that place a great deal of weight on autonomy and informed choice, it is difficult for these parents to understand why their wishes are denied by the medical community. This is especially so when it is clear that nothing can be done to either extend the lives of anencephalic infants or to alleviate their defect, and that lives could be saved if donation were permitted. The desire of parents to donate their children's organs when combined with the increasing demand for such donors requires a close consideration of the ethical case against the use of anencephalic infants for organ and tissue procurement.[4]

Public Trust and the Determination of Death

Recently, an effort was made to amend existing California state law governing the definition of death to allow for organ and tissue procurement from anencephalic infants.[9] The proposed modification of existing state law involved the redefinition of anencephaly as adequately fulfilling the criteria for the occurrence of brain death.

This effort failed. Critics of the proposed legislative reform argued that anencephalics often were born with some brain activity and, as such, could not be defined as dead. To do so risks undermining public faith and confidence in the validity of the brain death definition of death for both children and adults.[9] The social price of altering current definitions of brain death, a loss of public confidence and trust in the medical profession, is seen by many as too great a price to pay in order to gain access to a relatively small number of anencephalies who might serve as the source of organs and tissues.

Concerns about the loss of public trust engendered by efforts to redefine death to include anencephaly are not merely theoretical. Occasional stories do appear in the popular press of persons declared dead by medical professionals who confound their caregivers by suddenly regaining consciousness, talking, or moving. In late December, 1986 the *Sunday Times* of London (England) carried a front page story with the headline, "Brain Dead Donors Still Alive."[10] It does not take more than a few stories of this sort, whether entirely accurate or not, to convince the public that those involved in organ procurement cannot be trusted to accurately and honestly diagnose death.

Public mistrust of physicians and their honesty in declaring death is a possible reason why some Americans do not carry organ donor cards. Some people believe that if such a card is found on their person they may not, if they become sick or injured, receive all possible aggressive measures to extend their lives.

Great efforts have been made by the transplant community to educate the public about the definition of death and the criteria used to make such a determination. However, fears inspired by books such as *Coma* and misreports of brain death determinations as happened in the American press when Swedish hockey star Pelle Lindbergh was fatally injured in an automobile accident, when added to concerns about the impact pressures to contain costs will have on the provision of medical care for the severely ill and injured, have led the public to distrust physicians and other health care providers. There is doubt, especially among the poor and minority groups, as to whether transplant teams can be trusted to protect the interests of the dying if there has been an indication of a desire to serve as an organ donor by means of a donor card.

Whatever the merits of the effort in California to redefine death to include anencephalic infants, it must be realized that public confidence in matters pertaining to organ and tissue procurement is enormously fragile. Confusion as to the definition of anencephaly or misleading analogies between anencephalic infants and adults in permanent vegetative states, coma, or those who are demented as well as terminally ill could lead to serious harms in the willingness of individuals or families to consider organ donation from either children or adults.

The Moral Status of the Fetus

A further factor complicating the discussion of the morality of using anencephalic infants as organ and tissue sources is the growing concern for the fetus that is much in evidence in Western societies. Neonatologists have been successful in pushing back the boundaries of birth-weight at which a premature infant can be rescued via intensive medical interventions. American federal and state law has recently been revised to require that all possible efforts be made to save the lives of newborns unless they are born dead or dying.[11]

In a number of cases, pregnant women who have suffered brain death have been maintained on artificial life-support in order to facilitate the delivery of their fetuses. In other instances, women have been forced to undergo invasive medical interventions intended to preserve the lives of their fetuses despite possible risks to the welfare of the mother.[12] In at least one instance, a woman was charged with murder for engaging in behaviors believed to have caused the death of her child *in utero.*

These cases, when seen in the light of the ongoing debate about the morality of abortion, reveal the level of concern that American and other societies currently exhibit about the moral standing and welfare of unborn children. These concerns are readily extended to anencephalic infants and, consequently, make it highly unlikely that public policy will be modified so as to view children born with some brain activity and spontaneous heartbeat and respiration as dead and, consequently, suitable for use as organ or tissue sources.

Death and the Definition of Donorship Eligibility

Historically, the attempt to revise older conceptions of death involving the cessation of spontaneous heartbeat or respiration were closely linked to the need to obtain organs and tissues for transplantation.[8] The transplant community was in the forefront of earlier efforts aimed at securing legislation which recognized brain death, the total and irreversible cessation of all brain activity, as the valid definition of death. Donor eligibility is, as a result, inextricably linked in the minds of the medical and legal communities in most Western

nations with the determination of death using a brain death definition of that state.

But need organ donation be confined only to those who have been pronounced dead by competent medical authorities? Historically, organ and tissue donation has been permitted from at least one group of persons who were not dead. Donations between living related donors and their family members have long been viewed as both ethical and legal as long as the donation is based upon voluntary, free, and informed consent and the donation itself does not cause permanent harm or disfigurement to the donor. Both bone marrow and kidneys have been and continue to be obtained from living related donors.

Donations of blood, plasma, and sperm are also allowed between living persons. Western societies permit donations when the risk to the donor is slight, the tissues involved are renewable, and when those making the donation are mentally competent to do so. There has been some interest in recent years of extending the pool of living donors to include nonrelated donors in areas such as bone marrow and kidney transplantation.[13]

The moral basis for the inclusion of some persons who are unquestionably alive as organ and tissue donors is the belief that medicine, whether in procuring organs and tissues or for any other purpose, should respect and enhance the autonomy of the individual patient. Social utility cannot be allowed to override individual autonomy with respect to medical research, therapy, or the procurement of organs and tissues. Since, however, competent adults can make autonomous, free, and voluntary choices concerning organ and tissue donation in ways consistent with individual autonomy, legal experts and ethicists have held that some forms of donation by living human beings are permissible.

If one carefully examines the reason behind allowing live human beings to make donations of organs or tissues, a number of key values emerge. It is clear that such donations are viewed as minimally threatening to the life and well-being of the prospective donor. Moreover, it is also assumed that such donations are freely and voluntarily made without coercion or misinformation.

The reasons underlying the legal and ethical permissibility of some forms of donation by living human beings reveal important facts about the kinds of values that are held to be worthy of respect in the area of transplantation. Persons ought not be assisted or encouraged by medical professionals to make choices that will result in more than a minimal risk to their well-being for the purposes of assisting others. Moreover, the decision to donate ought to be a product of deliberative, informed and voluntary choice. The ethics of live donation would seem to indicate that whatever the benefits to be derived from obtaining organs and tissues from any source, autonomy, freedom, rationality, and respect for individual well-being must be given great weight.

With the exception of some types of tissue and organ donation by living human beings, the definition of donorship is inextricably linked in both the mind of the public and the medical profession with the definition of death. But why is this so?

Why is it that, for the most part, only those who are dead are seen as eligible to be tissue or organ donors? Part of the answer is based on pragmatic considerations.

Historically, the largest potential pool of potential donors for most transplantable organs and, thus, the one of most concern to those involved in organ and tissue transplantation has been cadavers. There have been many disputes and arguments about what sorts of policies ought to govern the use of cadavers.[14]

In general, the policies that have been adopted toward donorship in Western societies have been those that are understood to be most respectful of the wishes of the deceased or, in lieu of an expression of intent to donate, the voluntary, informed choice of family members. But if the aim of restricting donation to either the dead or a small sub-group of the living has been to prevent uncoerced, involuntary donation, as well as disfigurement or serious physical harm, then it might be argued that there are many individuals who are not at present viewed as eligible to serve as donors but who are not at any risk of suffering any of these harms. Perhaps law and regulation ought to be broadened to include such persons as eligible candidates for organ procurement.

Consider, for example, those persons who are in a primary vegetative state. They lack the abilities and capacities to be coerced or forced into donation. Nor do they have the capacity for sentience or self-awareness that would allow them to suffer anxiety, pain, or loss of vitality should they be used as donors. If such persons have voiced no prior objection to donation, and if the diagnosis of permanent coma is completely reliable, is there any reason for not classifying such individuals as prospective organ and tissue donors? Why is it necessary to wait until total brain death has occurred before procurement can be commenced?

Similarly, persons who have suffered brain death but who might wish to be kept maintained on artificial life-support for the purposes of tissue or organ harvesting might be used as a continuous source of organs or tissues. Proposals for "farming" so-called neomorts occasionally appear in the medical literature and the popular press,[15] but little systematic effort has been made to examine the morality of such proposals. If it is the case that the moral bases for procurement are to assure respect for autonomous choice, voluntarism, and deliberative rationality while at the same time preventing serious harm to the donor,[8] what are the grounds for resisting the creation of a pool of neomort donors?

It has also been suggested that it might be possible to use as tissue or organ sources those persons for whom resuscitative measures had been initiated but for whom they were not successful. In other words, instead of confining donorship to those who die in a hospital setting, the category of eligible donor might be extended to include those pronounced dead on arrival at a hospital but who nonetheless might have undergone sufficient medical interventions to allow harvesting of organs or tissues.

These macabre categories of tissue and organ sources raise the obvious question of why it is that someone must die in a hospital setting and in many countries be pronounced dead by medical authorities having no connection to the transplant team in order to be considered eligible as a cadaver source of organs or tissues. Does it make any moral sense to limit the category of donor eligibility to those who are dead according to medical opinion?

In great measure the answer seems to be that it violates our collective moral sensibilities to treat a human being solely as a tissue or organ source.[12] Most moral theories hold that it is wrong to treat someone only as a means and not an end. Slavery and prostitution are held to be morally repugnant by many on the grounds that they treat human beings only as vehicles or means for accomplishing ends that others desire or want. To permit cadaveric organ and tissue procurement from those who are in a permanent vegetative state or who are being maintained artificially solely for the purpose of harvesting tissues and organs appears to violate the maxim that we ought always to treat people as ends, not means. This is so even when they may have consented in advance to just such a use. Social institutions that would allow persons to consent to their ongoing use in tissue or organ farms in advance of their deaths, or which would see those arriving at the hospital door as nothing more than collections of harvestable tissues exhibit the sort of disrespect for persons that those in the transplant field wish to avoid and which many members of the general public find repugnant.

A further reason for confining cadaver organ and tissue procurement to those declared dead in a hospital setting by competent medical experts is that such a restriction reassures the public. Organ and tissue donation are considered only when there is absolutely no chance of continuing or restoring life. Restricting donation to those for whom death has been pronounced by experts having no connection to transplantation has in the past been used to assure the public that every effort was made to continue life. Restricting eligibility for donorship to the dead guaranteed that respect for the individual and his or her rights would not be outweighed by the benefits that might be obtained by harvesting organs and tissues useful to others. Insisting that only those who have been declared dead in hospital settings can be eligible for donation reinforces the value that Western societies wish to place on respect for the rights of the individual as against the needs or desires of society.[16]

The analysis of the moral reasons underlying the ways in which donorship eligibility is currently understood, that we ought to treat human beings as ends worthy of respect and not merely as means to the ends of other persons, that the medical profession should do nothing that will cause serious harm or injury to those in their care, and that the medical profession must remain vigilant in respecting autonomous, voluntary, and deliberative choice among all other values, reveals much of interest in considering the status of anencephalic infants as donors. For it is not evident that using such children as tissue or organ sources, that extending the definition of donor eligibility to include such children will violate any of these key moral requirements with respect to transplantation.

The Anencephalic Infant as a Source of Organs and Tissues

It is an accepted fact within medical science that nothing can be done to preserve the lives of children born with anencephaly. Even in the United States, where concerted legislative and regulatory efforts have been made to protect the welfare of infants born prematurely or with severe impairments, exceptions are permitted for the non-treatment of anencephalic infants.[11] American law has recognized that the severity of the impairment and the nature of the organ involved requires a special acknowledgment of the uncertain moral status of such infants.

Moreover, it is an equally accepted fact that anencephaly is a condition which prohibits the existence of any sort of sapient, cognitive life on the part of those afflicted with this defect. Anencephalic infants lack the neurologic capacity to feel pain, to be aware of the world, to communicate in any way with others, and to have any sense of their existence in the world.

If these facts are valid, then it would seem difficult to defend the exclusion of anencephalic infants from eligibility as tissue or organ sources. No doubt it seems bizarre to permit the harvesting of organs and tissues from human beings who manifest spontaneous cardiac function or respiration. But is this any more odd or bizarre than allowing organ procurement from adults whose cardiac function or respiration is being assisted by mechanical means?

It is difficult to see how children born with anencephaly could be harmed or injured in any way by allowing them to serve as organ donors. Since these children cannot live, cannot make choices or even have wishes or desires, and lack the means to be aware of pain or to suffer in any way, it is difficult to imagine how they could be harmed in any way.

Perhaps, it might be argued, despite the fact that anencephalic infants cannot be harmed or injured, they ought not to be used as tissue or organ sources on the grounds that to do so would still violate the principle that human beings ought not be treated solely as a means to advance the ends of others. Respect for each human being would prohibit including anencephalies as donors on the same grounds that we feel consternation at proposals to create neomort wards where dead bodies can be continuously harvested for organs and tissues.

The difficulty with such an argument is that it presupposes that it is membership in the human species that is deserving of respect rather than some property or aspect of humanness that generates the obligation to view individuals as ends and not means. If one maintains that it is humanness which is deserving of respect in and of itself and not some property or attribute such as sentience, consciousness, or self-awareness that we ordinarily associate with humanness, then it becomes difficult to know where to draw the line with respect to humanness.

To some extent, moral repugnance concerning neomort wards or the use of those in a permanent vegetative state as donors is based on a respect for what such persons once were. But anencephalic infants lack the capacity to ever possess any of the properties associated with even a minimal quality of existence.

Respect for the human body is not inconsistent with allowing the dissection of such a body for medical purposes. We do not prohibit dissection of bodies or the dissection of parts of bodies on the grounds that these things are human and therefore cannot be treated solely as the means to the welfare or well-being of others. All we ask is that the materials be used in a respectful and dignified manner by those who are licensed to use them for legitimate medical purposes.

The prohibition against using human beings solely as means to advance the interests or desires of others is based on a conception of humanness that is connected to a desire to respect the capacity for autonomy and choice rather than mere humanness. As those who have argued that we ought to modify our ethical stance toward animals have insisted,[17] it is not so much species membership that confers moral standing on a human being, but the capacities and abilities that human beings have to have some sort of mental life that merit respect. If this is true, and if anencephalic infants lack any possible hope of having the capacities and abilities that are minimally necessary for a mental life of any sort to exist, then it becomes difficult to know how to interpret the desire to respect the interests of such children. Those who wish to respect the dignity of all human beings must show why such a principle is violated when it is not extended toward children who lack any possible means of having interests.

Ironically, anencephaly is easier to diagnose than is death in a child. Thus, if the other reason for confining organ and tissue procurement to the dead is to assure that they will receive maximal care from those responsible for providing it, then there would appear to be stronger moral grounds for using anencephalics as tissue and organ sources than there are for using children diagnosed as brain dead. The diagnosis of anencephaly is 100% accurate.[18] The diagnosis of brain death in young children is not.

The fact that anencephalic infants lack the minimal capacities and abilities requisite for generating a duty of respect for their humanness does not thereby allow those in medicine to do anything they like with such children. The interests and sensibilities of parents and of society must still be taken into account in considering whether or not such children should be used as tissue or organ sources. But it ought to be realized that prohibitions against their use have little to do with the desire to respect the interests and desires of other persons.

If the parents of an anencephalic infant wish to donate their child as a tissue or organ source, and if this can be accomplished in a manner that does not violate the sensibilities and values of the medical profession or society concerning the treatment of human materials, then it would seem desirable to amend existing laws governing organ procurement to include anencephalies as possible organ and tissue sources. This ought not to be done by extending the definition of death to include anencephaly. Brain death has little if anything to do with the medical condition of such children, and the accuracy and certainty of diagnosis and prognosis associated with brain death are unnecessary in assessing the condition of anencephaly itself. Anencephaly is a far more reliable guide to prognosis than is brain death.

If society believes that the benefits from using anencephalic infants as tissue and organ donors outweigh the costs to the sensibilities of society concerning procurement, and if parents are willing to give their free, informed, deliberative consent to donation, then it would seem appropriate to create a special class of eligible donor—anencephalics. Existing laws ought to be modified to allow organ and tissue procurement from those pronounced dead in a hospital setting by competent medical authorities having no connection to a transplant program, *or* those children diagnosed as anencephalic by competent medical authorities and whose parents consent to such a use.

References

1. Oshima S, Ono Y, Kinukawa T, et al: *J Urol* 132:546, 1984.

2. Caplan AL: *JAMA* 254:3339, 1985.

3. Mahowald M, Silver J, Ratcheson R: *Hastings Cent Rep* 17:9, 1987.

4. Caplan AL: *Bioethics* 1:119, 1987.

5. Fishman PS: *Neurology* 36:389, 1986.

6. Elwood JM, Elwood JH: *Epidemiology of Anencephalus and Spina Bifida*. New York, Oxford, 1980.

7. President's Commission for the Study of Ethical Problems in Medicine and Biomedical and Behavioral Research: *Defining Death*. Washington, DC, Government Printing Office, 1981.

8. Caplan A, Bayer R: *Ethical, Legal and Policy Issues Pertaining to Solid Organ Procurement*, (October). Hastings-on-Hudson, NY, Hastings Center/ Empire BlueCross Blue Shield, 1985.

9. Capron A: *Hastings Cent Rep* 17:5, 1987.

10. Potts S: *Hastings Cent Rep* 17:2, 1987.

11. Murray T, Caplan A, (eds): *Which Babies Shall Live?* Clifton, NJ, Humana Press, 1985.

12. Annas G: *Hastings Cent Rep* 16:13, 1986.

13. Spital A, Spital M: *Arch Intern Med* 145:1297, 1985.

14. Caplan AL: *Hastings Cent Rep* 13:23, 1983.

15. Gaylin W: *Harper's Magazine* (September):34, 1974.

16. Veatch R: *The Patient as Partner*. Bloomington, IN, Indiana University Press, 1987.

17. Caplan AL: *Ann NY Acad Sci* 406:159, 1983.

18. Ashmead G, Ashmead J: *Postgrad Obstet Gynecol* 6:1, 1986.

Chapter 15

Use of Anencephalic Newborns as Organ Donors

Position Statement

Canadian Paediatric Society

Organ transplantation for infants and children with life-threatening illnesses has become very successful. However, this success is limited by a serious shortage of suitable donor organs. A variety of approaches to improve organ donation rates have been undertaken in adults but these approaches cannot be applied widely to paediatric patients because of physical limitations governing organ suitability and size. These limitations caused widespread discussion in the late 1980s and 1990s about considering the anencephalic infant as an organ donor, including the possibility of altering the standard brain death criteria to apply to the anencephalic infant and of donation of anencephalic infant organs before death[1,2,3,4,5]. The potential to save the lives of infants dying from cardiac, renal and liver disease, and the desire to give meaning and benefit to the anencephalic infant's family were presented as justification for changes in the medical standards and the law concerning death and organ donation from anencephalic infants[6,7].

Official statements from the Canadian Paediatric Society (CPS) (1990) and the American Academy of Pediatrics (1992) affirmed that anencephalic infants were not appropriate organ donors and rejected arguments advocating modification of the medical criteria of brain death and legal standards of pronouncement of death[8,9]. This updated CPS statement presents current information for clinicians supporting the previous CPS position that did not support the use of anencephalic infants as organ donors in the clinical setting.

Organ Transplantation in Infants

Organ transplantation is now an integral part of life-saving therapy for infants with serious illness, including cardiac, hepatic and renal disease. The increasing success resulting from improved surgical techniques and intensive care expertise, and progress in transplantation immunology and therapy have resulted in a serious organ donor shortage for infants. Due to organ size restrictions, this shortage has not been alleviated by strategies to increase donation rates or by increasing living related donation, as occurs in older children and adults.

The same ethical principles and medical criteria for transplantation in adults and older children apply to infants, either as recipients or as donors. Ethical principles require that the potential organ donor be declared brain dead or pronounced somatically dead before organ donation using standard cardiorespiratory criteria—the 'dead donor rule.' The process of discussion must be consistent with the standards of surrogate informed consent[10]. Parents, as the surrogate decision-makers for infants, must be fully informed of the risks to themselves, the potential infant donor and the recipient of involvement in the organ donation process. The benefits of saving another infant's life and of giving the death of their infant some spiritual meaning may influence parents to agree to the donation of their infant's organs. Similarly, most parents of dying infants may consider the benefit of organ transplantation to outweigh any risks. To avoid any subtle coercion, physicians involved in organ transplantation should not be involved in consent discussions with parents of potential organ donors. Physicians must be aware of the serious potential for parents to be coerced into organ donation. Ongoing evaluation of such cases should be undertaken to ensure that the benefits and risks to the infants, families and society are justified.

Organ Donation from Anencephalic Newborn Infants

Anencephaly is a central nervous system abnormality that is characterized by congenital absence of the forebrain, skull and scalp. Some rudimentary forebrain tissue may exist and a functioning brainstem is usually present. Most anencephalic infants die within days or weeks without life-supporting interventions[2,7]. One infant, 'Baby K,' lived for 2.5 years as a result of aggressive life support[11].

Use of anencephalic infant organs for transplantation gained widespread publicity in the late 1980s after the Loma Linda Medical Centre reported a successful newborn heart transplant using a Canadian anencephalic infant, 'Baby Gabriel,' as the organ donor. In 1989, Loma Linda reported a study[6] of 12 anencephalic infants who were supported

with intensive care measures for one week to facilitate declaration of brain death. Successful organ donation did not occur from any of the infants. The study authors concluded that anencephalic infants could not be used as organ donors without legal and medical changes to regulate brain death and organ donation. At the time of the writing of this statement, these changes have not occurred.

Infants with anencephaly require the same respect for life given to other human beings.

As with other newborns, the standard medical criteria and ethical principles for organ donation and transplantation must be applied to anencephalic infants when they are considered as potential donors. Organ donation may only be considered if the anencephalic infant has satisfied the criteria for brain death or somatic death as applied to other human beings. Physicians should ensure that the same ethical standards applied to other organ donors are used for infants with anencephaly.

Experience from individual cases and the Loma Linda study identified specific problems with the process of organ donation from anencephalic infants under the current medical and legal standards[3,6]. First, anencephalic infants will not usually satisfy the standard brain death criteria because of adequate brainstem function that maintains spontaneous respiration and heart rate after birth. Second, by the time brain death or somatic death has been declared, the organs will have undergone ischemic damage, making them unsuitable for transplantation. This occurs because cardiovascular and respiratory functions deteriorate gradually in anencephalic infants before a terminal event. Third, the use of life support does not improve the chance of successful organ donation from anencephalic infants. While organ function may be maintained with life support, as brainstem function deteriorates, multisystem organ failure develops before sudden death.

In 1994, the American Medical Association (AMA) Council on Ethical and Judicial Affairs stated an opinion supporting the use of anencephalic infant organs for transplantation before death of the anencephalic infant, as long as parental consent requirements were met and other safeguards were satisfied[12]. This radical departure from the 'dead donor rule' was subsequently supported by an AMA Council report[13] in 1995 explaining the rationale for this opinion. The AMA Council report expressed the hope that public consensus would result in changes to the law to allow organ donation from living anencephalic infants. Such a development in public opinion has not occurred due to legal and ethical concerns and recent medical developments.

Ethical concerns opposing organ donation from living anencephalic infants include the following[14,15]:

- application of similar arguments in favour of organ donation from other seriously brain-damaged living patients;
- serious risk of loss of public trust in transplantation programs;
- serious deleterious effects on families and staff involved in such cases; and
- risk of loss of public respect for the intrinsic value of all human life.

The current AMA Policy[16] affirms the 'dead donor rule' but supports the use of medical therapy and mechanical ventilation to sustain organ viability until death is declared.

New medical developments have greatly decreased the potential benefit from using anencephalic infants as organ donors. First, the widespread use and improved diagnostic accuracy of routine prenatal ultrasound has been associated with increased prenatal diagnosis of anencephaly and subsequent high rates of pregnancy termination. Second, folate fortification of food and preconceptual folate supplementation has significantly decreased the incidence of neural tube defects including anencephaly. As a result, the number of anencephalic infants born at term has decreased so much that the potential benefit from attempts to use their organs for transplantation is minimal[17,18,19,20]. Finally, the major indication for neonatal heart transplantation, hypoplastic left heart syndrome, is now commonly treated by Norwood staged surgery rather than by transplantation, in part because of organ donor shortage, but also because of long-term concerns about morbidity after transplantation[21].

In recent years, discussion of organ donation from anencephalic infants has diminished with the exception of occasional case reports and theoretical discussion[22,23,24].

Recommendations

- Organ donation from anencephalic infants should not be undertaken due to the serious difficulties surrounding the establishment of brain death in these infants and the lack of evidence to date supporting successful organ transplantation.
- There should be no alteration or modification of standard infant brain death criteria to include infants with anencephaly.
- Families who request the opportunity to donate organs from their infant with anencephaly should have information and educational material provided that

explain why this practice is not supported. The option of tissue and stem cell donation should be discussed using the ethical principles and medical practices applied to other donors.

- The practice of using medical therapy and mechanical ventilation to maintain organ function pending the declaration of death in infants with anencephaly is not supported.

Acknowledgements

This position statement was reviewed by the CPS Fetus and Newborn Committee during development.

Bioethics Committee (2004–2005):

Members: Drs Laura Arbour, Children's and Women's Health Centre of British Columbia, Vancouver, British Columbia (1998–2004); Paul Byrne, Stollery Children's Hospital, Edmonton, Alberta (1999–2004); Conrad Fernandez, IWK Health Centre, Halifax, Nova Scotia; Christine Harrison, The Hospital for Sick Children, Toronto, Ontario (chair, 1999–2005); Bryan Magwood, Health Sciences Centre, Winnipeg, Manitoba; Saleem Razack, The Montreal Children's Hospital, Montreal, Quebec; Jonathan Tolkin, Bloorview MacMillan Centre, Toronto, Ontario (board representative); Ellen Tsai, Kingston General Hospital, Kingston, Ontario.

Principal author: Dr Paul Byrne, Stollery Children's Hospital, Edmonton, Alberta.

(The recommendations in this statement do not indicate an exclusive course of treatment or procedure to be followed. Variations, taking into account individual circumstances, may be appropriate.)

References

1. Fost N. Organs from anencephalic infants: An idea whose time has not yet come. *Hastings Cent Rep* 1988; 18:5–10.

2. Shewmon DA. Anencephaly: Selected medical aspects. *Hastings Cent Rep* 1988; 18:11–9.

3. Rothenberg LS. The anencephalic neonate and brain death: An international review of medical, ethical, and legal issues. *Transplant Proc* 1990; 22:1037–9.

4. Welch GW. The infant with anencephaly. *N Engl J Med* 1990; 323:615.

5. Ashwal S, Peabody JL, Schneider S, Tomasi LG, Emery JR, Peckham N. Anencephaly: Clinical determination of brain death and neuropathologic studies. *Pediatr Neurol* 1990; 6:233–9.

6. Peabody JL, Emery JR, Ashwal S. Experience with anencephalic infants as prospective organ donors. *N Engl J Med* 1989; 321:344–50.

7. Shewmon DA, Capron AM, Peacock WJ, Schulman BL. The use of anencephalic infants as organ sources. A critique. *JAMA* 1989; 261:1773–81.

8. Rosenberg HC; Canadian Paediatric Society, Bioethics Committee. Transplantation of organs from newborns with anencephaly. *CMAJ* 1990; 143:12–3.

9. American Academy of Pediatrics, Committee on Bioethics. Infants with anencephaly as organ sources: Ethical considerations. *Pediatrics* 1992; 89:1116–9.

10. Canadian Paediatric Society, Bioethics Committee. Treatment decisions for infants and children. *Paediatr Child Health* 2004; 9:99–103. www.cps.ca/english/statements/B/b04–01.htm (Version current at June 13, 2005).

11. In re Baby "K", 1G F3d 500 (4th Cir 1994).

12. American Medical Association, Council on Ethical and Judicial Affairs. *Code of Medical Ethics: Current Opinions with Annotations.* Chicago: American Medical Association, 1994:162.

13. American Medical Association, Council on Ethical and Judicial Affairs. The use of anencephalic neonates as organ donors. *JAMA* 1995; 273:1614–8.

14. Arnold RM, Youngner SJ. The dead donor rule: Should we stretch it, bend it, or abandon it? *Kennedy Inst Ethics J* 1993; 3:263–78.

15. Sytsma SE. Anencephalics as organ sources. *Theor Med* 1996; 17:19–32.

16. American Medical Association. Anencephalic neonates as organ donors. www.ama-assn.org/ama/pub /category/8450.html (Version current at June 13, 2005).

17. Gucciardi E, Pietrusiak MA, Reynolds DL, Rouleau J. Incidence of neural tube defects in Ontario, 1986–1999. *CMAJ* 2002; 167:237–40.

18. Liu S, Joseph KS, Wen SW, *et al.* Fetal and Infant Health Study Group of the Canadian Perinatal Surveillance System. Secular trends in congenital anomaly-related fetal and infant mortality in Canada, 1985–1996. *Am J Med Genet* 2001; 104:7–13.

19. Mathews TJ, Honein MA, Erickson JD. Spina bifida and anencephaly prevalence – United States, 1991–2001. *MMWR Recomm Rep* 2002; 51(RR-13):9–11.

20. Persad VL, Van den Hof MC, Dube JM, Zimmer P. Incidence of open neural tube defects in Nova Scotia after folic acid fortification. *CMAJ* 2002; 167: 241–5.

21. Chang RK, Chen A, Klitzner TS. Clinical management of infants with hypoplastic left heart syndrome in the United States, 1988–1997. *Pediatrics* 2002; 110: 292–8.

22. Parisi F, Squitieri C, Carotti A, Di Carlo D, Gagliardi MG. Heart transplantation on the first day of life from an anencephalic donor. *Pediatr Transplant* 1999; 3:92–4.

23. Pasquerella L, Smith S, Ladd R. Infants, the dead donor rule, and anencephalic organ donation: Should the rules be changed? *Med Law* 2001; 20:417–23.

24. Walters J, Ashwal S. Masek T. Anencephaly: Where do we now stand? *Semin Neurol* 1997; 17:249–55.

Part III

Sale of Cadaveric or Live Organs

Daniel P. Reid

Thus far, the chapters presented have examined the implications of the legal and ethical framework surrounding organ donation from (almost?) cadavers and the use of anencephalic infants as potential pediatric organ sources. In a manner similar to Zaner's suggestion that parents of children with anencephaly should be able to direct the destination of their child's care and the use of their organs, there are those who argue that the sale of human organs should be viewed with the same respect for personal autonomy. Also, notice that as the sale and purchase of organs is considered, many of the chapters presented in this part deal with the empirical in addition to the theoretical.

While the sale of kidneys is not currently legal in the United States, Ghods and Savaj examine the established system for the sale of kidneys in Iran. In 1988 Iran legalized this practice and saw such positive results that by 1999 the kidney transplant waiting list had been eliminated and 50 percent of patients with end-stage renal disease (ESRD) were living with successful grafts. The success of the Iranian model, however, does not necessarily imply success elsewhere, nor did it come without an accompanying strenuous ethical debate.

In assessing the ethical dilemmas in a potential organ market in the United States, Halpern et al. borrow heavily from the ideas of Ghods and Savaj. It is noteworthy, however, that Halpern et al. were unable to find evidence for major concerns in organ sales. In a cross-sectional survey of commuters in an East Coast metropolitan area, results showed that the offer of payment did not alter perception of the risks involved with donation, nor did they create undue or unjust inducement to donate.

Rothman and Rothman explore a rationale for these results by examining the "extrinsic" and "intrinsic" incentives for donation. According to the definitions they lay out, the offer of monetary compensation represents an extrinsic incentive toward donation and should be avoided. They pull from the previous work of the economist Uri Gneezy, presupposing that extrinsic incentives can crowd out intrinsic incentives, such as the feeling of doing one's duty or altruism toward others. To reach an ethically sustainable market, they show that a balance of incentives must be established, such that the extrinsic incentives do not overshadow a donor's altruism and right of self-determination, and such that the incentive does not unnecessarily target the least well-off groups. The authors ultimately conclude that the implications for social relationships of transforming body parts into commodities are unknown and might bring unintended negative consequences.

Unfortunately, this protection of disadvantaged classes is not a global reality, made visible through Leigh Turner's assessment of the practice of commercial organ transplant in the Philippines. Framed by government and private organizations as "medical tourism," the Philippines and other Asian countries offer for-profit organ transplantations. These organs are purchased from impoverished donors, often for less than $2,000, and then sold for about $25,000 per transplant. This potential for exploitation is a major target of criticism of those who oppose the sale of organs. Turner continues on to expound on the other risks and shortcomings of allowing the less fortunate in society to take part in organ markets.

The ethical necessity to protect donors on a systemic level raises the question of Danovitch and Leichtman whether organ markets are a "Trojan Horse." Their greatest concern is that kidney selling would distort and undermine the altruism and common citizenship on which our whole organ donation system currently relies. Further, they discuss the count-

less other problems inherent to such a system. Ultimately, they seek an answer to the question, is changing the focus of organ donation from altruism to profit an unpardonable transgression of public trust?

Moving away from the issue of creating financial incentives for living donors, Mayrhofer-Reinhartshuber and Fitzgerald analyze what the results of a system that put a price on cadaveric organs would be. They present ways in which providing financial compensation for donation of the organs of deceased patients can increase the organ supply. Through analysis using cognitive dissonance theory, they reason that next of kin may be more willing to consent to donation if money is being offered.

The myriad views presented here on the topic of organ markets provide insights into the ethical dilemmas that develop when the merits of organ donation are seen in dollars and cents instead of in moral, emotional, and legally enforced altruism. Each chapter presents an extensive list of references. These are excellent sources for suggested further reading on the topic of the sale of organs, including how a monetary value for organs might be established and how different proposed and effected structures of the organ market might be and in fact have been developed.

Chapter 16

Iranian Model of Paid and Regulated Living-Unrelated Kidney Donation

Ahad J. Ghods and Shekoufeh Savaj

Abstract

Since the 1980s, many countries have passed legislation prohibiting monetary compensation for organ donation. Organ donation for transplantation has become altruistic worldwide. During the past two decades, advances in immunosuppressive therapy has led to greater success in transplantation and to increased numbers of patients on transplant waiting lists. Unfortunately, the altruistic supply of organs has been less than adequate, and severe organ shortage has resulted in many patient deaths. A number of transplant experts have been convinced that providing financial incentives to organ sources as an alternative to altruistic organ donation needs careful reconsideration. In 1988, a compensated and regulated living-unrelated donor renal transplant program was adopted in Iran. As a result, the number of renal transplants performed substantially increased such that in 1999, the renal transplant waiting list was completely eliminated. By the end of 2005, a total of 19,609 renal transplants were performed (3421 from living related, 15,356 from living-unrelated and 823 from deceased donors). In this program, many ethical problems that are associated with paid kidney donation also were prevented. Currently, Iran has no renal transplant waiting lists, and >50% of patients with end stage renal disease (ESRD) in the country are living with a functioning graft. In developed countries, the severe shortage of transplantable kidneys has forced the transplant community to adopt new strategies to expand the kidney donor pool. However, compared with the Iranian model, none of these approaches has the potential to eliminate or even alleviate steadily worsening renal transplant waiting lists.

In the past three decades, advances in immunosuppressive therapy and organ transplant technology have improved patient and graft survival rates in renal transplant recipients. Available data show that renal transplantation, not dialysis, has become the treatment of choice for ESRD[1]. Because transplantation significantly prolongs patient survival and improves the quality of life compared with dialysis therapy, the number of patients who ask for a renal transplant rather than dialysis has steadily increased. Unfortunately, the supply of transplantable kidneys has been much less than the demand. As a consequence, the number of patients who are on renal transplant waiting list for deceased-donor transplantation has increased continuously, and each year, thousands of patients die while waiting for renal transplantation.

The main reason for this increasing number of patients who are on the renal transplant waiting list is the steady growth of a patient population that needs renal replacement therapy worldwide. At the end of 2001, approximately 1,479,000 people were alive in the world just because they had access to dialysis and renal transplant facilities. This number increased to 1,783,000 by the end of 2004. The major factors that contribute to this continuous growth in the number of patients with ESRD has been explained by universal aging of populations, higher life expectancy of treated patients with ESRD and increasing access to dialysis and renal transplantation facilities of a generally younger patient population from developing countries.

The effective strategies to prevent increasing numbers of patients with ESRD or new treatment modalities to be either superior or alternative to dialysis and renal transplantation are not expected to be available at least in the upcoming decade[2,3].

Since the 1980s, many countries have passed legislation prohibiting monetary compensation for organ donation for transplantation. All organ donations have become altruistic, meaning that there are no financial incentives to people who are willing to have their organs or organs of their deceased family members used for transplants. An ethical consensus has developed around the world that there should be no payment for transplantable organs from either living or deceased individuals. Unfortunately, the altruistic supply of organs has been less than adequate, and the results of this altruistic system have met with limited success. During the past two decades, several approaches have been adopted to increase altruistic organ donations, but the gap between supply and demand has worsened over time. Some experts believe that the use of self-interest (i.e., financial incentives) to shape human behavior is much better understood than the use of altruism. Only under certain and limited circumstances does the human being show willingness for uncompensated transfers and generosity toward others, whereas the forces of self-interest are basic for almost all of our daily activities. This is the main reason that efforts to use altruism for organ donation have met limited success and why by providing financial incentives to organ sources, it is expected that the number of available organs for transplantation will increase[4,5].

Because the organ shortage has become more severe worldwide, some from the transplant community believe that altruism alone is not enough to satisfy the needs of the thousands of patients who are on renal transplant waiting lists and that providing some financial incentives or social benefits is necessary to increase the number of deceased or living organ donations. Some transplant clinicians also believe that prohibition of all forms of financial incentives to organ sources should not be considered an ethical attitude[6].

In 1988, a compensated and regulated living-unrelated donor renal transplant program was adopted in Iran. As a result, the number of renal transplant centers and renal transplantations that were performed rapidly increased such that by 1999, the renal transplant waiting lists in the country was eliminated successfully[7,8]. By the end of 2005, a total of 19,609 renal transplants were performed. This approach eventually was named the Iranian model renal transplant program. Currently, Iran has no renal transplant waiting lists, and >50% of patients with ESRD in Iran are living with a functioning graft.

In this article, first we review the backgrounds, characteristics, results, and ethical issues surrounding the Iranian model paid kidney donation program showing how the renal transplant waiting list in Iran has been eliminated successfully. Finally, we briefly discuss other strategies that have been adopted around the world to increase organ donation, including transplantable kidneys.

Background and Development of the Iranian Model

Iran, in ancient Greek sources called "Persia" or "The Land of Aryans," had a higher degree of civilization during the entire period of the first millennium B.C. and now is a developing country located in the Middle East between the Caspian Sea and the Persian Gulf. It covers 1,648,000 km^2 and has 68 million inhabitants. Iran's gross domestic product per capita is $7219 USD with a total health expenditure of 6% of its gross domestic product. The prevalence of patients with ESRD in Iran is approximately 25,000, or 370 patients per million.

The first renal transplantation was performed in Iran in 1967. From 1967 to 1988, the number of patients who were undergoing dialysis steadily increased, but the renal transplantation program severely lagged in growth in comparison with dialysis. Between 1967 and 1985, only approximately 100 renal transplants were performed. Since 1980, because of very limited renal transplant activity in the country, the Ministry of Health started allowing dialysis patients to receive transplants abroad with governmental funds. Any dialysis patient who had a letter of acceptance from a transplantation unit abroad was accepted as a transplant candidate and all travel and transplant expenses were paid. As a result, a large number of patients who were undergoing dialysis and wishing to receive a transplant created a long renal transplant waiting list at the Ministry of Health. Between 1980 and 1985, more than 400 of these patients traveled to European countries and some to the United States using governmental funds and received a renal transplant. The majority of these transplants were performed in the United Kingdom from living-related donors. In 1985, the high expense of renal transplantation abroad and the increasing number of patients who were on the renal transplant waiting list prompted health authorities to establish renal transplant facilities inside the country. Two renal transplant teams were organized, and between 1985 and 1987, a total of 274 renal transplants from living-related donors were performed[7,8].

In 1988, a large number of patients with ESRD needed renal transplant but had no living-related donor. The deceased-donor organ transplantation program had not been established, and it did not seem as though it would be started effectively any time in the near future. The patients had created a long renal transplant waiting list at the Ministry of Health to travel abroad with governmental funds for transplantation. Transplantation of so many patients abroad was very expensive and understandably unaffordable. Therefore, a government-funded, -regulated, and -compensated living-unrelated donor renal transplantation program was adopted in 1988. As a result, the number of transplant teams increased from two to 25. The number of renal transplantations that were performed increased rapidly such that by 1999, the renal transplant waiting list was eliminated[7,8]. By the end of 2005, a total of 19,609 renal transplantations were carried out (3421 from living-related donors, 15,365 from living-unrelated donors, and 823 from deceased donors). Figure 1 shows the annual number of

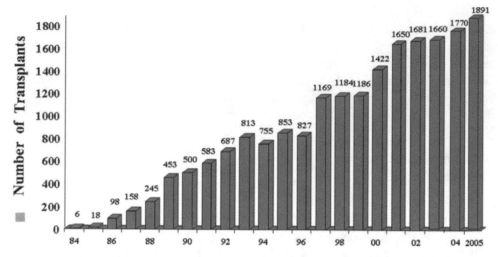

Figure 1. Annual number of renal transplants performed in Iran from 1984 to 2005.

renal transplants that were performed in Iran from 1984 to 2005. Renal transplant activity in Iran has reached 28 renal transplants per million per year. More than 78% of all renal transplants have been from living-unrelated donors.

Characteristics of the Iranian Model

In the Iranian model renal transplant program, during evaluation of all renal transplant candidates, the transplant physician emphasizes the advantages of living-related donor compared with living-unrelated donor renal transplant and recommends renal transplantation from a living-related donor. He also discusses the scarcity of deceased-donor kidneys in the country. If the patient has no living-related donor or the potential donor would not be willing to donate a kidney, then the patient is referred to Dialysis and Transplant Patients Association (DATPA) to locate a suitable living-unrelated donor. (Only a transplant center at Shiraz University with

active deceased-donor liver and kidney transplantation program asks all renal transplant candidates to wait up to 6 months for possible deceased-donor renal transplantation.) Those who volunteer as living-unrelated donors also contact DATPA. All members of DATPA are patients who have ESRD and receive no incentives for finding a living-unrelated donor or for referring the patient and donor to a renal transplant team (Figure 2).

Currently, there are 302 dialysis units, 25 transplant centers, and 79 DATPA offices all over the country. There is no role for a broker or an agency in this program. All renal transplant teams belong to university hospitals, and the government pays all of the hospital expenses of renal transplantation. After renal transplantation, the living-unrelated donor receives an award and health insurance from the government. A majority of living-unrelated donors also receive a rewarding gift (arranged and defined by DATPA before transplantation) from the recipient or, if the recipient is poor, from one of the charitable organizations.

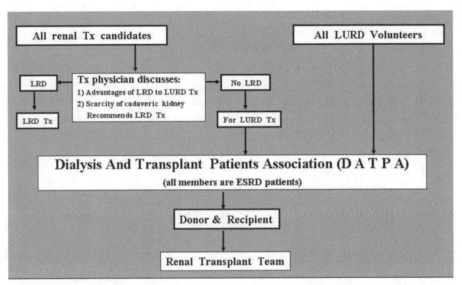

Figure 2. Role of Dialysis and Transplant Patients Association (DATPA) on paid kidney donation program. LURD, living-unrelated donor; LRD, living-related donor; Tx, transplantation.

The government also provides essential immunosuppressive drugs such as cyclosporine Neoral and mycophenolate mofetil to all transplant recipients at a greatly subsidized and reduced price. Charitable organizations also are very active in providing these drugs or in paying any expenses of renal transplantation to poor patients. Renal transplant teams receive no incentives from the recipient or from the government's award. The program is under the close scrutiny of the transplant teams and the Iranian Society for Organ Transplantation regarding all ethical issues. To prevent transplant tourism, foreigners are not allowed to undergo renal transplantation from Iranian living-unrelated donors. Also, they are not permitted to volunteer as kidney donors to Iranian patients. Foreigners can receive a transplant in Iran, but the donor and the recipient should be from the same nationality, and authorization for such transplantation should be obtained from the ESRD Office of the Ministry of Health[7,8].

Donor and Recipient Evaluation

The donor and the recipient evaluations in all transplant centers are very similar. In our transplantation unit at the Hashemi Nejad Kidney Hospital in Tehran, the selection and the preparation of all potential renal transplant recipients and living kidney donors are carried out by complete clinical and psychological evaluation as well as by performing appropriate laboratory tests and imaging. Recently, the European Best Practice Guidelines for Renal Transplantation and the Amsterdam Forum on the Care of the Live Kidney Donor Medical Guidelines are being used for this purpose[9,10]. From 1986 through 2000, for all living kidney donors, a voluntary consent was assessed by the "Donor Selection Panel," which consists of nephrologists, transplant surgeons, and members of nursing staff to exclude the possibility of pressure being exerted for kidney donation. Since 2000, the evaluation and the selection of potential donors and recipients has been carried out independently, first by transplant nephrologists, then by members of the surgical team. In selecting living-related donors, priority is given to the donor who has a better HLA match with the recipient. For living-unrelated donor transplants, HLA matching is not practical because the Iranian model is a directed kidney donation program, so any donor who is ABO compatible with the patient is accepted for evaluation.

Immunosuppressive Drugs

Before 1996, the available immunosuppressive drugs consisted of cyclosporine Neoral, generic azathioprine, and prednisone. Since 1996, mycophenolate mofetil has been used increasingly instead of azathioprine and by 2004 has almost replaced it. The government imports and greatly subsidizes these essential immunosuppressive drugs (Neoral, CellCept, azathioprine, and prednisone) and makes those available to all transplant recipients in a very reduced price. All patients with ESRD including renal transplant recipients belong to a group of patients called "Patients with Special Diseases" and are eligible for a government-provided medical insurance. As a result, the majority of transplant recipients receive these immunosuppressive drugs free. The remaining patients pay for these drugs a little money per month. If a transplant recipient is poor and could not afford the drugs, then the charitable organizations will pay for it. This is one of the reasons that all patients, either poor or rich, have equal access to renal transplantation in Iran. For high-risk cases (*e.g.*, those undergoing a second transplant, those with previous high panel reactivities), induction therapy with anti-thymocyte globulin and rarely with IL2 receptor antibodies is carried out. Antirejection therapy consists of methylprednisolone (1 g/d) for 3 to 5 days and anti-thymocyte globulin in patients with steroid-resistant rejection. IL2 receptor antibodies, tacrolimus, sirolimus, and OKT3 are neither subsidized by the government nor covered by insurance and so are very expensive and are used very rarely. As a result, individualization and tailoring of immunosuppressive therapy remains very limited.

Demographics and Outcome Data of Renal Transplantations

Unfortunately, there is no national transplant registry in Iran to report the short- and long-term results of transplantation in all transplant recipients and kidney donors. Most renal transplant teams report their own results as single-center experiences[11,12,13]. The ESRD Office of Iran has only demographic data but lacks the short- and long-term results of transplantation, so the results from the Hashemi Nejad Kidney Hospital (a pioneering transplant center and one of the largest in Iran) are given next as an example for the whole country. Between April 1986 and January 2006, a total of 1995 renal transplants were performed in this hospital. A total of 496 (25%) were from living-related donors, and the remaining 1499 (75%) were from living-unrelated donors. A total of 743 (37%) recipients were female, and 1252 (63%) were male. Their ages ranged from 8 to 68 yr. In one of our studies we reported a significant gender disparity in living-unrelated (paid) kidney donors (91% male, 9% female; age range 21 to 37 yr.)[14].

In a recent data analysis, the overall patient survival rates were 93.8, 87.8, and 76% and the overall graft survival rates were 90.4, 75.4, and 52.8% at 1, 5, and 10 yr., respectively. There were no significant differences in graft survival rates between recipients of one HLA haplotype–matched living-related donor and living-unrelated donor recipients (*P* = 0.35). In living-unrelated donor renal transplant recipients, the patient survival rates were 93.9, 87.1, and 72.2% and the graft survival rates were 90.5, 74.4, and 48.8% at 1, 5, and 10 yr., respectively (Figure 3).

Elimination of the Renal Transplant Waiting List

The Iranian model of regulated paid kidney donation has eliminated the renal transplant waiting list in the country. In Iran, as in other developing countries, the prevalence of patients with ESRD is markedly lower compared with the prevalence of patients who are on renal replacement therapy in developed countries. A major cause of this is the many patients who are from villages and small towns and do not receive a diagnosis and are not referred for dialysis therapy. There also is no adopted restricting policy for accepting patients with ESRD for renal transplantation;

however, the low prevalence of patients with ESRD results in fewer numbers of transplant candidates. This is the main reason that the renal transplant waiting list was eliminated quickly and successfully in Iran. At the end of 2004, the prevalence of patients with ESRD was 2045 per million people (pmp) in Japan, 1505 pmp in North America, 585 pmp in Europe, 380 pmp in Latin America, 370 pmp in Iran, and 190 pmp in the Middle East (3). As expected, in countries with higher ESRD prevalence values, more patients are on renal transplant waiting lists, and this is why a renal transplant activity of 25 to 28 pmp has eliminated the renal transplant waiting list in Iran, whereas much higher renal transplant activities have not done so in North America and European countries.

Ethical Issues Surrounding the Iranian Model

The ethical issues that are related to the Iranian model of paid kidney donation are

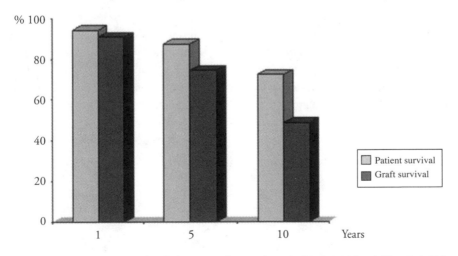

Figure 3. Results of 1499 living-unrelated donor renal transplants in Hashemi Nejad Hospital–Tehran. u, patient survival; f, graft survival.

presented in two parts. In the first part, the ethical issues that support the Iranian model are discussed, showing that the many ethical problems that arise from paid kidney donation have been prevented in this transplantation model. In the second part, several ethical problems that still remain in Iranian model are mentioned, emphasizing that public education and further governmental funding for living paid kidney donors and providing some social benefits to them will make the Iranian model ethically more acceptable. At that time, the revised form of this kidney donation model can be implemented at least in some developing countries to prevent many patient deaths and suffering[15].

Ethical Issues Supporting the Iranian Model

As mentioned, there is no role for a broker or an agency in this transplantation program. The association for patients with ESRD is a charitable organization and receives no incentives from donors or recipients. The government pays for all hospital expenses of renal transplantation. The medical and surgical fees for transplantation are greatly lower compared with the fees for similar services.

All transplant candidates who are poor receive renal transplantation. The elimination of renal transplant waiting lists means that all patients with ESRD, either rich or poor, have equal access to renal transplant facilities; otherwise, many poor patients would remain on the renal transplant waiting list. The main reason for this equal access is the active role of charitable organizations that pay for many expenses of renal transplantation that the poor patients cannot afford. One of the arguments against paid kidney donation is that the kidney donors are almost poor and illiterate, whereas the majority of recipients are educated and

wealthy. We previously conducted a study on 500 renal transplant recipients and their living-unrelated donors to determine which socioeconomic classes are receiving transplants more from paid kidney donors[16]. All of these donors and recipients were grouped according to their level of education, which showed no significant differences. In this study, 6.0% of living-unrelated donors were illiterate, 24.4% had elementary school education, 63.3% had a high school education, and 6.3% had university training. Corresponding levels in their 500 recipients were 18.0, 20.0, 50.8, and 11.2%, respectively. Then they were grouped according to whether they were poor, rich, or middle class. The results showed that 84% of paid kidney donors were poor and 16% were middle class, and of their recipients, 50.4% were poor, 36.2% were middle class, and 13.4% were rich. So >50% of kidneys from paid donors were transplanted into patients from poor socioeconomic class. This finding is a clue against commercialism in the Iranian model renal transplant program.

The paid kidney donation model did not inhibit the establishment of a deceased-donor organ transplantation program. Since April 2000, when legislation that was passed by parliament accepting brain death and deceased-donor organ transplantation, the annual number of cadaveric kidney, liver, and heart transplants has increased steadily in the country. In 2000, only 1.8% of all renal transplants were from deceased donors. This increased to 12% in 2004 and 2005 (Figure 4).

This slow increase in deceased organ donation is due to infrastructural deficiencies and cultural barriers in the country as well as to administrative incapabilities of health authorities rather than being all because of availability of the paid kidney donation program. This program probably has eliminated

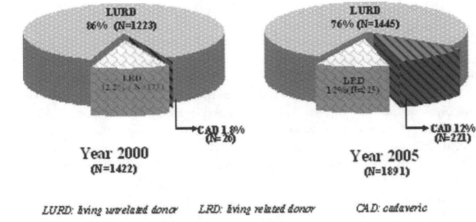

Figure 4. Sources of kidney donations in Iran in 2000 and 2005.

the many coercive living-related donor renal transplants. Before 1988, almost all renal transplants in Iran were from living-related donors. Since adoption of this transplantation model, the number of living-related donor transplants has decreased (in 2005, only 12% of all renal transplants were from related donors). We believe that this decreasing number has been due partly to elimination of coercive living-related donor transplants and partly to availability of the paid kidney donation program. Because of cultural reasons, coercive living-related donor renal transplants are common in most developing countries, including Iran; we believe that with a compensated and regulated living-unrelated donor renal transplantation program in place, it may be more ethical to perform a paid renal transplantation from a volunteer living-unrelated donor than from a living-related donor or spouse who is under some degree of family pressure or with emotional coercion.

The Iranian model of paid kidney donation also has eliminated the many illegal and commercial renal transplants. Before 1988, a number of patients who had no living-related donors traveled to India, where they received paid renal transplants. The majority of these bought transplants were associated with transmission of hepatitis and surgical complications. Several other patients traveled together with their unrelated donors to European countries and received a transplant. In a few of these cases, the transplant documents were prepared carefully as though the kidneys were being given altruistically by living-related donors. The adoption of the legalized and compensated living unrelated donor renal transplant program in 1988 eliminated the need for Iranian patients for commercial or illegal paid transplants abroad. Shortly after adoption of the Iranian model of kidney donation, several wealthy patients from Arabic countries came to Iran and received transplants from Iranian paid donors. Transplantations were performed by surgeons who, unfortunately, had no accurate understanding of ethical issues regarding organ transplantation. A kidney market for transplant tourism was nearly to flourish in the country. As a result, the Iranian Society for Organ Transplantation made a regulation and sent it to the Ministry of Health and transplant centers that no foreigners are allowed to undergo renal transplantation from Iranian kidney donors. This amendment prevented the development of transplant tourism in Iran.

We previously conducted a study on nationality of transplant recipients and kidney donors in 1881 consecutive renal transplants in our center. Nineteen (1%) recipients were refugees, and 11 (0.6%) were other foreign nationals who received kidneys from living-related donors or from living-unrelated donors of the same nationality. Of 1881 renal transplant recipients, 18 (0.9%) also were Iranian immigrants (residing abroad for years) who came and received kidneys from Iranian paid donors. Transplantation of these 18 patients was true transplant tourism. The scale of this form of transplant tourism is very small (<1%) in the Iranian model; however, it is under ethical evaluation[17].

During the past two decades, because of 23 yr. of civil war in Afghanistan (1978 to 2001) and 8 yr. of the Iran-Iraq war (1980 to 1988), Iran has hosted approximately 0.5 million Iraqi refugees in its western provinces and approximately 2.5 million Afghan refugees in its eastern provinces and major urban centers. The majority of these refugees have lived outside camps, having access to the Iranian labor market and a number of government services such as dialysis and renal transplant facilities. In June 2004, we conducted a study to investigate the access of Afghan refugees to Iranian transplant centers as kidney donors and recipients[18]. At that time, 1.6 million refugees still remained in Iran. This study showed that 241 refugees had ESRD (179 were undergoing dialysis, and 62 had renal transplantation in Iran). Kidney donors for these 62 transplant recipients were living-related donors in nine, spouses in two, Afghani living-unrelated

donors in 50, and deceased-donor kidney in one. Afghan refugees are among the poorest people in the world. In >15,000 living-unrelated donor renal transplantations performed in Iran, no refugee had donated a kidney to an Iranian patient. This study concluded that transplantation of all refugees in need and the absence of their use as kidney donors to Iranian patients proffer strong evidence against commercialism and a reason to believe that the Iranian model renal transplantation is practiced with ethical standards. There also is no doubt that by adoption of the Iranian model of regulated paid kidney donation, we have prevented many patient deaths and suffering in the country.

Ethical Problems Still Remaining in the Iranian Model

Because the amount of governmental donor award (approximately $1200 USD) is not enough to satisfy the majority of kidney donors, recipients provide rewarding gifts to donors. If the recipient is poor, then the rewarding gift is provided by charitable organizations. This also results in directed paid kidney donation, meaning that the transplant candidate and the volunteering kidney donor meet each other in a DATPA meeting for arrangement of rewarded gifting to be paid to the donor after transplantation. Providing sufficient financial incentives and some social benefits to each living-unrelated donor by the government will eliminate rewarding gifts and will make the Iranian model a non-directed paid kidney donation program whereby the donors and the recipients will not see and know each other at least before transplantation. All transactions for financial incentives will be carried out by organ procurement organizations (OPO). The OPO will receive all governmental donor award budgets as well as all charitable donations. The donor will donate a kidney to the OPO and will receive all defined financial incentives from the OPO. Because of lack of administrative expertise in health authorities, this approach has not yet been tested in the Iranian kidney donation model.

Unfortunately, the financial incentives to kidney donors in the Iranian model neither have enough life-changing potential nor have enough long-term compensatory effect, resulting in long-term dissatisfaction of some donors. However, providing adequate financial incentives to kidney donors and awarding some social benefits to them will eliminate almost all long-term dissatisfaction. Some opponents have sensationalized that the majority of Iranian paid kidney donors have been poor and have remained poor after kidney donation. As mentioned, in the Iranian model of paid kidney donation, not only the majority of donors (84%) but also the majority of transplant recipients (50.4%) also is from poor socioeconomic class. This national program is not adopted to upgrade the socioeconomic class of kidney donors and is very different from commercial transplants that are carried out in other countries.

The only social benefit that is awarded to Iranian kidney donors is health insurance. Providing more legal and social benefits to paid kidney donors, in addition to financial incentives, will satisfy them better in the long term. When an unrelated donor donates a kidney to a patient with ESRD, the intent also is to save or improve the life of another member of society. Therefore, the society should feel an obligation to provide compensation for this service. There are some legal and social items of benefits for war-injured veterans in each society. Several of these items can be legalized and offered to each kidney donor in

addition to financial incentives as a token of appreciation and compensation by society[19].

Public education also is necessary to show the minimal risk of kidney donation and better outcome of living-related donor renal transplantation to increase the number of transplants from living-related donors. In one of the pioneering renal transplant centers in Tehran, laparoscopic live-donor nephrectomy is being taught and performed with encouraging results to increase the number of live kidney donations especially from related donors[20].

The cadaveric renal transplant activity can be increased substantially in the country if the health authorities give higher priority to the deceased-donor organ donation program. In the Shiraz University transplant center, where deceased-donor organ procurement is in higher priority as a result of an active liver transplant program, the number of cadaveric renal transplantations is the highest in the country[21]. Finally, there is a need for establishment of a donor registry to study the long-term medical and socioeconomic consequences on all living kidney donors.

Other Reasons for Adopting and Continuing Regulated Paid Kidney Transplantation in Iran

Use of Altruism Has Failed to Alleviate Organ Shortage

In the 1980s, the shortage of transplantable organs was less severe than it is today, and the majority of transplant experts were optimistic that altruistic organ donation would be an effective strategy for alleviating or even eliminating organ shortage. This was the main reason that legislation prohibiting monetary compensation passed and organ donation became altruistic[4,5]. Now, after two decades, it has become evident that considerable efforts to provide a sufficient supply of organs through altruism have met with limited success. Because the severe organ shortage has resulted in many patient deaths, a number of transplant experts have been convinced that providing financial incentives to organ sources as an alternative to altruistic organ donation needs careful reconsideration[22,23].

For example, in 2001, several legislative proposals were submitted to the US Congress to promote organ donation. These proposals called for a donor medal of honor and a tax credit or tax refund upon donation of an organ from a living or deceased person. However, several influential senior experts in transplantation have urged the US Congress to retain the prohibition of monetary compensation for organ donation[24]. Nevertheless, the previous severe condemnations by some ethicists against paid kidney donation is softening gradually; it is possible that some type of compensated living-unrelated donor renal transplantation also may be legalized in the United States or other developed countries in the future.

Renal Transplantation from Living-Unrelated Donors Is Steadily Increasing Worldwide

Because it has been shown that the outcome after living-unrelated donor renal transplants is the same as after one haplotype-matched living-related kidney transplants and superior to the outcome after deceased-donor renal transplants[25], in the United States, the number of renal transplants from living donors increased by 257%, from 1812 in 1988 to 6473 in 2003. Kidney donation increased substantially in all living donor groups, but the greatest increase was in altruistic, nonspousal living-unrelated donors. It is interesting that the percentage of living donors who were either spouse or unrelated to the recipient increased from 5% in 1988 to 33% in 2003[26]. In other countries, such as Canada, the number of living-unrelated kidney donors also has increased[27]. Because the number of uncompensated living-unrelated donors has been very limited in Iran, the paid kidney donation program has been adopted to use this viable source of transplantable kidneys.

Proposals of Some Ethicists Regarding Shortage of Transplantable Kidneys Are Disappointing and Unacceptable

Even though so many patients worldwide die or suffer on dialysis needing renal transplantation, there still are many ethicists from developed and developing countries who are against compensated renal transplantation. These ethicists who support only altruistic organ donations have proposed that in developed countries, the solution is to increase renal transplant activity by accepting marginal donors or by passing presumed consent law, but the renal transplant waiting list is increasing steadily in developed countries, and many patients continue to die while waiting for a renal transplant. In the United States, the number of patients who are on the renal transplant waiting list increased from 23,604 in 1988 to 80,492 in 2003. The number of patients who died while waiting for a renal transplant also increased from 1133 (4.8%) in 1988 to 3944 (4.9%) in 2003[28]. In developing countries, the proposals of most transplant ethicists have been mainly to establish a Western model for deceased-donor organ transplantation with high renal transplant activity, but many infrastructural deficiencies (along with cultural barriers) in these countries prevent such a large-scale cadaveric renal transplantation program. Second, they propose to increase further living-related donor renal transplants, which surely will result in transplantation with coercion, particularly in female donors, a situation that is more unethical than the use of paid living kidneys. In a study by Muthusethupathi et al.[29] from India, in 125 first-degree related donor renal transplantations, 66% of kidney donors but only 17% of recipients were female.

Results of the Iranian Model of Paid Kidney Transplantation Are Encouraging

As mentioned, the patient and graft survival rates are the same as the results from conventional transplant centers. The donor morbidity and mortality also are comparable to international data. In more than 18,000 live-donor nephrectomies that were performed in Iran, there have been four (0.02%) perioperative donor mortalities in the whole country. This mortality rate is similar to what has been reported from the world's large series[30,31,32]. The major and minor perioperative complications reported from our center were 1.5 and 8.5%, respectively[33]. The long-term risks of kidney donation have not been studied in our center. There is a need for donor registry and funding. Only a few European transplant centers have living kidney donor registries. In the United States, even though more than four times the number of Iran live kidney donations are performed each year, the live kidney donor registry and the long-term outcome data in all living kidney donors are lacking. Some studies have shown the lower risk for long-term mortality compared with an age- and gender-matched background population. This increased survival is not surprising because kidney donors are positively selected and screened for disease[34]. However, the effect of kidney donation on the long-term outcome of living donors has always been studied in terms of increased renal death or renal morbidities. A long-term follow-up on a large number of living donors is necessary to ensure, for example, that kidney donation and drop of GFR has not predisposed living donors to increased cardiovascular events.

Regulated Paid Kidney Transplantation Has Prevented Illegal and Commercial Transplantations in Iran

Currently, all transplant candidates and their families are well informed that one's quality of life with a renal allograft is greatly improved over living with chronic dialysis[1] and that renal transplantation from living-unrelated donors is superior to that of deceased-donor transplants[25]. It also has been shown that the shorter the period on dialysis, the better the patient and graft survival rates[35]. For these reasons, many patients with ESRD want to receive a transplant quickly from living donors, rather than wait for years to receive a deceased-donor kidney. Some patients from developed countries are traveling abroad to buy kidneys from strangers in developing countries. Because of the shortage of transplantable kidneys and facing long waiting lists, some patients also have turned to Internet sites that offer the matching with living-unrelated kidney donors. Several patients have received transplants from donors that they found through www.MatchingDonors.com[36].

Iranian Model Is Very Different from Commercial Transplantations Carried out Elsewhere

Unfortunately, much of the transplant community's experience with paid kidney transplantation is from centers that have approached it with little regard to ethical standards. Before 1995, several thousand unregulated paid renal transplants were performed in India each year. The kidneys were sold by middlemen to wealthy patients who came not only from India but also from overseas. Poor donors were exploited by brokers and transplant teams, who received a major part of the money that came from the kidney sale. Almost all of these transplants were performed in private back-street clinics with incomplete donor and recipient evaluation and resulted in high incidence of surgical complications and transmission of infections[37,38].

The Iran model of a regulated transplant program involves paid kidney donation, but the ethical aspects are strictly enforced by the transplant teams and the Iranian Society of Organ Transplantation.

Other Successful Strategies for Expanding the Kidney Donor Pool

The rapidly increasing number of patients who are on renal transplant waiting lists has forced the transplant community to look at new strategies to increase the number of transplantable kidneys. These strategies are as follows: Encouraging live-donor renal transplantation (from genetically related and emotionally motivated donors); passing presumed consent law; use of extended criteria (marginal) and non–heart-beating deceased donors (NHBDD); performing ABO-incompatible, paired-exchange renal transplantations; and accepting non-directed kidney donations. All of these strategies have been effective in expanding the kidney donor pool on a limited scale, but compared with Iranian model, none of these approaches has the potential to eliminate or even alleviate renal transplant waiting lists.

By using several strategies, the number of kidney transplants from living and deceased donors markedly increased during the past two decades. In the United States, the significant increase in renal transplant activity was due to the use of kidneys from living-related and living-unrelated donors. Renal transplants from living donors increased by 257%, from 1812 in 1988 to 6473 in 2003[26]. The largest increase was in kidney transplants from spouses and living-unrelated donors. The spousal transplants that led to the increase in unrelated donor renal transplants grew from 1995 to 2000. Since 2000, this has stabilized at approximately 700 transplants per year. The substantial increase was in the number of non-spousal, unrelated donor transplants, which grew by 1600%, from 73 in 1994 to 1250 in 2003[39]. The deceased-donor renal transplants increased only by 34%, from 7284 in 1988 to 9765 in 2003[26]. Nearly all of this modest increase came from acceptance of marginal or extended-criteria donors (ECD). However, the ECD renal transplants are associated with poorer outcomes. Even the ECD renal transplantation is no longer a rapidly growing source; it increased in the United States from fewer than 200 in 1988 to only 1200 in 2002[40].

The use of NHBDD has grown since the report of their effectiveness was published[41]. The rate of NHBDD kidney transplants varies from one country to another. This number increased in the United States from 106 in 1995 to 414 in 2003[26]. In Japan, the number of renal transplants from deceased donors is small, and most of these are from NHBDD (of 1324 deceased-donor kidney transplants, 45 were from heart-beating deceased donors and 1274 were from NHBDD)[42]. In The Netherlands, during the past decade, the number of NHBDD kidney transplants has increased remarkably. Surprising, the number of heart-beating kidney transplants has diminished at the same rate, so the total number of annual renal transplants from deceased donors has remained the same. In Germany, transplantation from NHBDD is prohibited[43].

In countries such as Spain, Austria, Belgium, and Singapore, with "presumed consent" legislation, the rate of organ donation and kidney transplantation has increased substantially. This law mandates that every adult individual who dies is a potential donor unless during his life he specifically declines to participate[44]. The proposal of presumed consent was not tested for its effectiveness in the United States and many other countries because it is considered against the autonomy of families of deceased donors.

Currently, the Spanish model, which was established in 1989, is the most successful deceased-donor organ donation program. The success of the Spanish model is not due to passing presumed consent law in Spain, because relatives of all potential donors must be approached and they can refuse organ donation. The success and the uniqueness of the Spanish model is its realistic approach of providing hospitals with specific budgets for organ donation and mandating the placement of trained staff who are responsible for the donation process[45].

Most of these staff are physicians, mainly intensive care unit specialists, and they belong to the staff of the hospital. They generally continue in their medical role, but as transplant coordinators, their main objective is to improve the organ donation rate. There also is increasing attention to enhance public education about organ donation. Since 1989, the Spanish model has increased dramatically the number of organ donors. This model has been so effective that the organ donation rate has increased by >100% in 10 yr.[46]. However, the Spanish model has not eliminated or alleviated renal transplant waiting lists.

As a result of the severe shortage of transplantable kidneys, some transplant centers now are performing ABO-incompatible living-donor renal transplants. This type of renal transplantation is costly, limited in number, and associated with more acute rejection episodes compared with ABO-compatible renal transplants[47].

Some transplant centers also are accepting volunteering altruistic strangers who are willing to donate a kidney to anyone who is in need. The large experience with a non-directed kidney donor program belongs to the University of Minnesota group. From 1997 to 2003, they received calls from 362 individuals for kidney donation. After a careful evaluation, only 23 (6%) finally were accepted and donated kidneys[48]. In most developed countries, several of these strategies are being used to increase the kidney donor pool, but in none of these countries have renal transplant waiting lists been eliminated.

Currently, much of the research activities are focused, and funding is spent on xenotransplantation, genetic engineering of organs, and human embryonic stem cell studies that all have the potential to revolutionize organ transplantation by making a sufficient number of transplantable organs available. Unfortunately, none of these approaches is expected to be applicable in clinical transplantation in the upcoming decade. Until that time, the adoption of some regulated models of paid organ donation similar to the Iranian model can eliminate successfully renal transplant waiting lists and save many lives.

Acknowledgment

The authors wish to acknowledge the leadership role of Dr. Iradj Fazel in Iranian Model kidney donation and in establishing cadaveric organ transplantation in Iran.

References

1. Schnuelle P, Lorenz D, Trede M, Van Der Woude FJ: Impact of renal cadaveric transplantation on survival in end-stage renal failure: Evidence for reduced mortality risk compared with hemodialysis during long-term follow-up. *J Am Soc Nephrol* 9:2135–2141, 1998.

2. Moeller S, Gioberge S, Brown G: ESRD patients in 2001: Global overview of patients, treatment modalities and development trends. *Nephrol Dial Transplant* 17: 2071–2076, 2002.

3. Grassmann A, Gioberge S, Moeller S, Brown G: ESRD patients in 2004: Global overview of patient numbers, treatment modalities and associated trends. *Nephrol Dial Transplant* 20: 2587–2593, 2005.

4. Mahoney JD: Should we adopt a market strategy to organ donation. In: *The Ethics of Organ Transplantation*, edited by Shelton W, Balint J, Amsterdam, Elsevier Science, 2001, p. 65–88.

5. Ghods AJ: Governed financial incentives as an alternative to altruistic organ donation. *Exp Clin Transplant* 2: 221–228, 2004.

6. Ghods AJ: Without legalized living unrelated donor renal transplantation many patients die or suffer—Is it ethical? In: *Ethical, Legal, and Social Issues in Organ Transplantation*, edited by Gutmann T, Daar AS, Sells RA, Land W, Lengerich, Pabst Science Publishers, 2004, pp 337–341.

7. Ghods AJ: Renal transplantation in Iran. *Nephrol Dial Transplant* 17: 222–228, 2002.

8. Ghods AJ, Ossareh S, Savaj S: Results of renal transplantation of the Hashemi Nejad Kidney Hospital–Tehran. In: *Clinical Transplants 2000*, edited by Cecka JM, Terasaki PI, Los Angeles, UCLA Tissue Typing Laboratory, 2001, pp 203–210.

9. The EBPG Expert Group on Renal Transplantation: European best practice guideline for renal transplantation (part 1). *Nephrol Dial Transplant* 15[Suppl 7]: 3–39, 2000.

10. A Report of the Amsterdam Forum on the Care of the Live Kidney Donor: Data and medical guidelines. *Transplantation* 79 [Suppl 6]: S53–S66, 2005.

11. Fazel I: Renal transplantation from living related and unrelated donors. *Transplant Proc* 27: 2586–2587, 1995.

12. Mehraban D, Nowroozi A, Naderi GH: Flank versus trans-abdominal living donor nephrectomy: A randomized clinical trial. *Transplant Proc* 27: 2716–2717, 1995.

13. Taghavi R: Does kidney donation threaten the quality of life of the donor? *Transplant Proc* 27: 2595–2596, 1995.

14. Ghods AJ, Nassrollahzadeh D: Gender disparity in a live donor renal transplantation program: Assessing from cultural perspectives. *Transplant Proc* 35: 2559–2560, 2003.

15. Ghods AJ: Should we have live unrelated donor renal transplantation in MESOT countries? *Transplant Proc* 35: 2542–2544, 2003.

16. Ghods AJ, Ossareh S, Khosravani P: Comparison of some socioeconomic characteristics of donors and recipients in a controlled living unrelated donor renal transplantation program. *Transplant Proc* 33: 2626–2627, 2001.

17. Ghods AJ, Nasrollahzadeh D: Transplant tourism and the Iranian model of renal transplantation program: Ethical considerations. *Exp Clin Transplant* 2: 351–354, 2005.

18. Ghods AJ, Nasrollahzadeh D, Kazemeini M: Afghan refugees in Iran model renal transplantation program: Ethical considerations. *Transplant Proc* 37: 565–566, 2005.

19. Ghods AJ: Changing ethics in renal transplantation: Presentation of Iran model. *Transplant Proc* 36: 11–13, 2004.

20. Simforoosh N, Basiri A, Tabibi A, Shakhssalim N: Laparoscopic donor nephrectomy—An Iranian model for developing countries: A cost-effective no-rush approach. *Exp Clin Transplant* 2: 249–253, 2004.

21. Malek-Hosseini SA, Salahi H, Bahador A, Roozbeh J, Raees Jalali GA, Mehdizadeh AR, Razmkon A: Cadaveric renal transplantation at southern Iran (Shiraz) organ transplant center [Abstract]. *Exp Clin Transplant* 2[Suppl]: 104, 2004.

22. Matas AJ: The case for living kidney sales: Rationale, objection and concerns. *Am J Transplant* 4: 2007–2017, 2004.

23. Friedman EA, Friedman AL: Payment for donor kidneys: Pros and cons. *Kidney Int* 69: 960–962, 2006.

24. Delmonico FL, Arnold R, Scheper-Hughes N, Siminoff LA, Kahn J, Youngner SJ: Ethical incentive—no payment—for organ donation. *N Engl J Med* 346: 2002–2005, 2002.

25. Gjertson DW, Cecka JM: Living unrelated donor kidney transplantation. *Kidney Int* 58: 491–499, 2000.

26. Rosendale JD: Organ donation in the United States: 1988–2003. In: *Clinical Transplants 2004*, edited by Cecka JM, Terasaki PI, Los Angeles, UCLA Tissue Typing Laboratory, 2005, pp 41–50.

27. McAlister VC, Badovinac K, Fenton SSA, Greig PD: Transplantation in Canada: Review of the past decade from the Canadian organ replacement register. In: *Clinical Transplants 2003*, edited by Cecka JM, Terasaki PI, Los Angeles, UCLA Tissue Typing Laboratory, 2004, pp 101–108.

28. Davies DB, Harper A: The OPTN waiting list, 1988–2003. In: *Clinical Transplants 2004*, edited by Cecka JM, Terasaki PI, Los Angeles, UCLA Tissue Typing Laboratory, 2005, pp 27–40.

29. Muthusethupathi MA, Rajendran S, Jayakumar M, Vijayakaumar R: Evaluation and selection of living related kidney donors: Our experience in a government hospital. *J Assoc Physicians India* 46: 526–529, 1998.

30. Matas AJ, Bartlett ST, Leichtman AB, Delmonico FL: Morbidity and mortality after living kidney donation, 1999–2001: Survey of United States transplant centers. *Am J Transplant* 3: 830–834, 2003.

31. Johnson EM, Remucal MJ, Gillingham KJ, Dahms RA, Najarian JS, Matas AJ: Complications and risks of living donor nephrectomy. *Transplantation* 64: 1124–1128, 1997.

32. Hartmann A, Fauchald P, Westlie L, Brekke IB, Holdaas H: The risk of living kidney donation. *Nephrol Dial Transplant* 18: 871–873, 2003.

33. Ghods AJ, Savaj S: Iranian experience with live kidney donors outcome [Abstract]. *Exp Clin Transplant* 2[Suppl]: 64–65, 2004.

34. Fehrman-Ekholm I, Elinder CG, Stenbeck M, Tyden G, Groth CG: Kidney donors live longer. *Transplantation* 64: 976–978, 1997.

35. Meire-Kreisch HU, Port FK, Ojo AO, Rudich SM, Hanson JA, Cibrik DM, Leichtman AB, Kaplan B: Effect of waiting time on renal transplant outcome. *Kidney Int* 58: 1311–1317, 2000.

36. Frieden J: Live organ donors sought via Internet. *Intern Med News* 38: 1–6, 2005.

37. Chugh KS, Jha V: Commerce in transplantation in third world countries. *Kidney Int* 49: 1181–1186, 1996.

38. Goyal M, Mehta RL, Schneiderman LJ, Sehgal AR: Economic and health consequences of selling a kidney in India. *JAMA* 288: 1589–1593, 2002.

39. Cecka JM: The OPTN/UNOS renal transplant registry. In: *Clinical Transplants 2004*, edited by Cecka JM, Terasaki PI, Los Angeles, UCLA Tissue Typing Laboratory, 2005, pp 1–16.

40. Cecka JM: The OPTN/UNOS renal transplant registry 2003. In: *Clinical Transplants 2003*, edited by Cecka JM, Terasaki PI, Los Angeles, UCLA Tissue Typing Laboratory, 2004, pp 1–12.

41. Kootstra G, Ruers TJM, Vroemen JPAM: The non-heart-beating donor: Contribution to the organ shortage. *Transplant Proc* 18: 1410–1412, 1986.

42. Teraoka S, Nomoto K, Kikuchi K, Hirano T, Satomi S, Hasegawa A, Uchida K, Akiyama T, Tanaka S, Babazona T, Shindo K, Nakamura N: Outcome of kidney transplants from non-heart-beating deceased donors as reported to the Japan Organ Transplant Network from April 1995–December 2003: A multi-center report. In: *Clinical Transplants 2004*, edited by Cecka JM, Terasaki PI, Los Angeles, UCLA Tissue Typing Laboratory, 2005, pp 91–102.

43. Cohen B, Smits JM, Haase B, Persijn G, Vanrenterghem Y, Frei U: Expanding the donor pool to increase renal transplantation. *Nephrol Dial Transplant* 20: 34–41, 2005.

44. Abouna GM: Ethical issues in organ transplantation. *Med Princ Pract* 12: 54–69, 2003.

45. Belitsky P, Nashan B, Kiberd B, West K, Legare JF, Keough-Ryan T, Watt K: The year in review 2004—Organ donation. In: *Clinical Transplants 2004*, edited by Cecka JM, Terasaki PI, Los Angeles, UCLA Tissue Typing Laboratory, 2005, pp 273–276.

46. Miranda B, Vilardell J, Grinyo JM: Optimizing cadaveric organ procurement: The Catalan and Spanish experience. *Am J Transplant* 3: 1189–1196, 2003.

47. Tanabe K, Tokumoto T, Ishida H, Toma H, Nakajima, Fuchinoue S, Teraoka S: ABO-incompatible renal transplantation at Tokyo Women's Medical University. In: *Clinical Transplants 2003*, edited by Cecka JM, Terasaki PI, Los Angeles, UCLA Tissue Typing Laboratory, 2004, pp 175–181.

48. Jacobs CL, Garvey C, Roman D, Kahn J, Matas AJ: Evolution of a non-directed kidney donor program. In: *Clinical Transplants 2003*, edited by Cecka JM, Terasaki PI, Los Angeles, UCLA Tissue Typing Laboratory, 2004, pp 283–291.

Chapter 17

AN EXCERPT FROM

Regulated Payments for Living Kidney Donation: An Empirical Assessment of the Ethical Concerns

Scott D. Halpern, Amelie Raz, Rachel Kohn, Michael Rey, David A. Asch, and Peter Reese

Abstract

Background: Although regulated payments to encourage living kidney donation could reduce morbidity and mortality among patients waiting for a kidney transplant, doing so raises several ethical concerns.

Objective: To determine the extent to which the 3 main concerns with paying kidney donors might manifest if a regulated market were created.

Design: Cross-sectional study of participants' willingness to donate a kidney in 12 scenarios.

Setting: Regional rail and urban trolley lines in Philadelphia County, Philadelphia, Pennsylvania.

Participants: Of 550 potential participants, 409 completed the questionnaire (response rate, 74.4%); 342 of these participants were medically eligible to donate.

Intervention: Across scenarios, researchers experimentally manipulated the amount of money that participants would receive, the participants' risk for subsequently developing kidney failure themselves, and who would receive the donated kidney.

Measurements: The researchers determined whether payment represents an undue inducement by evaluating participants' sensitivity to risk in relation to the payment offered or an unjust inducement by evaluating participants' sensitivity to payment as a function of their annual income. The researchers also evaluated whether introducing payment would hinder altruistic donations by comparing participants' willingness to donate altruistically before versus after the introduction of payments.

Results: Generalized estimating equation models revealed that participants' willingness to donate increased significantly as their risk for kidney failure decreased, as the payment offered increased, and when the kidney recipient was a family member rather than a patient on a public waiting list ($P < 0.001$ for each). No statistical interactions were identified between payment and risk (odds ratio, 1.00 [95% CI, 0.96 to 1.03]) or between payment and income (odds ratio, 1.01 [CI, 0.99 to 1.03]). The proximity of these estimates to 1.0 and narrowness of the CIs suggest that payment is neither an undue nor an unjust inducement, respectively. Alerting participants to the possibility of payment did not alter their willingness to donate for altruistic reasons ($P = 0.40$).

Limitation: Choices revealed in hypothetical scenarios may not reflect real-world behaviors.

Conclusion: Theoretical concerns about paying persons for living kidney donation are not corroborated by empirical evidence. A real-world test of regulated payments for kidney donation is needed to definitively show whether payment provides a viable and ethical method to increase the supply of kidneys available for transplantation.

Primary Funding Source: None.

The insufficient supply of transplantable kidneys from traditional donors after neurologic determination of death (1–2) has prompted increasing use of kidneys from the following types of donors: donors after circulatory determination of death (3), donors with risk factors for harboring transmittable infections (4), expanded-criteria donors (that is, those with risk factors, such as older age or hypertension) (5), and living donors related or unrelated to the recipient (6–7).

Unfortunately, despite these efforts to increase the pool of kidneys, the median time to transplantation, number of patients on the waiting list, and number of patients who die while waiting for an organ continue to increase (8). Thus, for the past decade, ethicists and members of the transplant community have debated the approach of paying healthy persons to become living donors (9–17). International black markets in organs are almost universally condemned because safeguards to protect donors are largely absent, brokers rather than donors may commandeer most of the payments, and such systems almost invariably entail wealthy travelers purchasing organs from poor natives (18–19). By contrast, a less well-resolved ethical debate regards a regulated national market for kidneys in which donors receive payment according to a fixed and transparent schedule, organs are allocated according to standard criteria, and standards are set and monitored to ensure appropriate longitudinal care for donors (14, 20).

The potential benefits of such a regulated market are clear. Compared with lifelong dialysis, kidney transplantation from deceased donors substantially increases quality-adjusted life expectancy and is cost-saving (21–22). Because kidney transplantation from living donors produces greater benefits (6), particularly when done before recipients initiate dialysis (7), even large payments (for example, $100,000) are estimated to be a cost-effective way to increase the supply of kidneys available for transplantation (8, 23).

However, at least 3 concerns exist with regulated payments for living kidney donation. First, payments may represent undue inducements—payments might alter a person's perception of the risks associated with donation, thereby preventing a fully informed decision to sell a kidney. Second, payments may represent unjust inducements—payments might preferentially influence lower-income persons, thereby creating a market in which organs are acquired from poor persons and provided to those with sufficient financial and social resources to be listed for transplantation. Third, payments may dissuade altruistic donation or cause potential altruistic donors to request payment.

In this study, we did not aim to assess the conceptual strengths and weaknesses of these concerns, but rather we used empirical methods to determine the extent to which these concerns might manifest if a regulated market for kidneys were established in the United States.

Discussion

We found no evidence that any of the 3 main concerns with a regulated system of payments for living kidney donation would manifest if such a market were established. Providing payments did not dull persons' sensitivity to the risks associated with donor nephrectomy, suggesting that payment does not represent an undue inducement—one that would make rational choice difficult. Furthermore, providing payments did not preferentially motivate poorer persons to sell a kidney, suggesting that payment does not represent an unjust inducement—one that would put substantially more pressure on poorer persons than on wealthier persons.

Similar to real-world observations from Iran's partially regulated kidney market (39–40), we found that poorer persons were more likely than wealthier persons to consider donation to an unrelated donor. However, contrary to both our hypotheses and concerns expressed about the Iranian market (40), we found that poorer persons were more willing to donate independent of payment (Figure 3 [Editors' note: Figure has been omitted.]). Even after restricting our analyses to the poorest and wealthiest participants, we found no evidence that payment influenced these 2 groups differently. This result is consistent with previous observations that payment does not preferentially motivate clinical research participation among poor persons (25). Thus, our results do not corroborate concerns about the ethics of payment per se, but rather they suggest that poorer persons may contribute disproportionately to the supply of organs with or without payment. Reasons for these behaviors, perhaps including differences in the opportunity costs of donating among richer and poorer patients, merit future study.

We also found no evidence that introducing monetary incentives would "crowd out" a person's altruistic incentives to donate. This result is consistent with a previous public survey that found that payments would encourage kidney donation for monetary reasons far

more commonly than it would discourage donation for altruistic reasons (41). Together, these studies cast substantial doubt on the concern that offering payments would undermine altruistic donation. They suggest that systems allowing payment for kidney donors would produce more transplantable organs than systems barring it.

Our study has several strengths. First, by experimentally manipulating the presentation of factors associated with donation decisions within participants, we forced persons to reveal their preferences and presumed behaviors (26–27). This approach contrasts with questionnaires that merely query stated preferences. Second, our study had substantial power to detect even minimal statistical interactions between payment and income and between payment and risk, as reflected by the narrowness of the CIs (42) surrounding the point estimates of these interactions. Thus, it is unlikely that we did not detect a true effect of payment as either an undue or an unjust inducement. Third, the high response rates to the survey and component items reduce the possibilities of important nonresponse biases. Fourth, the validity of the results is suggested by the low proportion of internally inconsistent responses (24, 37).

An important limitation of our study is that participants' responses to hypothetical offers may not reflect the decisions they would make if they were truly offered payment for a kidney. For example, hypothetical offers of payment may be insufficient to blunt a person's perception of risk, but real money might do just that. However, it seems unlikely that our study failed to detect real effects of money because participants clearly paid attention to and were influenced by money. We found that larger payments encouraged donation in general, and, as expected, payments were particularly important when participants contemplated donating to strangers. Furthermore, the experimental presentation of structured vignettes has been shown to produce valid results in other settings (43). Nonetheless, evaluating responses to hypothetical situations can take us only so far; ultimately, the effects of payment will need to be tested in natural settings.

Another possible limitation of the study regards the diversity of participants. Our sample contained a greater percentage of highly educated persons than expected from the general public. However, we found no relation between education and any outcome measure, and none of our results changed when analyses were restricted to the least-educated members of the sample. Similarly, it is possible that we did not enroll persons at the very extremes of the U.S. income distribution. However, our sample included roughly equal proportions of participants in each of the 6 predetermined income brackets, and we found unchanged results when we limited analyses to the highest versus lowest brackets.

Finally, some might believe our study is limited in that we did not address the views that payment for kidney donation is intrinsically unethical because it represents "commodification" of the body or that introducing payments for organs could have broader social ramifications, such as curtailing a person's general selflessness. However, these arguments apply equally to payments for surrogate motherhood or clinical research participation—activities that carry similar if not greater risks than kidney donation (11) yet are legal in most nations. Thus, regardless of the merits of these arguments, regulated kidney sales are difficult to challenge on these grounds.

Our study adds evidence to what has been a largely theoretical debate about the propriety of paying persons to become living kidney donors. The results both corroborate predictions that payments could effectively increase the supply of transplantable kidneys (8, 14) and cast doubt on intuitions that payments would be undue or unjust, or would undermine a person's otherwise altruistic behaviors (10, 16). Because participants' responses to our questionnaires did not carry real-world consequences, our results are insufficient to support the establishment of a national system of regulated payments for kidney donation. Instead, because these and other empirical results counter theoretical concerns about regulated payments, we recommend proceeding with a highly controlled and geographically limited test of such payments that is explicitly designed to detect both intended and unintended consequences of real-world payments for living kidney donation.

Acknowledgment: The authors thank Thomas R. Ten Have, PhD, and Mark Cary, PhD, for their assistance in the design and analysis of this study.

Grant Support: By a Greenwall Foundation Faculty Scholar Award in Bioethics (Dr. Halpern), the National Institutes of Health (Dr. Reese; grant K23–078688–01), and internships from the University of Pennsylvania Center for Bioethics (Ms. Raz, Ms. Kohn, and Mr. Rey).

References

1. Guadagnoli E, Christiansen CL, Beasley CL. Potential organ-donor supply and efficiency of organ procurement organizations. *Health Care Financ Rev.* 2003; 24:101–10.

2. Sheehy E, Conrad SL, Brigham LE, Luskin R, Weber P, Eakin M, et al. . Estimating the number of potential organ donors in the United States. *N Engl J Med.* 2003; 349:667–74.

3. Weber M, Dindo D, Demartines N, Ambühl PM, Clavien PA. Kidney transplantation from donors without a heartbeat. *N Engl J Med.* 2002; 347:248–55.

4. Halpern SD, Shaked A, Hasz RD, Caplan AL. Informing candidates for solid-organ transplantation about donor risk factors. *N Engl J Med.* 2008; 358:2832–7.

5. Port FK, Bragg-Gresham JL, Metzger RA, Dykstra DM, Gillespie BW, Young EW, et al. . Donor characteristics associated with reduced graft survival: an approach to expanding the pool of kidney donors. *Transplantation.* 2002; 74:1281–6.

6. Chkhotua AB, Klein T, Shabtai E, Yussim A, Bar-Nathan N, Shaharabani E, et al. . Kidney transplantation from living-unrelated donors: comparison of outcome with living-related and cadaveric transplants under current immunosuppressive protocols. *Urology.* 2003; 62:1002–6.

7. Mange KC, Joffe MM, Feldman HI. Effect of the use or nonuse of long-term dialysis on the subsequent survival of renal transplants from living donors. *N Engl J Med.* 2001; 344:726–31.

8. Becker GS, Elias JJ. Introducing incentives in the market for live and cadaveric organ donations. *J Econ Perspect.* 2007; 21:3–24.

9. Boulware LE, Troll MU, Wang NY, Powe NR. Public attitudes toward incentives for organ donation: a national study of different racial/ethnic and income groups. *Am J Transplant.* 2006; 6:2774–85.

10. Delmonico FL, Arnold R, Scheper-Hughes N, Siminoff LA, Kahn J, Youngner SJ. Ethical incentives—not payment—for organ donation. *N Engl J Med.* 2002; 346: 2002–5.

11. Friedman AL. Payment for living organ donation should be legalised. *BMJ.* 2006; 333:746–8.

12. Hippen BE. In defense of a regulated market in kidneys from living vendors. *J Med Philos.* 2005; 30:593–626.

13. Israni AK, Halpern SD, Zink S, Sidhwani SA, Caplan A. Incentive models to increase living kidney donation: encouraging without coercing. *Am J Transplant.* 2005; 5:15–20.

14. Matas AJ. The case for living kidney sales: rationale, objections and concerns. *Am J Transplant.* 2004; 4:2007–17.

15. Radcliffe-Richards J, Daar AS, Guttmann RD, Hoffenberg R, Kennedy I, Lock M, et al. . The case for allowing kidney sales. International Forum for Transplant Ethics. *Lancet.* 1998; 351:1950–2.

16. Rothman SM, Rothman DJ. The hidden cost of organ sale. *Am J Transplant.* 2006; 6:1524–8.

17. Veatch RM. Why liberals should accept financial incentives for organ procurement. *Kennedy Inst Ethics J.* 2003; 13:19–36.

18. Scheper-Hughes N. Keeping an eye on the global traffic in human organs. *Lancet.* 2003; 361:1645–8.

19. Goyal M, Mehta RL, Schneiderman LJ, Sehgal AR. Economic and health consequences of selling a kidney in India. *JAMA.* 2002; 288:1589–93.

20. Matas AJ. Design of a regulated system of compensation for living kidney donors. *Clin Transplant.* 2008; 22:378–84.

21. Schnitzler MA, Lentine KL, Burroughs TE. The cost effectiveness of deceased organ donation [Letter]. *Transplantation.* 2005; 80:1636–7.

22. Schnitzler MA, Whiting JF, Brennan DC, Lentine KL, Desai NM, Chapman W, et al. . The life-years saved by a deceased organ donor. *Am J Transplant.* 2005; 5:2289–96.

23. Matas AJ, Schnitzler M. Payment for living donor (vendor) kidneys: a cost-effectiveness analysis. *Am J Transplant.* 2004; 4:216–21.

24. Halpern SD, Berns JS, Israni AK. Willingness of patients to switch from conventional to daily hemodialysis: looking before we leap. *Am J Med.* 2004; 116:606–12.

25. Halpern SD, Karlawish JH, Casarett D, Berlin JA, Asch DA. Empirical assessment of whether moderate payments are undue or unjust inducements for participation in clinical trials. *Arch Intern Med.* 2004; 164:801–3.

26. Ryan M, Farrar S. Using conjoint analysis to elicit preferences for health care. *BMJ.* 2000; 320:1530–3.

27. Ryan M, McIntosh E, Shackley P. Methodological issues in the application of conjoint analysis in health care. *Health Econ.* 1998; 7:373–8.

28. Fehrman-Ekholm I, Dunér F, Brink B, Tydén G, Elinder CG. No evidence of accelerated loss of kidney

function in living kidney donors: results from a cross-sectional follow-up. *Transplantation*. 2001; 72:444–9.

29. Soneji ND, Vyas J, Papalois VE. Long-term donor outcomes after living kidney donation. *Exp Clin Transplant*. 2008; 6:215–23.

30. Ibrahim HN, Foley R, Tan L, Rogers T, Bailey RF, Guo H, et al. . Long-term consequences of kidney donation. *N Engl J Med*. 2009; 360:459–69.

31. Young A, Karpinski M, Treleaven D, Waterman A, Parikh CR, Thiessen-Philbrook H, et al. Differences in tolerance for health risk to the living donor among potential donors, recipients, and transplant professionals. *Kidney Int*. 2008; 73:1159–66.

32. Zeger SL, Liang KY. Longitudinal data analysis for discrete and continuous outcomes. *Biometrics*. 1986; 42:121–30.

33. Heyman J, Ariely D. Effort for payment. A tale of two markets. *Psychol Sci*. 2004; 15:787–93.

34. Localio AR, Margolis DJ, Berlin JA. Relative risks and confidence intervals were easily computed indirectly from multivariable logistic regression. *J Clin Epidemiol*. 2007; 60:874–82.

35. Byar DP, Piantadosi S. Factorial designs for randomized clinical trials. *Cancer Treat Rep*. 1985; 69: 1055–63.

36. Kerry SM, Bland JM. The intracluster correlation coefficient in cluster randomisation. *BMJ*. 1998; 316:1455.

37. Phillips KA, Maddala T, Johnson FR. Measuring preferences for health care interventions using conjoint analysis: an application to HIV testing. *Health Serv Res*. 2002; 37:1681–705.

38. Census Bureau. State and county quick facts: Philadelphia County, Pennsylvania. Accessed at http://quickfacts.census.gov/qfd/states/42/42101.html on 22 January 2010.

39. Ghods AJ, Savaj S. Iranian model of paid and regulated living-unrelated kidney donation. *Clin J Am Soc Nephrol*. 2006; 1:1136–45.

40. Harmon W, Delmonico F. Payment for kidneys: a government-regulated system is not ethically achievable. *Clin J Am Soc Nephrol*. 2006; 1:1146–7.

41. Jasper JD, Nickerson CA, Hershey JC, Asch DA. The public's attitudes toward incentives for organ donation. *Transplant Proc*. 1999; 31:2181–4.

42. Goodman SN, Berlin JA. The use of predicted confidence intervals when planning experiments and the misuse of power when interpreting results. *Ann Intern Med*. 1994; 121:200–6.

43. Peabody JW, Luck J, Glassman P, Dresselhaus TR, Lee M. Comparison of vignettes, standardized patients, and chart abstraction: a prospective validation study of 3 methods for measuring quality. *JAMA*. 2000; 283:1715–22.

Chapter 18

The Hidden Cost of Organ Sale

Sheila M. Rothman and David J. Rothman

Abstract

The idea of establishing a market for organs is now the subject of unusual controversy. Proponents emphasize the concept of autonomy; opponents invoke fairness and justice. The controversy, however, has given sparse attention to what it would mean to society and medicine to establish a market in organs and to the intended and unintended consequences of such a practice. This article addresses these issues by exploring the tensions between 'extrinsic' and 'intrinsic' incentives, suggesting that donation might well decline were financial incentives introduced. It also contends that social relationship and social welfare policy would be transformed in negative ways and that a regulated market in organs would be extraordinarily difficult to achieve. Finally, it argues that organ sale would have a highly detrimental effect on medicine as a profession.

Introduction

The idea of establishing a market for organs, although certainly not new, is now attracting unprecedented support. Much of the enthusiasm comes from members of the transplant community, but it is also favored by a growing number of economists and bioethicists who believe that the sale of body parts has become 'morally imperative.' To be sure, the practice is explicitly prohibited by U.S. law, rejected by the guidelines of almost every national and international transplant society and opposed by many commentators. But never before has a market solution been so vigorously endorsed.

Almost every article advocating legalization opens by noting the shortfall in organs (over 50,000 people await a kidney), and the resulting increase in morbidity and mortality. At the same time, the number of living donors has increased dramatically (they now provide more than half of all kidneys for transplantation), to the benefit of recipients and apparently without harm to themselves. Thus, as one transplant surgeon has observed: 'Discussing organ sales simply does not feel right, but letting candidates die on the waiting list (when this could be prevented) does not feel right either' (1–3).

Ethics has occupied a central place in the debate over the sale of kidneys, with two key principles vying for primacy. Proponents emphasize the concept of autonomy—the right of persons to sell their body parts, free of heavy-handed paternalism. Opponents invoke standards of fairness and justice; the poor will sell their kidneys to the rich, engendering systematic exploitation. What has been relegated to the margins, however, is full consideration of the implications of such a system for medicine and for society. Proponents flatly assert that sale would increase the supply and not reduce the rate of altruistic donation. They posit that such a market could be effectively regulated and that sellers would benefit greatly from the financial windfall. But these claims are not well substantiated and may prove wrong. No less important, they fail to take into account the many other possible effects of allowing a market in organs (4,5).

Because the intended and unintended consequences of policy change cannot be easily predicted, this analysis is put forward in tentative, even speculative, terms. The aim is to raise considerations that may have been glossed over, to highlight the possibilities that have not been imagined, and to prompt second thoughts about postulates that seem obvious. The intent is not to persuade one side or the other that these projections will inevitably be realized but to encourage both sides to deepen and widen the scope of their concerns. Just as studies of the possible impact of legislation on the environment are mandated, so the likely impact of legalization of organ sale warrants consideration.

Crowding Out

Advocates think it self-evident that market incentives will yield more organs for transplantation. 'People are more likely to do something if they are going to get paid for it' (6). And sellers will not drive out donors. Whatever financial incentives exist, siblings and parents will continue to donate to loved ones.

These expectations, however, may be disappointed. Since the 1970s, a group of econo-mists and social psychologists have been analyzing the tensions between 'extrinsic incentives'—financial compensation and monetary rewards, and 'intrinsic incentives'—the moral commitment to do one's duty. They hypothesize that extrinsic incentives can 'crowd out' intrinsic incentives, that the introduction of cash payments will weaken moral obligations. As Uri Gneezy, a professor of behavioral science at the University of Chicago School of Business, observes: 'Extrinsic motivation might change the perception of the activity and destroy the intrinsic motivation to perform it when no apparent reward apart from the activity itself is expected' (7–12). Although the case for the 'hidden costs of rewards' is certainly not indisputable, it does suggest that a market in organs might reduce altruistic donation and overall supply.

Perhaps the most celebrated analysis of the tension between intrinsic and extrinsic incentives is Titmuss' work in blood donation. His book, *The Gift Relationship* (1971), argued that the 'commercialization of blood represses the expression of altruism (and) erodes the sense of community.' Payment undermined the altruistic motivations of would-be blood donors. Titmuss supported his hypothesis by comparing blood donation in the United States and the United Kingdom. Analyzing data from England and Wales over the period 1946–1968, where the sale of blood was prohibited, Titmuss found that the percentage of the population who donated blood and the amount of blood donated steadily increased. By comparison, in the United States, where the sale of blood was allowed, donations declined. Because U.S. data were more fragmentary, Titmuss drew as best he could on a variety of sources, including surveys, municipal statistics and comments by medical experts and blood bank officials. Nevertheless, he confidently concluded: The data, 'when analyzed in microscopic fashion, blood bank by blood bank area by area, city by city, state by state,' revealed 'a generally worsening situation' (12).

Following Titmuss' lead, other studies have tried to buttress the empirical case for crowding out. One intriguing experiment turned an Israeli day care center into a research site. It was not unusual for some parents to arrive late to pick up their children; center administrators complained but levied no penalties. The researchers first took a baseline measure of the frequency of lateness and then had the center post a notice on its bulletin board: 'The official closing time . . . is 1600. Since some parents have been coming late, we . . . have decided to impose a fine. . . . NIS 10 ($2.50) will be charged every time a child is collected after 1610. The fine will be calculated monthly, and is to be paid with the regular monthly payment.' Although one might have predicted that late pickups would decline, the number actually increased. And even when several weeks later the researchers had the center cancel the late charge, the higher level of lateness persisted.

To explain these outcomes, the researchers proposed that in the prefine days, parents interpreted the extra time that the teacher spent taking care of the children as 'a generous, nonmarket activity'; they did their best to arrive on time because the teacher was considerate and should 'not be taken advantage of.' Once the fine was levied, the added time of child care had a price and parents believed they could purchase it as often as necessary. 'When help is offered for no compensation in a moment of need, accept it with restraint. When a service is offered for a price, buy as much as you find convenient.' Moreover, the lateness

persisted after the elimination of the charge because there was no reverting to the older norm once the charge had been levied: 'Once a commodity, always a commodity' (10).

Another research team divided a group of teenagers who had been volunteering to collect contributions for disabled children into three different cohorts: one was not paid for their service, the second was paid a small amount, and the third was paid a more substantial amount. Using the total funds that each group collected as the outcome measure, they found that the best returns came from the volunteers, the next best from the substantially paid, and the least from the lowest paid. Financial incentives, the investigators concluded, proved less effective than moral commitments (13–15).

Still others have highlighted the potential conflict between extrinsic and intrinsic rewards by framing the following question: You see an older man hauling two boxes of bottles to the recycling center on a rainy afternoon. Knowing that the center does not reimburse for bottles, you admire his commitment to environmental concerns. Now imagine that the recycling center reimburses at a nickel a bottle and you witness the same scene. Might your admiration turn to pity and stigma replace esteem? Might you consider the older man to be very cheap or poverty stricken because he is returning bottles? Indeed, would you yourself be more or less likely to recycle where you paid for the items (11)?

None of these exercises are without important methodological weaknesses. The Israeli day care center may not have made the fine severe enough. Had the lateness penalty been $50 or $100, not $2.50, extrinsic incentives might have worked better. By the same token, had the teenagers been very well paid for their services, the reimbursed groups might have outperformed the volunteers. These points notwithstanding, the literature on the hidden cost of rewards raises the prospect of a market crowding out donation. Rather than donate and run the risks of surgery and future complications, family and friends might opt to purchase an organ; and if the market is as efficient as proponents claim, the purchased organ would be equally sound. This outcome is precisely what anthropologists have found in developing countries where organ sale is routine. In India, for example, recipients did not want to ask family members to donate and family members preferred to purchase (16).

The same dynamic might occur here were organ sale permitted. Moral incentives are now very well established in federal and state laws and an ethos of altruism is emphasized by transplant teams. A new federal act (2004) and some dozen states now allow reimbursement for donor travel, lost wages and living expenses (17). But no one permits financial gain. Altering the rules by introducing financial incentives might undermine the system, discourage donation, and reduce supply. To counter this possibility, proponents might point to the sale of sperm and egg and argue that opening a market in these body parts did not bring deleterious consequences. However, egg and sperm are not analogous to kidneys. For one, there was no tradition of altruism in sperm collection. Common practice was for students, usually medical students, to give their sperm for nominal sums. Second, clinics have not relied heavily on the altruism of family and friends for egg donation, perhaps because of reluctance among some would-be recipients to have the biological mother so prominent a figure in the child's life (18,19). Thus, the sale of egg and sperm does not

directly speak to the tension between extrinsic and intrinsic reward.

Confronting these potential negative outcomes, yet other proponents have suggested that organ sale be introduced on an experimental basis so its impact could be closely monitored. Select several states or a region to serve as laboratories and were the total number of organs to decline, the experiment in sale would be ended. But even this approach would not be free of risk. As suggested in the Israeli day care center research, there may be no going back. Once a commodity, always a commodity.

Social Relations and Kidney Sale

What impact might organ sale have on day-to-day social interactions? Let us make a few preliminary assumptions. The purchase price for an organ would have to be nontrivial. One calculation, based on cost savings were transplantation to more completely replace dialysis, sets the figure at $275 000 per kidney (20). For sake of argument, let us divide that number by a little more than half and use a price of $125 000. Because government policy would have to strongly favor such an arrangement, let us also presume that the sum would be tax free.

Would sellers be attracted? Undoubtedly. They would likely come from the lower class and lower-middle class, although at this price some in the middle class might participate as well. It is doubtful that anyone with significant means would sell a kidney even for a substantial sum.

The removal of the kidney would leave an indelible mark in the form of a scar. Were the procedure done laparoscopically, it would be small and not easily distinguished from other surgical interventions. Still, it would be visible, if not to strangers then to intimates. Evidence of the sale would thus be written on the body and speak to moral character. It would point not to heroism and generosity of spirit (intrinsic reward) but to desperation and avariciousness (extrinsic reward). In fact, a study conducted in Iran found that kidney sellers suffered extreme shame in their community (21). In the United States, the opprobrium might be even greater. Historians of punishment, for example, have proposed that the practice of public torture was abandoned in the 18th century not because the punishments were ineffective, but because citizens shared new and acute sensibilities about bodily integrity, which the spectacle of dismemberment violated (22). Although a surgical scar does not rise to this level, it may still be asked whether we are ready to countenance the signs of kidney sale.

The everyday consequences of an organ market might create other problems. If kidney sale brought a payment of $125 000 tax free, it would make financial sense to undergo the procedure sooner rather than later. For someone at age 21, investing $125 000, perhaps in a mutual fund, would likely double the sum by age 30. Should one then boast of the sale to a prospective partner? At what point in a relationship would one relate the fact? Would it be presented as having the means for a down payment on a starter home? Would the partner be obliged to sell a kidney in the future to enable a move to a still larger home? Should one anticipate inquiries from prospective in-laws on whether you have yet sold your kidney? Should one anticipate such questions from bill collectors (in India this is not hypothetical), or from welfare or unemployment officers or from attorneys in bankruptcy proceedings? Should one also anticipate parents asking an 18-year-old to sell a kidney to offset substantial college tuition costs, or later, wedding costs?

In sum, the implications for social relationships of transforming body parts into commodities are unknown and might bring unintended negative consequences. As Margret Radin, a professor of law, has astutely observed: 'The law both expresses and works to form and evolve cultural characteristics and commitments. . . . "Preferences" bring law into being, but law also makes and changes "preferences".' Because there is feedback between law and culture, we might come to regret the legalization of kidney sale (23).

The Myth of the Regulated Market

Proponents offer very different models for a market in organs, making it difficult to know precisely what is being advocated. Some would restrict compensation to cadaveric organs and give credits to families who agree to the removal. Others, including a committee of the American Medical Association, endorse a futures market in organs: they would compensate would-be donors for agreeing to organ removal upon death (24–29). Still others urge a regulated market among living vendors but provide almost no details (1,6,20). Mostly everyone rejects a public auction with the kidney going to the highest bidder; the preference is for distribution by a central, UNOS-like organization, permitting individuals to sell but not to purchase an organ (30–32). Such compromises, it should be noted, are inconsistent with proponents' attachment to the market. After all, people are even more likely to do something if they are very well paid for it—so why not permit auctions?

Whatever the proposed system, regulation may not be readily accomplished. Once a market is lawful, half-way measures that allow for sellers but not for buyers might prove inoperative. Effectively regulated markets typically involve so-called 'natural monopolies' wherein entry points can be effectively policed. (Think of electric power, telephone service and railroads.) By contrast, in kidney sale, with almost everyone eligible to enter the market, oversight will not be easily established or maintained. So too, as most students of regulated markets are quick to admit, change almost inevitably carries unintended consequences. Deregulate the market in energy trading and Enron scandals occur; deregulate the telephone market and the communications industry is transformed; deregulate the savings and loan business and corruption breaks out. Hence, the question must be asked: since practices may develop in ways that cannot be predicted or controlled, are we ready to live with a system that makes kidneys a commodity?

Who May Sell?

With significant sums available to kidney vendors, the question of eligibility assumes new importance. Medical selection criteria for sellers would almost certainly come under intense pressure, with physicians urged to discount potentially disqualifying characteristics (from hypertension to a history of substance abuse). Would-be sellers might also withhold information on present habits or past personal and family medical histories, following the market maxim of let the buyer beware.

Some proponents would restrict sale to U.S. citizens (31,32), but the limitation seems neither logical nor appropriate. Why penalize green card holders or long-term residents? Or for that matter, tourists or illegal immigrants?

Since the goal is to maximize the number of organs and since kidney sale ostensibly benefits the vendor, why exclude anyone? Why should not the poor of Bombay enjoy an option given to the poor of Appalachia? Why deprive a patient of a kidney because the seller must travel? The end result, however, might give new meaning to the lines of Emma Lazarus engraved on the Statue of Liberty: 'Give me your tired, your poor . . . the wretched refuse of your teeming shore.'

The Impact on Medical Professionalism

Allowing kidney sale would pose fundamental challenges to professional medical ethics and doctor-patient relationships (33). Currently, in the practice of living organ donation, donor altruism mitigates, although does not entirely eliminate, the principle of 'do no harm.' In the pioneering days of living donation, surgeons like Joseph Murray were deeply troubled about the morality of 'maiming' one person (in his case, one twin) for the benefit of another (34–36). This concern was overcome only by emphasizing the deep emotional ties between donor and recipient. The psychological damage to a twin, proscribed from saving his brother's life, reset the risk-benefit calculus and justified the surgeon's intervention. But a strictly commercial transaction offers no mitigating circumstances. The physician unavoidably becomes an accessory to a patient's incomegenerating activity, a circumstance almost without precedent. Although surgical techniques have improved, risks still remain, so medicine would have to qualify the principle of 'do no harm' because of a dollar amount.

Upward Mobility through Kidney Sale

One claim frequently made to justify kidney markets is that the sums paid to vendors will redound to their economic benefit. The bioethicist Robert Veatch recently retracted his long-held opposition to sale, arguing that because American society has so neglected the poor, objections must be put aside. Social welfare programs are so inadequate that it is wrong to oppose a measure that might assist them (37). The empirical question, however, is whether organ sale would actually benefit the poor or, to the contrary, bring even more deleterious effects.

The best data comes from the third world. In India, as Goyal et al. have documented, 87% of kidney sellers reported a deterioration of health status and one third, a decrease in family income. Of 292 persons who sold a kidney to pay off debts, 74% still had debts 6 years later, and those in poverty increased from 54% prior to the sale to 71% after the sale (38). These findings are reinforced by Cohen's in-depth interviews with 30 sellers and their families in Madras. Although they were attempting to pay off debts, he found that 'sellers are frequently back in debt in a few years.' He also discovered that debt collectors became more aggressive in 'kidney selling zones,' making a system of sale self-reinforcing (16).

To be sure, the American experience might be different, with the economic returns from sale promoting property mobility. But kidney sale might also have a negative impact on social welfare policy. Some proponents have argued, for example, that kidney sellers should receive lifetime health insurance, and in this way move the country closer to national health insurance. But legalized kidney sale might have the very opposite effect.

If you want health insurance, sell your organ. Surely this is not the most promising method for accomplishing a more just distribution of health-care benefits. Were there no organ shortage, no one would propose kidney sale as a way of equalizing economic conditions.

Conclusion

However lamentable the consequences of the shortage of organs, kidney sale might turn out to be counterproductive. It might not produce the increase in organs that proponents anticipate. More, it might engender conditions inimical to professional medical practice and social cohesion.

Acknowledgments: This work was supported by a Robert Wood Johnson Foundation Investigator Award in Health Policy Research to the authors and by the Samuel and May Rudin Foundation. The views expressed are those of the authors and imply no endorsement by either foundation. We are especially grateful to Natassia Rozario for her outstanding research assistance.

References

1. Matas AJ. The case for living kidney sales: Rationale, objections and concerns. *Am J Transplant* 2004; 4: 2007–2017.

2. Taylor JS. *Stakes and Kidneys: Why Markets in Human Body Parts Are Morally Imperative.* Burlington, VT: Ashgate Press, 2005.

3. Cherry MJ. *Kidney for Sale by Owner: Human Organs, Transplantation, and the Market.* Washington, DC: Georgetown University Press, 2005.

4. Milmoe Mccarrick P, Darragh M. Incentives for providing organs. *Kennedy Inst Ethics J* 2003; 13:53–64.

5. Delmonico FL, Arnold R, Scheper-Hughes N, Siminoff LA, Kahn J, Yougner SJ. Ethical incentives— not payment for organ donation. *N Engl J Med* 2002; 346: 2002–2005.

6. Gill MS, Sade RB. Paying for kidneys: The case against prohibition. *Kennedy Inst Ethics J* 2002; 12: 17–45.

7. Fehr E, Falk A. Joseph Schumpeter lecture: Psychological foundations of incentives. *Eur Econ Rev* 2002; 46:687–724.

8. Deci EL. Effects of externally mediated rewards on intrinsic motivation. *J Pers Soc Psychol* 1971; 18: 105–115.

9. Frey BS, Jegen R. Motivation crowding theory. *J Econ Surv* 2001; 15:589–611.

10. Gneezy U, Rustichini A. A fine is a price. *J Legal Stud* 2000; 29:1–17.

11. Gneezy U. *The W Effect of Incentives.* The University of Chicago Business School, 2003.

12. Titmuss RM. *The Gift Relationship: From Human Blood to Social Policy.* New York: Vintage Books, 1971.

13. Frey BS, Gotte L. *Does pay motivate volunteers? In: Working Paper Series No 7. Institute for Empirical Economic Research.* University of Zurich, 1999.

14. Gneezy U, Rustichini A. Pay enough or don't pay at all. *Q J Econ* 2000; 115:791–810.

15. Freeman RB. Working for nothing: The supply of volunteer labor. *J Labor Econ* 1997; 15: S140–S166.

16. Cohen L. Where it hurts: Indian material for an ethics of organ transplantation. *Daedalus* 1999; 128: 135–165.

17. UNOS Transplant Living Website. Financial aspects: State tax deductions and donor leave laws. Retrieved January 19, 2006 from, http://www.trans plantliving.org/livingdonation/financialaspects/statetax .aspx

18. Braverman AM, Corson SL. A comparison of oocyte donors' and gestational carriers/surrogates' attitudes towards third party reproduction. *J Assist Reprod Genet* 2002; 19.10:462–469

19. Schover LR, Rothmann SA, Collins RL. The personality and motivation of semen donors: A comparison with oocyte donors. *Hum Reprod* 1992; 7.4: 575–579.

20. Matas A, Schnitzler M. Payment for living donor (vendor) kidneys: A cost-effectiveness analysis. *Am J Transplant* 2003; 4:216–221.

21. Zargooshi J. Quality of life of Iranian kidney "donors." *J Urol* 2001; 166:1790–1799.

22. Spierenburg P. *The Spectacle of Suffering* Cambridge: Cambridge University Press, 1984.

23. Radin MJ. *Contested Commodities: The Trouble with Trade in Sex, Children, Body Parts and Other Things.* Cambridge: Harvard University Press, 1996.

24. Peters TG. Life or death: The issue of payment in cadaveric organ donation. *J Am Med Assoc* 1991; 265:1302–1305.

25. Peters TG. A stand in favor of financial incentives in organ recovery. *Dial Transplant* 2002; 31:4–5, 322, 324–325.

26. Transplantation and immunology letter. *Transpl Immunol* 1992; VIII.

27. Cohen R. *Increasing the supply of transplant organs: The virtues of a futures market.* George Washington Law Rev 1989–1990; 58:1–50.

28. Harris CE, Alcorn SP. To solve a deadly shortage: Economic incentives for human organ donation. *Issues Law Med* 2001; 16:213–233.

29. American Medical Association Council on Ethics and Judicial Affairs. Financial incentives for organ donation. *Arch Intern Med* 1995; 155:581–589.

30. Harris J, Erin C. An ethically defensible market in organs: A single buyer like the national health service is an answer. *Br Med J* 2002; 325:114–115.

31. Savulescu J. Is the sale of body parts wrong? *J Med Ethics* 2003; 29:138–139.

32. Erin C, Harris J. An ethical market in human organs. *J Med Ethics* 2003; 29:137–138.

33. Kahn JP, Delmonico FL. The consequences of public policy to buy and sell organs for transplantation. *Am J Transplant* 2004; 4:78–180.

34. Moore FD. Three ethical revolutions: Ancient assumptions remodeled under pressure of transplantation. *Transplant Proc* 1988; 20 (1 Suppll):1061–1067.

35. Murray JE. *Surgery of the Soul: Reflections of a Curious Career.* Canton, MA: Science History Publications, 2001.

36. Delmonico FL. Interview with Joseph Murray. *Am J Transplant* 2002; 2:803–806.

37. Veatch R. Why liberals should accept financial incentives for organ procurement. *Kennedy Inst Ethics J* 2003; 1:19–36.

38. Goyal M, Mehta RL, Schneiderman LJ, Sehgal AR. Economic and health consequences of selling a kidney in India. *J Am Med Assoc* 2002; 288:1589–1593.

Chapter 19

Commercial Organ Transplantation in the Philippines

Leigh Turner

Countries throughout Asia promote themselves as leading destinations for international travelers seeking inexpensive healthcare. India, Indonesia, Malaysia, Singapore, the Philippines, and Thailand are all trying to attract greater numbers of what their promotional campaigns call "medical tourists."[1] Government tourism initiatives, hospital associations, medical tourism companies, and individual hospitals advertise hip and knee replacements, spinal surgery, cosmetic surgery, and other medical procedures.[2] In contrast to most nations marketing treatments to international patients, the Philippines differentiates itself by selling "all inclusive" kidney transplant packages. Patients from other countries travel to the Philippines and receive kidneys purchased from poor individuals.[3]

The Philippines' market in kidney transplants is connected to widespread poverty in urban slums and outlying rural areas.[4] Organ brokers target inhabitants of poor communities. Although trafficking in persons and organ brokering is illegal in the Philippines, the country's trade in kidney transplants is well known and attracts only sporadic attention from local law enforcement agencies.

Within the United States, nearly 105,000 individuals are wait-listed for organ transplants.[5] Of this population, more than 78,000 patients need kidney transplants. The gulf between the number of individuals requiring renal transplants and the number of kidneys available for transplantation is large and growing. Public awareness campaigns promoting organ donation, increased use of kidneys from living-related and living-unrelated donors, and expanded criteria for use of kidneys procured from deceased donors have not closed the gap between supply and demand. Other countries face a similar gulf between demand for organs and supply of organ transplants.

In response to the scarcity of organs available for transplantation, underground economies or "black markets" have emerged in several countries. Organ brokers connect international patients with sufficient funds to poor individuals willing to exchange kidneys for cash. Persons engaging in commercial organ transplantation have purchased organs in such countries as India, Pakistan, the Philippines, and China.[6] In China, organs were taken from executed prisoners. Hearts, livers, lungs, and kidneys were all advertised on Internet sites and sold to international patients. In most other countries where commercial transplants are available, kidneys are bought from living providers.

Due to changes in legislation and regulatory enforcement, it is now much more difficult for foreign patients to purchase kidneys in China and several other jurisdictions where commercial sales of organs occurred. Pakistan and India now have legislation prohibiting buying and selling human organs. Though legislative reforms have driven commerce in organs underground, commercial transplants still occur in both countries.[7] In 2006, China curtailed the number of foreign patients purchasing organ transplants at Chinese medical facilities.[8] In contrast, commercial organ transplantation persists in the Philippines.

The situation in the Philippines is complex. Some transplant professionals and government representatives oppose the country's permissive attitude toward commercial organ transplantation.[9] Other physicians and government officials want to increase the number of international patients purchasing kidney transplant packages at hospitals in the Philippines.[10] These individuals see commercial organ transplantation as a revenue generator for medical facilities trying to attract patients from other countries.

There are several ways in which trade in organs is condoned and promoted by government bodies and transplant physicians in the Philippines. The Philippine Information Agency, a branch of the Philippine government, advertises that kidney transplants are available in the Philippines for $25,000.[11] The "Philippine Health and Wellness and Medical Tourism Roadshow" a public–private initiative involving government representatives, physicians, and hospital representatives, travels to other countries and promotes the Philippines' "medical tourism" program.[12] Transplant physicians and government representatives are members of the delegation. Seeking to attract customers from the Middle East, the Philippines has also hosted Saudi Arabian delegates interested in increasing the

number of Saudi citizens purchasing kidney transplants at Philippine hospitals.[13]

Commercial organ transplantation in the Philippines is facilitated by the Internet. At least 13 websites promote kidney transplants in the Philippines. "Medical tourism" companies, hospitals, and individual organ brokers all market kidney transplants at Philippine medical facilities. Commercial organ transplants occur in both government hospitals and private medical centers. Prices for kidney transplants range from $18,941 to over $85,000. Most facilities charge $65,000 to $85,000. Expenses cover "donors' fees," tests, screening, organ transplantation, and accommodations in hospital rooms and hotels located near local transplant facilities.

When someone sells a kidney in the Philippines, he or she typically earns no more than $2,000. Organ brokers encounter little difficulty finding impoverished individuals willing to exchange kidneys for cash. Many poor individuals decide that selling a kidney is their only way to escape from a world of slums and shanties.

Proponents of commercial markets in organ transplants argue that poor individuals should be free to sell kidneys. They should be "at liberty" to choose between the risks associated with selling a kidney and the risks of keeping two kidneys while remaining impoverished. Advocates of commercial organ transplantation deny that purchasing a kidney from a poor person constitutes a form of exploitation or involves coercion. Rather, they argue that permitting a market in organs promotes choice and freedom. Defenders of this line of reasoning note that poor individuals often earn money by engaging in risky or physically debilitating forms of labor. In the Philippines, for example, some individuals endure backbreaking work as poorly paid day laborers and others scrabble for a living by combing through garbage dumps in search of items they can sell or exchange. Why, defenders of commercial organ transplants wonder, should we prohibit someone from selling a kidney if the transaction can enable the person to escape from poverty? This argument, built on the rhetoric of choice and the assumption that individuals experience economic benefits from selling a kidney, does not map onto what is known about the consequences of allowing poor individuals to exchange kidneys for cash.

Commercial organ transplantation poses significant dangers to both transplant recipients and poor individuals who attempt to alleviate impoverishment by exchanging kidneys for cash. Individuals who sell kidneys are particularly vulnerable to harm.[14] Most individuals do not experience long-term economic benefits or improved life circumstances when they sell a kidney.[15] Organ brokers commonly pay substantially less than what they promise.[16] They often charge fees for finding a buyer, extract rent money as sellers wait to have nephrectomies, and use other tactics to maximize earnings by reducing payments to individuals selling kidneys. These strategies mean that individuals selling a kidney often gain little from the transaction. Researchers exploring the sale of kidneys in India and Pakistan indicate that whatever profits are made commonly go to debt collectors. Kidney sales do not help sellers escape from penury.[17]

Once a kidney is removed the person selling the organ rarely receives adequate posttransplant care. Instead, he or she is released from the hospital without proper follow-up care. Some individuals experience infections and other complications postnephrectomy and must use earnings from kidney sales to purchase costly treatments.

Lack of proper care following nephrectomy

poses considerable risks to organ sellers. Poor individuals who sell a kidney often find that they cannot return to whatever form of livelihood previously enabled them to subsist. Dockyard workers, brick-kiln workers, rickshaw drivers, and other laborers often become too weak to perform demanding physical tasks. Rather than generating economic returns and increasing savings, selling a kidney can lead to further economic deprivation.

Under optimal conditions and with excellent medical care, removal of a kidney from a healthy donor involves little risk. However, when operations are conducted in unhygienic facilities, when clinicians are not motivated to offer proper medical care to individuals selling a kidney, and when organ sellers return to polluted, hazardous social environments, removal of a kidney puts individuals at increased risk of health problems.

Researchers studying kidney selling observe that individuals who sell organs often subsequently regret their decisions. Prior to selling a kidney they overestimate what they will gain from the transaction and underestimate the financial, social, and emotional costs they will incur. Postnephrectomy they discover that harms greatly outweigh benefits of selling a kidney.

Commercial organ transplantation is harmful not only to individuals selling kidneys. Studies investigating health outcomes for recipients of purchased organs also reveal serious problems with commercially acquired organs.[18] Both organ brokers and transplant physicians profit when someone buys an organ. The pressure to maximize earnings from commercial organ transplantation can lead to substandard selection of organ providers. Inadequate testing and screening of organs prior to transplantation places purchasers of kidneys at increased risk of serious infections.

International patients receiving commercial organ transplants have returned home with HIV, viral hepatitis, tuberculosis, malaria, and other infections.[19] Often, patients return with little documentation of the care they received abroad. Inadequate or nonexistent medical records hinder the capacity of caregivers to provide proper posttransplant care. Defenders of cross-border commercial organ transplants claim that ill individuals have "nothing to lose" by traveling overseas and buying an organ. To the contrary, purchasing an improperly screened or incompetently transplanted organ can have grievous consequences.

Proponents of the Philippines' commercial market in organ transplants claim that buying and selling kidneys benefits both individuals who sell kidneys as well as recipients of transplants. This utilitarian mode of analysis neglects basic ethical questions about whether organs ought to be purchased and sold through market mechanisms. In addition, it overstates benefits for buyers and sellers and underestimates the extent to which organ providers and organ recipients can be harmed through commercial organ transplantation.

Despite the harms associated with buying and selling kidneys in poorly regulated environments, the Philippine government encourages foreign patients to purchase organ transplants in the Philippines. Government websites tout the low cost of buying kidneys in the Philippines. Kidneys are available for purchase at government-run hospitals. Internet websites of hospitals and medical tourism companies enable organ brokers to connect buyers to sellers. Several companies claim that it takes less than two weeks to proceed from initial query to receiving a kidney transplant.

In response to international condemnation from human rights activists, persistent diplomatic efforts, and lobbying from leaders of national and international transplantation societies, several countries with underground economies in commercial organ transplantation have established laws and regulations intended to halt the buying and selling of human organs. Given the serious risk it poses to poor citizens of the Philippines and patients traveling from other countries, the organ transplant bazaar in the Philippines must also be closed for business.

Notes

1. Connell J. Medical tourism: Sea, sun, sand and . . . surgery. *Tourism Management* 2006; 27: 1093–100; Ramirez de Arellano A. Patients without borders: The emergence of medical tourism. *International Journal of Health Services* 2007; 37:193–8.

2. Turner L. "First world health care at third world prices": Globalization, bioethics and medical tourism. *Biosocieties* 2007; 2:303–25.

3. Romualdez A. Kidney disease and equity. *Malaya* 2007 Oct 23; Scheper-Hughes N. The ends of the body: Commodity fetishism and the global traffic in organs. *SAIS Review* 2002; 22:61–80.

4. Jimenez M, Bell S. Poorest Filipinos sell kidneys to Canadians. *National Post* 2001 Jun 5: A1; Derbyshire D. Inside the transplant tourist trade: The desperate men of One Kidney Island. *Daily Mail* 2007 Mar 12.

5. Figures obtained from Organ Procurement and Transplantation Network, available at http://www.optn.org/latestData/rptData.asp (last accessed 8 May 2008).

6. Cohen L. Where it hurts: Indian material for an ethics of organ transplantation. *Daedalus* 1999; 128:135–65; Scheper-Hughes N. Keeping an eye on the global traffic in human organs. *Lancet* 2003; 361:1645–8.

7. Muraleedharan V, Jan S, Prasad S. The trade in human organs in Tamil Nadu: The anatomy of regulatory failure. *Health Economics, Policy and Law* 2006; 1:41–57.

8. Woan S. Buy me a pound of flesh: China's sale of death row organs on the black market and what

Americans can learn from it. *Santa Clara Law Review* 2007; 413:413–40.

9. Araneta M. Doctors slam campaign to promote sale of organs. *Manila Standard Today* 2006 Nov 4.

10. Esquerra C. Filipino kidney is worth more—DOH official. *Inquirer* 2006 Oct 31.

11. Philippine Information Agency. RP conducts health, wellness and medical tourism roadshow in US. PIA press release, available at http://pia.gov.ph/?m512&sec5reader&rp53&?5p070602.htm&no521&date506/02/2007 (last accessed 13 February 2008).

12. Philippine Consulate General, Los Angeles Meets Members of Philippine Health, Wellness, Medical Tourism Roadshow. Department of Foreign Affairs press release; 2007 May 10, available at http://www.dfa.gov.ph/news/pr/pr2007/may/pr402.pdf (last accessed 8 May 2008).

13. Royal Embassy of Saudi Arabia Manila. Embassy News: Ambassador Wali Hosts Dinner for Saudi Medical Delegation; 2007 May 6, available at http://www.mofa.gov.sa/Detail.asp?InSectionID53050&InNewsItemID565860 (last accessed 8 May 2008).

14. Jha V. Paid transplants in India: The grim reality.

Nephrology, Dialysis, Transplantation 2004; 19:541–3; Naqvi S, Ali B, Mazhar F, Zafar F, Rizvi S. A socioeconomic survey of kidney vendors in Pakistan. *Transplant International* 2007; 20:934–9.

15. Goyal M, Mehata R, Schneiderman L, Sehgal A. Economic and health consequences of selling a kidney in India. *JAMA* 2002; 288:1589–93.

16. Jha V, Chugh K. The case against a regulated system of living kidney sales. *Nature Clinical Practice Nephrology* 2006; 2:466–7.

17. Rothman D. Ethical and social consequences of selling a kidney. *JAMA* 2002; 288:1640–1.

18. Prasad G, Shukla A, Huang M, Honey R, Zaltzman J. Outcomes of commercial renal transplantation: A Canadian experience. *Transplantation* 2006; 82(9): 1130–5; Canales M, Kasiske B, Rosenberg M. Transplant tourism: Outcomes of United States residents who undergo kidney transplantation overseas. *Transplantation* 2006; 82(12):1658–61.

19. Kennedy S, Shen Y, Charlesworth J, Mackie J, Mahony J, Kelly J, Pussell B. Outcome of overseas commercial kidney transplantation: An Australian perspective. *Medical Journal of Australia* 2005; 182:224–7.

Chapter 20

Kidney Vending

The "Trojan Horse" of Organ Transplantation

Gabriel M. Danovitch and Alan B. Leichtman

As physicians and nephrologists who are actively engaged in the evaluation and the treatment of kidney transplant candidates, recipients, and donors, we are concerned by what we see as a growing threat to the core values that have permitted organ transplantation to flourish during the last half century. Kidney vending, once considered taboo in "respectable" circles, is being debated with some frequency, and in this issue of *JASN*, specific proposals for implementation have been made. To his credit, Matas (1) presents his case in a rational and dispassionate manner. In the professional and lay press, however, there has been a disturbing change of tone. Those who oppose vending have been derided as "beancounters" and "high-minded moralists" (2); the current system has been described as a "failure" (3); routine psychological evaluation of donors has been described as "intrusive, demeaning" (4); the Institute of Medicine's caution against treating the body as if it were for sale (5) has been described as "outdated thinking" (6); and respected transplant professionals have been castigated in the national press because of their concern for the potential exploitation of donors (7).

There is a lot at stake. The altruistic impulses of living donors and of the families of deceased donors are on the auction block

and risk being displaced by the uncertainties of an unfamiliar market place. Matas seems unconcerned by this possibility, and to some proponents of organ vending, the anticipated demise of altruism in organ donation even comes as a blessing (2). To the detractors of our current altruism-based system, the acceptance by the general public of the difficult concepts (brain death, donation after cardiac death, living donation, etc.) that are at the core of our work is taken for granted, because the supply of donors has been inadequate for the need. Dollars will solve our problem: Put kidneys up for sale (valued at approximately $90,000 by Matas's estimate [8]) and there will be enough organs for everyone. Imagine: No more waiting lists. And it all will be "above board" and run by regional organ procurement organizations and professional panels that will vet donors, protect their health, allocate the kidneys, and administer the finances (1)—all done in a manner that is beyond reproach. We are skeptical.

Those who are opposed to organ vending have been described as being "timid" (6), as if they lived in some ivory tower divorced from the "real world," but it is that real world that is the source of our concern. Living kidney donation is a safe procedure, but even in the most experienced hands, it is never risk-free.

Safe donation, both for the donor and the recipient, requires honesty and openness about the potential donor's health, high-risk activities, and family history. Although it never can be taken for granted, in our current altruism-based system, openness generally can be presumed, and donors are compensated for the risk that they take by seeing the blossoming health of those they love or care for. In a vending system, in which regard for the recipient is divorced from the motivation for donation, powerful financial incentives for a donor not to be forthcoming about critical information could affect both their own health and that of the recipient (e.g., a distant history of a melanoma; an uncle on dialysis; high-risk sexual behavior, perhaps). Recipients of vended kidneys have been reported to suffer a high rate of infectious complications, not all of which could have been prevented easily by routine evaluation (9). Would specially trained investigators need to be included in the transplant team to ensure the accuracy of the paid donor's history and to ensure public safety? Because the risk that the kidney sellers would take is compensated only by dollars, how are they likely to feel about themselves when those dollars run out? Available studies from countries that sanction or do not control kidney selling suggest that the lump sum that the sellers receive has little impact on their long-term financial security, and many end up worse off, financially and otherwise (10). There is no reason to believe that kidney venders in the developed world would be protected from this outcome.

We are confident that Matas and other proponents of a kidney vending system in the United States do not want to see the abuse of kidney sellers that is so common in the third world. But who would the donors be if not the disadvantaged and the vulnerable among us? How could we be sure that paid donors were not being manipulated or even blackmailed? To avoid the evils of "transplant tourism," Matas and others have suggested that in a "regulated" vending system, the market would be confined to self-governing geopolitical areas such as nation states or the European Union (11). In the United States, would paid donors have to be citizens? Could legal residents or even illegal ones be permitted to sell their organs? We live in a world where many industrialized nations struggle, often unsuccessfully, to protect their own borders against illegal entry. With so much money at stake, how would these activities be policed? Other countries learn from the sophisticated organ transplant system that we enjoy in the United States. What example would we be setting if we permitted vending? Representatives of developing countries have repeatedly expressed well-grounded fear that such a change in policy would make it even more difficult for them to control corruption and criminal exploitation of donors (12,13).

Our greatest concern is that kidney selling would distort and undermine the altruism and common citizenship on which our whole organ donation system currently relies. The term "crowding out" describes the hypothesis that the moral commitment to do one's duty can be weakened by financial compensation and monetary reward (14). It is not easy for parents to accept kidneys from their children; or to watch their children donate to each other; or for patients to approach their family, spouses, or friends. If kidneys could be bought, particularly if the government or an insurance entity was paying, then the temptation or even demand not to expose the potential altruistic donor to the risk that is intrinsic to the process could be overwhelming; and it is not only altruistic living kidney donation that could suffer. The approach to recently bereaved family members, an already extraordinarily difficult and profoundly sensitive task, could be made considerably more difficult by their knowledge that organs could be purchased for large sums of money and the bodies of their loved ones left undisturbed. Deceased donation is the source not only of kidneys but also of hearts, livers, lungs, and pancreata. Displacement of altruistic deceased kidney donation by vending has the very real potential of endangering precious opportunities for life-saving and life-enhancing extrarenal donation.

These considerations are not merely theoretical, and two "natural experiments" provide some insight as to the forces at play. Before 1997, when the British transferred sovereignty to mainland China, living donors were the source of nearly 50% of all kidney transplants in Hong Kong. Since 1997, transplant candidates have traveled to China to purchase kidneys, and the number of living donor transplants in Hong Kong has fallen to only 15 to 20% of all kidney transplants performed there (H.K. Chan, Hong Kong Transplant Registry, personal communication, September 4, 2006). The relative ease with which Israeli kidney transplant candidates, until recently, traveled abroad to purchase kidneys has been accompanied by a reduction in living-related donation in Israel itself (T. Ashkenazi, Israeli Ministry of Health, personal communication, May 7, 2006).

As nephrologists, we do not savor the impact that a vending system could have on our work and our relationship with our donor patients. The evaluation of donors, both medical and surgical, is replete with clinical nuances. Careful assessment of risk and donor education are at the core of donor evaluation (15). The decision to progress with donation, although often clearcut may require refined clinical judgment by the medical team and critical thinking by the donor. The inclusion of major financial rewards for donation could well place tremendous pressure on transplant doctors to act against their best medical judgment. It is not difficult to imagine such scenarios: Might a donor surgeon, faced with a kidney with multiple vessels, elect to perform nephrectomy when he or she might otherwise have declined to do so because of the knowledge that the donor desperately needs the vending money? Might a nephrologist feel similarly pressured to approve a donor with mild hypertension, borderline proteinuria, or a history of kidney stones? Medical decision making is already difficult enough without its distortion by large financial rewards.

One of the arguments that repeatedly is made in favor of a vending system is that the current altruism-based system has stagnated and is impotent to address the burgeoning shortage of kidneys. We share the legitimate concern that lives are being lost while patients wait for a kidney (16). That concern in itself does not represent an argument in favor of vending, because it is quite unclear that a vending-based system would be effective and it could well be destructive (14). It is no longer true that the rates of deceased donor organ donation are static. To the contrary, the 3-mo average deceased kidney donation rate has risen 29% since January 1, 2001, and these increases have largely reflected increases in recovery of kidneys from standard criteria donors. Matas quotes Sheehy et al. (17) to contend that "even if every potential donor in the United States became an actual donor, there still would be a shortage of kidneys." This analysis, however, was limited to candidates for donation after brain death. It did not take into account multiple innovative endeavors to increase other sources of donor organs. These include living donor exchange (18), intended candidate donation (19), desensitization protocols for positive cross-match—and blood group—incompatible pairs (18), increased use of donors after circulatory determination of death (20), and increased use of extended-criteria donor kidneys (21). In the United States, perhaps the most promising endeavor of all is the so-called "Organ Donation Breakthrough Collaborative," whereby the best practices of the most successful organ procurement organizations are disseminated to less effective ones. An unprecedented impact on rates of deceased donation, from both extended- and standard-criteria donors, already can be recognized following the effort of the collaborative (22), and waitlist mortality rates seem to be falling. In 2004 alone, there was an increase in the number of deceased donors by 11% (23), and this trend is continuing (22). It is not "pie in the sky" to look forward to a reduction in the waiting list to acceptable levels if we continue to invest our best efforts, resources, and ingenuity. All of these new endeavors expand and exploit the altruism that has been the driving force of our success to date. They build on what we know rather than endanger what we have achieved. They do not reflect "lack of imagination" (2) or "doing nothing more productive than complaining" (3) as some eminent critics of our current system have suggested. We are unconvinced by Matas's somewhat blithe contention that they could flourish simultaneously with a vending system.

The general public is rightfully sensitive to any hint of injustice or malfeasance in our national transplant system. They are entitled to be, because they are not only the recipients of organs but also the source. The past two decades have seen organ transplantation become one of the great medical benefits to humankind. For this to happen, an extraordinary degree of trust has developed between the public and their transplant teams that must not be taken for granted. Kidney vending might seem like a tempting solution to the organ shortage, but like the Trojan horse of old, once we permit it within our gates, we may find that it brings destruction and not relief. We believe strongly that a bright future for organ transplantation requires that we foster altruism and not stifle it.

References

1. Matas A: Why we should develop a regulated system for kidney sales: A call for action! *Clin J Am Soc Nephrol* 1: 609–612, 2006.

2. Epstein R: Kidney beancounters. *Wall Street Journal* May 15, 2006.

3. Friedman EA, Friedman AL: Payment for donor kidneys: Pros and cons. *Kidney Int* 69:960–962, 2006.

4. Postrel V: Cash for kidneys. *Los Angeles Times* June 10, 2006.

5. Childress J, Liverman C (eds.): *Organ Donation: Opportunities for Action*, Washington, DC, National Academies Press, 2006.

6. Satel S: Death's waiting list. *New York Times* May 15, 2006.

7. Postrel V: Unfair kidney donations. *Forbes* 2006.

8. Matas A, Schnitzler M: Payment for living donor (vendor) kidneys: A cost-effectiveness analysis. *Am J Transplant* 4: 2116–2121, 2004.

9. Shukla A, PA, Fazio L, Pace K, Stewart R, Prasad R, Zaltzman J, Honer R: Commercial renal transplantation: A Canadian experience [Abstract]. *Am J Urol* 175[Suppl]:1457, 2006.

10. Goyal M, Mehta RL, Schneiderman LJ, Sehgal AR: Economic and health consequences of selling a kidney in India. *JAMA* 288: 1589–1593, 2002.

11. Harris J, Erin C: An ethically defensible market in organs. *BMJ* 325: 114–115, 2002.

12. Mani MK: Payment for donor kidneys. *Kidney Int* 70: 603, 2006.

13. Jha V, Chugh KS: The case against a regulated system of living kidney sales. *Nat Clin Pract Nephrol* 2: 466–467, 2006.

14. Rothman SM, Rothman DJ: The hidden cost of organ sale. *Am J Transplant* 6: 1524–1528, 2006.

15. Delmonico F: A report of the Amsterdam Forum on the care of the live kidney donor: Data and medical guidelines. *Transplantation* 79[Suppl]: S53-S66, 2005.

16. Casingal V, Glumac E, Tan M, Sturdevant M, Nguyen T, Matas AJ: Death on the kidney waiting list: Good candidates or not? *Am J Transplant* 6: 1953–1956, 2006.

17. Sheehy E, Conrad SL, Brigham LE, Luskin R, Weber P, Eakin M, Schkade L, Hunsicker L: Estimating the number of potential organ donors in the United States. *N Engl J Med* 349: 667- 674, 2003.

18. Montgomery RA, Simpkins CE, Segev DL: New options for patients with donor incompatibilities. *Transplantation* 82:164–165, 2006.

19. Delmonico FL, Morrissey PE, Lipkowitz GS, Stoff JS, Himmelfarb J, Harmon W, Pavlakis M, Mah H, Goguen J, Luskin R, Milford E, Basadonna G, Chobanian M, Bouthot B, Lorber M, Rohrer RJ: Donor kidney exchanges. *Am J Transplant* 4: 1628–1634, 2004.

20. Johnson SR: Donors after cardiac death: Opportunity missed. *Transplantation* 80: 569–570, 2005.

21. Cecka JM, Cohen B, Rosendale J, Smith M: Could more effective use of kidneys recovered from older deceased donors result in more kidney transplants for older patients? *Transplantation* 81: 966–970, 2006.

22. O'Connor K, Delmonico FL: Donation after cardiac death and the science of organ donation. *Clin Transpl* 16: 220–245, 2006.

23. Port FK, Merion RM, Goodrich NP, Wolfe RA: Recent trends and results for organ donation and transplantation in the United States, 2005. *Am J Transplant* 6: 1095–1100, 2006.

Chapter 21

Financial Incentives for Cadaveric Organ Donation

David Mayrhofer-Reinhartshuber and
Robert Fitzgerald

Abstract

One of the main obstacles of organ transplantation all over the world is the insufficient number of available cadaveric organs. Various attempts are considered to increase the consent rate. A financial incentive as a possibility to raise the number of procured organs is a very controversial topic. Arguments for and against financial incentives are presented as well as the different models.

Introduction

One of the main problems of organ transplantation is the shortage of donor organs. This is a result of an increasing demand in organs for donation on the one hand and a low donation rate on the other hand. In the Kingdom of Saudi Arabia in the year 2001 the donation rate was only less than 2.5 per Million Population[1]. In comparison Spain has a donation rate of 32 per million population. One of the reasons of the low donation rate is the high numbers of families who refuse to give their consent to the removal. In Saudi Arabia only 28.7% of the asked families gave their consent to the organ donation[1]—in Spain 76.6% of the asked families gave their consent[2].

Different attempts are considered to increase the consent rate to the donation request. These attempts can be differentiated between those before a possible donation and those during the donation process. Before organ donation the consent rate can be influenced by enhancing the public opinion and knowledge toward organ donation by the use of advertisement and school education programs. During the donation process attempts to increase donation rates are financial incentives or training of the requestor.

A financial incentive as a possibility to raise the consent rate is a very controversial topic with a few supporters and many opponents. A basic problem is that in most countries it is illegal at the time to acquire, receive, or transfer any human organ for valuable consideration for use in human transplantation. So the implementation of financial incentives cannot be carried out in most countries without a change of the established laws.

Arguments pro financial incentives

The main arguments of the supporters are that the established altruistic system has failed to meet the current needs and only financial incentives could raise the number of organ donors[3,4]. Lysaght and Mason compared the situation of organ donation with leaving fire-fighting in a big town to the same voluntary fire department that served the city well during early years[4].

Another argument in favour for financial incentives is that the donor respectively the relatives of the donor are the only ones not directly benefiting from the transplantation process. All other persons concerned like physicians, surgeons, nurses, or coordinators etc. get paid, the benefactor gets the organ and only the family of the donor gets nothing except a thank you.

Peters[3] and Lysaght and Mason[4] also argue, that the demands of other medical resources like plasma, sperm or eggs only can be satisfied by payment. Even medical schools buy cadavers for teaching purposes and pay participants in medical research projects.

Different models for financial incentives

Models about the form of financial incentives are multiple. The simplest straightforward form of a financial incentive is the payment of a lump sum as claimed by Peters[3] and by Lysaght and Mason[4] whereby the suggestions of the high of the amount vary between $1,000 and $20,000. Similar to a lump sum is the suggestion of a tax credit for giving the consent to organ donation. A different model of financial incentives is the reimbursement for funeral expense claimed by Delmonico et al.[5,6]. A small reimbursement should not evoke the impression of selling the organs but rather express appreciation for the donor and the donation. This form of financial incentives would not subvert the altruistic system but rather support and improve it.

Another suggestion for financial incentives regarded to be very ethical is a contribution to a charitable organization determined by the donor or the family of the deceased[6]. A model how a donor can opt-in the donation process while still alive is the a futures market system, whereby an individual agrees in advance to donation with payment to his beneficiaries or his estate taking place only after donation[7]. A big advantage of this model is that the decision to donate has not to be made in the difficult situation of the sudden death of a next of kin and the decision can be made by the donor himself and not by his relatives.

Arguments contra financial incentives

Opponents of financial incentives base their objection primarily on the argument that the altruistic donation model has not failed as much as it has not been fully promoted[7]. The consent rate can also be increased by additional information and advertisement to raise the public knowledge toward the organ donation or by training for the requestor. There is also the assumption that financial incentives would not raise the number of organ donors. In the public opinion financial incentives are not very popular. In a Gallup survey only 12% of the respondents reported increased willingness to donate under a donation system of financial incentives[6]. In another survey to the impact of funeral expense for organ donation only 1.87% of the asked answered that a small amount of 300$ would have a positive effect on their decision to donate[6]. Additionally, the risk that a policy of compensation could deter donation from those who would have consented altruistically. Protas[8] calculated in his article for the USA that if 50% of those now refusing consent would change their decision and 30% of those now consenting would refuse to do so if they should sell the organs the supply of the organs would be unchanged. The only thing that would change anyway would be the costs for the transplantation. In blood donation the system in America and Europe has changed from financial incentive to an altruistic donation system, because blood from paid donors was shown to have a higher rate of post transfusion infection. A reason for this was that paid donors who have an economic need for compensation were found to be untruthful about their medical history. The same caution would apply to the acceptability of organs recovered from compensated donors[6,9].

Another assumption against financial incentive is the fear of a slippery slope effect[10] that once a moral barrier is broken it would be difficult to contain abuses by regulation and law. A free market of human organs could develop where the demand regulates the price. In a free market the poor would be discriminated twice because they would not be able to afford organ transplantation on the one hand and on the other hand they would become the donors for the more wealthy due to their financial demands[10].

Why a psychological consideration of the organ donation and the impact of financial incentive?

Because financial incentives are not only a matter of ethics, medicine or economics but also of psychology! Psychological theories and knowledge can help to explain the decision making process of the next-of-kin and the factors influencing this process.

Most arguments of the supporters as well as the opponents of financial incentive are assumption and fears and nearly no empirically based data and theories. Therefore we want to introduce a well proven psychological theory, the "Theory of cognitive dissonance" developed by Festinger[11].

The basic elements of the theory of cognitive dissonance are cognitions that consist of opinions, notions and attitudes toward certain objects or acts. These cognitions can be in different relationship with each other, they can be consonant if one follows from one another

- e.g., Smoking can cause lung cancer— I do not smoke

They can be dissonant if they are controversial to one another

- e.g., Smoking can cause lung cancer— Smoking is very relaxing

Or they can be irrelevant to one another.

- e.g., Smoking can cause lung cancer— I love red cars

If there are positive and negative cognitions (dissonant) to a certain object or act this will result in a psychological uncomfortable feeling of inner suspense—the cognitive dissonance.

In the case of cadaveric organ donation a next-of-kin who has to make the decision if giving or refusing the consent will have various cognitions in favour and against the donation.

Possible cognitions for the consent to organ donation could be:

- I could save a life with my consent to the organ donation;
- I wish I could have an organ the time I need one

Possible cognition against consent to organ donation:

- I don't know if my deceased next-of-kin wanted to donate his organ
- Is my next-of-kin really dead?
- Is this the will of god?

In case of these dissonant cognitions cognitive dissonance will occur and the next-of-kin who has to make the decision will have an uncomfortable feeling of inner suspense.

To reduce the cognitive dissonance the next-of-kin has two possibilities:

- to add consonant cognition
- to reduce dissonant cognitions

As a result of this the attitudes toward the two possibilities change.

In our case if the next-of-kin has decided to give the consent to the donation of the organs he will add positive cognition toward the organ donation like:

- I think that the deceased relative would have wanted to help another person in need
- Helping another person is in the will of god.

Additionally negative cognitions are removed and therefore the cognitive dissonance—the uncomfortable feeling of inner suspense will disappear. As result of the organ donation the value of this act will be enhanced.

What happens if financial incentives would be given to the next-of-kin of the donor for their consent?

As starting point we have the consent to the donation what is mostly a dissonant decision because of the different cognition in favour and against the donation.

We now differ between the decision with a financial incentive and the decision without financial incentives.

Financial incentive in a higher amount would be a sufficient reason for the consent and therefore no change in attitudes toward the organ donation and the transplantation process would take place. If the consent is given without the motivation by financial incentives, no sufficient external reason exists. Therefore the cognitive dissonance only can be reduced by adding consonant cognitions and removing of dissonant cognitions and the value of organ donation and transplantation would enhance.

An explanation for these phenomena is that dissonant acts enhance the personal value toward the act, if there is not a sufficient external reason as explanation for the decision. Financial incentives in a high amount can be a sufficient external reason for a dissonant act and therefore no change in attitudes occur.

We conclude that next-of-kin who consent to organ donation without a financial incentive will enhance their attitude toward organ donation. Next-of-kin who consent to organ donation and are financial compensated won't enhance their attitudes toward organ donation.

This can in the long run in addition to the risk of a direct effect (sold your next-of-kin) affect adversely the public opinion toward organ donation and could counterproductively influence the consent rate. It remains open, if this would apply to a small reimbursement of the funeral expense, as this would not be a sufficient reason for organ donation.

References

1. http://www.scot.org.sa/brain-death.html
2. http://www.msc.es/ont/ing/f_data.htlm
3. Peters TG: Life or death. The Issue of Payment in Cadaveric Organ Donation. *Journal of the American Medical Association* 1991; 256:1302–1305.
4. Lysaght MJ, Mason J: The Case for Financial Incentives to Encourage Organ Donation. *ASAIO Journal* 2000; 46:253–256.
5. Delmonico FL, Arnold R, Scheper-Hughes N, Siminoff LA, Kahn J, Youngner S: Ethnical Incentives

—not Payment—for Organ Donation. *New England Journal of Medicine* 2002; 346:2002–2005.

6. Arnold R, Bartlett S, Bernat J, Colonna J, Dafoe D, Dubler N, Gruber S, Kahn J, Luskin R, Nathan H, Orloff S, Prottas J, Shapiro R, Ricordi C, Youngner S, Delmonico FL: Financial Incentives for Cadaver Organ Donation: An Ethical Reappraisal. *Transplantation* 2002; 73: 1361–1367.

7. Nelson EW, Childress JE, Perryman J, Robards V, Rowan A, Seely MS, Steriolf S, Swanson MR: *Financial Incentives for Organ Donation. A Report of the UNOS Ehtics Committee Payment Subcommittee* 1993. http://www.unos.org\Resources\bioethics_whitepapers_finance.htm.

8. Protas JM: Buying human organs–Evidence that money does not change everything. *Transplantation* 1992; 53:1371–1373.

9. Estelund T: Monetary blood donation incentives and the risk of transfusion-transmitted infection. *Transfusion* 1998; 38:874.

10. Pellegrino ED: Families' self-interest and the Cadaver's Organs: What Price Consent. *New England Journal of Medicine* 1991; 265:1305–1306.

11. Festinger L, Carlsmith JM: Cognitive Consequence of the forced Compliance. *Journal of Abnormal Social Psychology* 1959; 58:203–211.

Part IV

Other Strategies for Increasing the Number of Available Organs

Daniel P. Reid

Outside the simple yes option on driver's license applications, there are currently no other ways available to be considered an organ donor in the United States unless the next of kin wishes to donate after the death of a loved one. However, several new systems for increasing the number of available organs have been proposed, and some have been put into practice elsewhere.

Whyte et al. propose a variant on the current system used in the United States, which would work under the guise of "presumed consent." This means that individuals are assumed to want to be organ donors unless they have made formal declarations to the contrary. Also built into this system is an element of immediate and paramount veto power given to the family of the deceased. This system, they contend, gives health care professionals a better environment in which to "nudge" families toward donation, overcoming the "perception problems" of the current system such as misconceptions about quality of care, determination of death, and ultimate goals of the health care team in situations where organ procurement is an option. They argue against a mandated decision approach to organ donation because they believe this approach is not a "nudge" but a forceful intrusion into people's lives.

After looking at the flaws of the current system presented by Whyte et al., our attention is turned to Kennedy et al. who provide moral arguments in favor of the "presumed consent" system. Working from an easily acceptable starting point that increasing the supply of organs is a "good" deed, they show that the burden of proof is placed upon those who would rather maintain the current flawed system. To counter such arguments, they systematically address both the benefits of the system and the potential objections to it.

In order to move forward and develop ethically sound new systems, however, it is also necessary to examine historical objections. Aksoy addresses the concerns that Islamic scholars have expressed on using cadaveric organs without the donor's consent. He uses the cultural lens of Islam to address these concerns and show that the urgency and severity of the low organ supply are sufficient to support the harvesting of cadaveric organs without the donor's prior consent.

Under the current system of organ procurement in the United States, volunteering as a donor is not seen as a morally obligatory act but rather as laudable altruism. Thus, Chandler et al. propose a "priority system." They recommend that those who have previously registered as organ donors be rewarded with a status of higher priority for transplant reception, should they need one, over those who have not registered. Using Singapore and Israel as examples, they examine the issues of perception and reciprocity in organ donation schemes. They also recommend surveys of public opinion before a priority system be established here.

Analogous to the consideration of anencephalics for pediatric organs (see part II), prisoners on death row present an opportunity to increase the number of available organs. Caplan reviews the ethical quagmire that stands between prisoners and organ donation in his chapter. The general health of prisoners, methods of execution, the possible removal of organs as a method of capital punishment and the necessary involvement of medical professionals in peri- or postexecution transplantation each present major obstacles to the use of prisoners as sources of adult organs. It is of note that the recent use of this practice, specifically in China, has created an international backlash to this procedure.

Neades, on the other hand, returns to the topic of presumed consent and presents a systematic analysis of current opt-out systems in practice. Using Portugal, Norway, and Belgium as a sample of European countries using this system, she conducted a survey study of health care professionals in these countries to measure their responses to the presumed consent laws. In her final analysis, she identifies several key factors of the opt-out system that would need to be examined before implementing such laws in the United Kingdom.

Touching on a system that has seen great domestic success, Serur and Charlton present the idea of paired kidney donation. A major problem with transplantation under the current system is the lack of properly matched donors for those in need of an organ. Thus, by using a chain of recipients, each with a donor to match the next recipient, and with great coordination, these chains have been very successful, including one chain with sixty members, transplanting thirty kidneys. In the excerpted portion of their chapter, they examine the growth process of this practice, as well as the practical difficulties and ethical challenges that this system faces in reality.

Following Serur and Charlton, Wallis et al. continue on a similar path, examining, in the excerpt selected, the strengths and weaknesses of paired kidney donation. However, they use some slightly more empirical evidence in their analysis and specifically try to address problems of allocation and equity in paired donation schemes.

Finally, Fiore, in her chapter, the singular web-only news piece presented in this volume, introduces the idea that even when kidneys are considered to be "high risk," their use in transplantation still brings great benefit to their recipients. She discusses the outcome of a study into the two-year survival of recipients of these "high risk" kidneys. This supports her ultimate conclusion that, since there is such a dire situation in terms of kidney supply, rejecting as many kidneys as has been the case is neither necessary nor prudent.

While there are many potential alternative sources from which to draw transplantable organs, each system presents its own set of challenges. In order to find the most efficient and most ethical method for increasing the donor pool, each of these approaches must be analyzed critically. To that end the authors in this part have cited extensively from the works of others, and these references provide excellent background and follow-up to the approaches proposed here.

Chapter 22

Nudge, Nudge or Shove, Shove— The Right Way for Nudges to Increase the Supply of Donated Cadaver Organs

Kyle Powys Whyte, Evan Selinger, Arthur L. Caplan, and Jathan Sadowski

Abstract

Richard Thaler and Cass Sunstein (2008) contend that mandated choice is the most practical nudge for increasing organ donation. We argue that they are wrong, and their mistake results from failing to appreciate how perceptions of meaning can influence people's responses to nudges. We favor a policy of default to donation that is subject to immediate family veto power, includes options for people to opt out (and be educated on how to do so), and emphasizes the role of organ procurement organizations and in-house transplant donation coordinators creating better environments for increasing the supply of organs and tissues obtained from cadavers. This policy will provide better opportunities for offering nudges in contexts where in-house coordinators work with families. We conclude by arguing that nudges can be introduced ethically and effectively into these contexts only if nudge designers collaborate with in-house coordinators and stakeholders.

I n *Nudge: Improving Decisions About Health, Wealth, and Happiness*, Richard Thaler and Cass Sunstein (2008) defend nudges as useful tools for helping people make decisions that increase individual and societal savings and decrease unnecessary costs and harms. The behavioral economist (Thaler) and administrator of the White House Office of Information and Regulatory Affairs (Sunstein) apply their proposal to a range of problems, from obesity, to poor retirement planning, to getting out of bed on time. They also offer a proposal for solving a key problem in biomedical ethics. Thaler and Sunstein argue that mandating people to choose whether to donate their organs as a requirement for obtaining a driver's license would increase the amount of registered donors, while "imposing essentially no new burdens on taxpayers" and avoiding the political barriers that a policy of presumed consent might face (Thaler and Sunstein 2008, 178).

Thaler and Sunstein are wrong. The reason why is important in considering the merits of nudging people in various directions as a matter of public policy and the merits of mandated choice strategies more generally. Their defense of mandated choice, when considered as a nudge offered to people applying for driver's licenses, is not preferable to a policy of presumed consent or what we prefer to refer to as default to donation. The appropriateness of nudges depends both on understanding people's general cognitive biases and on accounting for the meaning they attribute to particular contexts. The latter is underexplored in *Nudge*. To show that this gap is of great importance, we clarify why the meaning perceived in situations is crucial for evaluating nudges, and therein explain why a policy of default to donation is preferable, despite the taint some attribute to presumptive policies (Smith 2010). We favor a policy of default to donation that is subject to immediate family veto power, includes options for people to opt out (and be educated on how to do so), and emphasizes the role of organ procurement organizations and in-house transplant donation coordinators creating better environments for increasing the supply of organs and tissues obtained from cadavers. We conclude by arguing that nudges can be introduced ethically and effectively into these contexts only if nudge designers collaborate with in-house coordinators, ethicists, and other relevant professionals and stakeholders.

What Is a Nudge?

Thaler and Sunstein's project in *Nudge* is to explore smart ways to improve our individual lives and the general welfare of society. They have in mind improvements in the sorts of values we all share: our health, wealth, and happiness. That is, we all want to find ways to become healthier, eliminate debt, plan well for retirement, adopt sustainable habits, fulfill resolutions, et cetera. But we often make bad decisions about how to get what we prefer, as is evidenced by rampant failure to stick to our diets or increase our retirement investments at pace with salary raises.

While these bad decisions impact individuals—and, when exercised in mass, society in general—government regulation is likely not going to be the best approach for correcting every problem area. Regulation can be costly and clunky. In some cases, the best solutions do not involve changing or introducing regulations at all (John et al. 2009; Lobel and Amir 2009).

People often make bad decisions as a consequence of predictable biases guiding their behavior. Consider food choices at a cafeteria buffet line, where it is tempting to put too much of the wrong foods on our plates. Sometimes we do this because we do not have enough time to make a selection. Other times we lack sufficient nutritional information about the options. In other instances, our minds are elsewhere, perhaps reflecting on earlier or future events. When conditions like these obtain, we tend to go for the foods that are most prominently displayed, or proceed without thinking carefully about whether the size of the plate is proportioned to our actual intake requirements. Even when we are free from these impediments, other complicating factors readily take hold. Sometimes we are so famished from hard work that heightened arousal trumps earlier promises to eat more healthily. In other cases we use food to reward hard work, even knowing that stacking our plate high is not good for us.

Thaler and Sunstein refer to predictable tendencies like these as cognitive biases, and claim that they guide our behavior in cases where we have to act quickly, lack sufficient information, and fail to anticipate what our feelings and moods will be. Their guiding thesis is that in situations like these it is neither necessary to create new incentives for people nor justifiable to restrict choices through an expensive government policy. Rather, the best course of action is to adjust the context within which people make choices, so as to make humans' predictable tendencies work for, rather than against, their preferences. This is where nudges come in.

Thaler and Sunstein define a nudge as "any

aspect of the choice architecture that alters people's behavior in a predictable way without forbidding any options or significantly changing their economic incentives" (Thaler and Sunstein 2008, 6). Nudges are thus changes in the choice context that work with our biases, and help prompt us, in subtle ways, to make decisions that leave us and, usually, society better off.

It is important to note that Thaler and Sunstein do not see nudges as normatively problematic forms of manipulation.[1] They emphasize ethical constraints that demarcate nudges from propaganda and advertising. In principle, nudges can only improve people's lives if they effect behavioral change that accords with preexisting preferences. In this sense, nudging is not just about determining what changes or calibrations of choice contexts will work with people's biases, but also about making sure the situation in which the problem occurs is one where a nudge can be effectively and subtly used, and that does not violate widely accepted ethical norms, including transparency and publicity. They tout these norms as ensuring that nudges are not exploitative.

In light of the ethical constraints, the idea of nudging people is prima facie appealing as an innovative way to promote positive personal and collective behavioral changes. But whether a nudge is right for solving a particular problem depends on whether the predictable biases can be identified and understood well enough for a nudge designer—who is referred to as a "choice architect"—to account for them. It also depends on whether the choice context can be calibrated in such a way as to work with cognitive biases. This last point is crucial because when nudges are offered, they change how people deal with information and situations. There remains an empirical question, in any given case, as to whether these changes simply work with identified biases (thus improving the decision outcome), or whether they are more causally efficacious, and actually change the meaning of the situation itself. If the latter arises, decision makers can respond differently to a nudge than choice architects have anticipated (Selinger and Whyte 2010).

These considerations suggest that the right nudge for a decision depends on what can be known both about decision makers' tendencies and about the aspects of the situation that will change or remain constant after a nudge is inserted. Both of these issues should be the basis of evaluating nudges proposed for biomedical and other problems. Thaler and Sunstein pay insufficient attention to the perceptual issues in proposing forced choice as a solution to organ donation.

Mandating (Nudging) the Choice to Donate

Thaler and Sunstein claim that one of barriers preventing more U.S. citizens from becoming organ donors is the "explicit consent" policy (2008, 178). The 2006 amendments to the Uniform Anatomical Gift Act (UAGA) strengthen an individual's right to opt in and choose to become a donor. Many people, however, do not record their decision to donate. In New York State in 2009 less than 11% of those at the Department of Motor Vehicles (DMV) indicated a willingness to donate (WSYR-TV 2011). Even when people do opt in by checking off "donor" on their driver's license, organ procurement organizations (OPOs) will often follow the negative wishes of the family of the deceased, overriding a recorded decision to donate (Healy 2006; Spital 1996; Thaler and Sunstein 2008).

Thaler and Sunstein focus on the issue of why willing donors tend not to opt in even when they can record their wishes on forms for obtaining driver's licenses. If one does not explicitly consent to donate on the form, the default setting is that one has not consented at all. Having to take pains to override this setting plays into people's predictable bias toward choosing options that require the least effort, especially in a setting like a DMV where they are just trying to get the license application process over with.

While the default setting cannot force anyone to do anything, it nevertheless "deters willing donors from registering" because it allows the pervasive human inclination for "inertia" to exert such a "strong influence" that people who wish to be organ donors fail to act in accordance with their preferences (Thaler and Sunstein 2008, 178–179). To lend some support to this point, they cite a study in Iowa that showed only 64% of residents who stated that they personally wanted to donate their organs "had marked their driver's license and only 36% had signed an organ donor card" (Thaler and Sunstein 2008, 178).

Another reason based on predictable biases has to do with how families identify a deceased relative's beliefs about organ donation when no evidence of explicit consent exists. In these situations, family members have to make a post hoc decision, often in the absence of a clear idea of what the deceased preferred. Faced with uncertainty, relatives may proceed cautiously and even prevent a passionate commitment to donate from being fulfilled.

Though not mentioned by Thaler and Sunstein, family consent remains a major barrier even when the deceased's wishes are recorded. Klassen and Klassen (1996) discuss how factors like the unexpectedness of a death can leave family members traumatized. Being

in such a condition may limit the possibility of careful consideration of the deceased's or family's wishes (see Siminoff et al. 1995; Spital 1996). Parents of young children may desire "to hold their child as support is withdrawn and heartbeat and respiration stop, and find that they cannot allow the child to be taken for procurement surgery" (Klassen and Klassen 1996, 71). Some families that express initial interest in organ donation cannot endure what is often a two-day wait until full brain death, and request that their relative be extubated before final determination of brain death (71).

Thaler and Sunstein contend that an alternative nudge is a policy of presumed consent, which structures the default setting so that inertia works with, rather than against, people's preferences, and where family members' biases may be excluded from weighing in on the decision. Presumed consent would mean that "all citizens" should be "presumed to be consenting organ donors" unless through some easily available means—such as checking an opt-out box when applying for a driver's license—they specify otherwise (Thaler and Sunstein 2008, 181–182). Not even family members would be able to override this presumption. To validate their proposal, they cite a 2003 study that shows 42% of people would choose to be organ donors under an opt-in scheme, while only 18% would opt out of organ donation if their consent was presumed (Thaler and Sunstein 2008, 178).

Although presumed consent is attractive to Thaler and Sunstein as a nudge, they back off from advocating for it. Some critics suggest that presumed consent runs a risk of public backlash against "government intrusion" into people's lives, while others claim that presumed consent is considered by many to be morally repugnant. Because presumption and implied consent are controversial ideas, Thaler and Sunstein predict that presumed consent policy will engender local conflict, including attempts by families of deceased potential donors to prevent organ removal from occurring (Thaler and Sunstein 2008, 182). With so many sensitive issues being triggered, they characterize presumed consent policy as impractical.

Thaler and Sunstein claim that mandated choice, another option they depict as a nudge, is a more viable way to increase organ donations. Instead of presuming consent, citizens will have to make an informed decision about their donation status as one of the requirements for getting something that they ordinarily need, such as a driver's license. Here the nudge is the change in choice context from opt in to having to decide to opt out or not. Moreover, the options could be presented alongside information about the rate of people who die because they are unable to receive a needed transplant. Such information would not serve to manipulate people who are deeply opposed to donating their organs. However, the information might make some people pause, especially those who would otherwise lack appreciation of why organ donation is important.

Spital (1996) gives additional reasons in support of mandated choice. The biases and delays associated with devastated family members and stressed hospital workers are eliminated. Mandated choice also "takes advantage of favorable public attitudes because all competent adults would decide about organ donation for themselves in a relaxed setting, where thinking is likely to be clear" (67). Requiring adults at least to consider this issue could increase public awareness of the great value of organ donation and "altruism and volunteerism" would be preserved (67).

Nudging through forced choice also avoids the political disputes that arise over proposals that forbid options, such as in routine removal, which grants the state ownership of citizens' organs once they are deceased, and thereby runs contrary to the widely endorsed principle that individuals should have appropriate latitude in determining what is to be done with their bodies (Hamer and Rivlin 2003). It also avoids the pitfalls of proposals that revolve around creating economic incentives (Satel 2009; Postrel 2010), such as can be found in living donation proposals that offer tax credits for kidneys (Thaler and Sunstein 2008, 179).

Thaler and Sunstein might well favor presumed consent over mandated choice in a less contentious world. They refrain from endorsing it for practical reasons. However, Thaler and Sunstein's support of mandated choice is perhaps even more problematic because it undermines the rationale behind nudging.

Nudges and Meaning

Is mandated choice really preferable to presumed consent? A crucial question that Thaler and Sunstein do not adequately explore is whether people's actual experience of the forced choice nudge of mandated choice changes the meaning of the situation, and perhaps does so in a way that complicates their predictions about its effectiveness. Indeed, Thaler and Sunstein do not discuss the importance of perceptions of meaning in the sorts of situations with which anyone who has been to a DMV will be all too familiar. Without understanding these perceptions, it may be difficult to nudge people as planned, they may be nudged toward a decision that is inconsistent with the rationale for the nudge or they may feel more shoved than nudged.

Thaler and Sunstein favor mandated choice in part because this option appears to give people a clear opportunity to express their preference about organ donation, without any adverse behavior modification arising from the interface of the driver's license application. What they overlook is that mandating choice in a DMV context causes stress that creates just the sort of problematic decision scenario from which nudges are supposed to rescue people. In this way, their version of mandated choice undermines the rationale for nudging.

Most people find the DMV to be either stressful or simply an unpleasant place to be. After waiting for a long time to be seen, it is easy to become tired, eager to leave, anxious, frustrated, and even angry. Because these strong, negative emotional states can incline people to poorly frame their choices, the DMV simply is not an appropriate place to make important decisions, such as whether to donate an organ.

Additionally, emotions may spike if DMV personnel are perceived to be hostile to organ donation or frustrated by anything that makes additional work for them. It could be the case that license applicants will feel uncomfortable and possibly suspicious if they perceive DMV personnel to be overly eager to see organ donation boxes marked. Very quickly, the experience of having to choose may feel like being forced to choose in a government or bureaucratic context replete with unknown personnel. Because such emotional states can influence the box that gets selected, context matters. While the issue of how context influences decision-making is raised, in principle, throughout *Nudge*, Thaler and Sunstein lose sight of it here.

Thaler and Sunstein also fail to consider whether people would be too afraid to check off the organ donation box out of concern that doing so would provide incentives for health care workers to provide them with limited treatment in order to obtain organs (Childress 2001). As Mary Ann Baily notes, this factor looms large in decision making about organ donation because "Many Americans don't trust the government or the health care system. Some already fear that signing a donor card may make physicians give up on them too soon, especially if the hospital is likely to lose money on their care" (Baily 2010).

If Baily is right, then mandated choice could actually minimize rather than expand the pool of available organ donors. Her observation serves as a good reminder that when it comes to understanding human decision making, emphasis on general cognitive biases, which is Thaler and Sunstein's main focus, should not come at the expense of ignoring how perceptions of meaning are sensitive to changes of context. Indeed, concern even exists about mandating a choice about donation in a context related to the operation of a motor vehicle. Some, rationally or not, may fear that they might bring about their own death through a motor vehicle accident by deciding to donate at the DMV.

Ultimately, negative perceptions about the DMV make it a very difficult place to secure consent to donation. While these considerations are based on subjective perceptions of DMVs, they are at least enough to undermine Thaler and Sunstein's presumption that a nudge could simply be inserted with any real chance of success. Our view is bolstered by the recent experience in China with mandated choice and organ donation at the DMV—an experience that revealed huge cultural resistance to making decisions in that setting (Manman 2011).

Even if concerns about the DMV setting could be overcome, would mandated choice do what nudges are supposed to do? The purpose of nudges is to help people make decisions in accordance with their preferences in situations where they lack the time and information, or are in an unanticipated emotional state. Mandated choice, in any form, would not actually nudge people already in such a situation. Rather, it actually forces people into such a situation. Individuals would be forced to record a decision in a context with limited time, limited information, no one able to answer questions, and without the capacity to consult with one's family or partner (if consulting them happens to matter to someone). Indecision due to lack of time was reported recently in Los Angeles after the state of California required driver's license applications to state their decision to donate (Mohajer 2011). This can turn into a bad combination because it puts choosers in the sorts of situations from which nudges are supposed to free us by working with our biases. Thaler and Sunstein's suggestion that information be provided also runs awry of what nudges are supposed to be about. Nudges do not provide information when it is lacking. Instead, they work with the biases that people inevitably lean on when they lack information (Hausman and Welch 2010).

To some degree, our formulation of the problem is shared by Childress, who describes mandated choice as overemphasizing the individualistic, rationalistic, and legalistic aspects of autonomy (Childress 2001, 14). Individuals are isolated from connections to family members and other trusted and beloved people whom they would want to be present when making an important decision regarding their death. The driver's license protocols also severely constrain people's ability to appeal for more information or support. Thaler and Sunstein describe the biases present in explicit consent as donor reluctance and the family members' stress. But the existence of these biases does not warrant creating nudges that force reluctant donors to choose while eliminating crucial decision-making support. To the contrary, an appropriate nudge should be designed around the premise that family or partners will almost always play a key role at the time of death.

It might be argued that this concern could be removed by allowing people to decide at home before they go to the DMV. This is also a problematic alternative. Reflecting on being able to donate is not a concern that would delay somebody's getting a driver's license or having it renewed. Furthermore, since there are penalties associated with not having a driver's license, an extension would constrain the chooser and further the problems just outlined. A similar outcome would arise if people were required to register a decision as part of filling out their tax forms. Despite the inevitability of death and taxes, having to record a decision on posthumous organ donation is not something that many would like to discuss in front of a tax professional. Nor could they expect competent counseling about this decision from someone in this line of work.

Our considerations demonstrate that the issue of how meaning is perceived in the organ donation context—from the significance of the DMV to filling out one's tax forms to the significance of familial presence—is underdeveloped in *Nudge*. As noted elsewhere, in every example that Thaler and Sunstein provide of a successful nudge, perceptions of meaning turn out to be irrelevant. The nudges they celebrate prompt behavior in highly restrictive contexts where conflicting values about place, profession, identity, and context do not exist or are unimportant (Selinger and Whyte 2010).

The organ donation example further helps us see that Thaler and Sunstein have a tendency to rely on studies that exclude contextual, perceptual, and interpretive variables. When they describe the study that supports their position on the problems facing explicit consent, they emphasize the fact that researchers obtained their data through an online survey "that asked people, in different ways, whether they would be willing to be donors" (Thaler and Sunstein 2008, 180). What Thaler and Sunstein leave unaddressed are questions concerning the completeness of the study (i.e., does it also inquire into people's views on the trustworthiness of health care workers, DMV staff?) and the potential differences in attitude that can distinguish thinking about organ donation from a computer located outside of the DMV, and making a personal commitment for or against organ donation while inside a DMV. Our criticisms here could explain why some studies question the success of mandated choice. In Virginia and Texas, driver's license applications are required to record people's decision to donate. Virginia includes the options to donate, not donate, or not decide at all. After 6 months, "45% percent registered as nondonors, 24% were undecided, and only 31% registered as donors" (Klassen and Klassen 1996, 72). Evidence from a similar policy in Texas suggests that mandated choice is problematic: 80% refused to be donors (Siminoff and Mercer 2001; Siminoff and Sturm 2000).

Conclusion: Toward a New Default to Donation Policy

There are a number of worries that have been raised about nudging through presumed consent. Most hinge on the failure of such a policy to give appropriate emphasis to individual autonomy. But a richer notion of defaulting to donation that is sensitive to context and meaning can meet these concerns.

Additionally, as Thaler and Sunstein and others emphasize, family members' will to decide immediately following the death of their relative basically spells practical or political failure for presumed consent policies. Another concern expressed by many (Childress; Thaler and Sunstein) is that presumed consent would be perceived as an attack on the rights of individuals (quoted in Phillips 2006, 169). These concerns are similar to those that have been raised more generally with nudges that change defaults (see Bovens 2009; Nagel 2011; Rizzo and Whitman 2008).

We do not see any of these concerns as being fatal for a presumed consent policy. Instead, we see opt-out systems as facilitating the rescue of people who are in need of organs.[2] To gain public support, a presumed consent policy ought to give an explicit decision-making role to family members, protect individual rights, and take steps to address the difficult emotional circumstances that surround sudden and often unexpected death. Default to donation can accomplish these goals. In our conception of default to donation, patients would still be able to record their wishes and have them respected. Registries would be constructed for those wishing not to donate and these would have to be consulted prior to organ procurement. Family members could override the presumption to donate in any case where a deceased person did not make their wish known in writing. Family members' overriding recorded wishes would be discouraged, but they would gain more authority than they have now to control donation in lieu of a written directive. Opt out policies in some nations leave family members the right to object (Chouhan and Draper 2003; Zink and Wertlieb 2006).

Will default to donation produce more organs to rescue those who need them? Belgium's passing of a presumed consent policy was followed for the next 5 years by a 114% increase in the number of kidneys available for transplantation. Nothing remotely similar occurred in geographically similar countries without a default to donation policy. Denmark actually experienced a decrease in donation rates after it adopted an expressed-consent, opt-in policy in 1986, despite that fact that its previous rate of cadaveric organ procurement under the older default to donation policy was one of the highest in the world at the time. Donation rates in Singapore also rose after passing a presumed-consent policy (Chouhan and Draper 2003, 157). More recently, Abadie and Gay (2006) argue that presumed-consent legislation (even when families get to make the final decision) has "a positive and sizeable effect on organ donation" rates (Abadie and Gay 2006, 599). They found that "countries with presumed consent legislation have higher organ donation rates" (600) based on a data set from 22 countries over a 10-year period.

At least three states, Delaware, Colorado, and New York, have considered modifying their laws to presumed-consent stances (Nytimes.com 2010). These efforts quickly fizzled out. However, they were not default to donation approaches. No serious educational campaign was mounted to inform the public about how a default to donation system would work, the guarantees that would be put in place to protect choice, the role to be played by families and partners, and the lack of any evidence in the European experience that any person's or family's right to decline has been abused or ignored. Given the clear obligation to make more organs available and the coolness with which organized religion and many political bodies have received proposals for using economic incentives (Associated Press 2008; UN/COE 2009), the best option for

modifying public policy would seem to be trying a default to donation approach.

If developed further, the default to donation policy we propose includes ideas for how to work with distressed family members in order to ensure that those who would ordinarily support donation will actually be permitted to do so upon their death. Here, specific nudges could be developed for these contexts to advance this aim. These nudges will only work with respect to cadaver donation if their focus is shifted away solely from individuals and toward figuring out the best ways to respond to the tragic situations in which family members find themselves (Israni et al. 2005). It is these situations where individuals find themselves to be lacking in time and information and to be in emotional states that cloud decision making. Approaches like nudges that aim at improving family members' decision making are highly appropriate and are based on the idea that family involvement is integral in many cases. One possible way of exploring such approaches is through improving the decision-making environments that family members encounter in hospitals. An in-house coordinator (IHC) from an OPO could be a crucial factor for creating an environment for family members that is more conducive to organ donation. Sociological research shows that acts of altruism usually do not happen in a vacuum. There tends to be a "strongly institutionalized aspect, with staffed organizations working to produce contexts in which [altruism] can happen" (Healy 2004, 389–390). Hospitals may not have dedicated OPO staff members. Instead, they make use of regional representatives who are only called in once a potential donor becomes available. Having an unknown professional address family members at the moments of the most intensive dread and trauma certainly does not promote the altruistic environments that are needed. A better option for promoting careful thinking and altruistic preferences is for hospitals and OPOs[3] alike to consider increasing the number of trained IHCs. This approach has proven especially successful in Spain (Agence France-Presse 2010; UN/COE 2009). The interactions between IHCs and family members are also situations where nudges could be researched. IHCs, OPOs, and choice architects, among others, should explore collaboratively what nudges are possible in these contexts. These collaborations would also expand on literatures that have raised critical issues regarding the early involvement of IHCs. We emphasize that developing possible nudges for these contexts should not be attempted by any one person, but through a collaborative process that would gradually yield results that could be introduced into practice.

Our default to donation policy attends to individual rights and autonomy, education on how to opt out, and the involvement of family members. As just described, we also see IHCs as one possible way of creating local approaches to improving family members' decision-making environments. This latter aspect of our default to donation policy falls in line with what we know about IHCs and organ donation. Empirical data suggest that hospitals with a dedicated IHC experience much higher consent and conversion rates.[4] One study compared rates from before the IHC was present (Salim et al. 2007), pre-IHC, 1998–2001, and after the IHC was present, post-IHC, 2002–2005. The study stated, "Post-IHC was associated with a significantly higher consent rate (52% vs. 35%, $p < 0.01$), a significantly higher conversion rate (50% vs. 34%, $p<.01$), and a 17% increase in organs donated compared with Pre-IHC"(1411).

These comparative percentages show that the presence of a dedicated IHC had a large effect on the overall number of organs donated. A different study (Shafer et al. 2003) showed very similar increases in organs donated once at least one IHC was placed inside of a hospital. "The use of IHCs, based directly in the hospital, resulted in significant increases in donor referral, consent, and conversion rates across all racial and ethnic groups, with the largest increases noted in minority populations" (1331).

The presence of an IHC and other improvements in OPOs[5] certainly are not nudges. But they are environmental changes to the situations that family members find themselves in when confronted by the death of their relatives. The problem is that we often unintentionally set up decision contexts that promote bad decisions. Nudges are worth considering for situations of distress, grieving, and trauma that incline family members to decide not to donate their relatives' organs when they would have under better circumstances. Though unintentional, the decision contexts do the same thing as nudges, only they do not improve people's decisions.

If we agree that the shortage of available organs is a problem, that some people who wish to be donors are not, that radical shifts toward compensation are not in the offing, and that part of the problem with presumed consent is the failure to engage the ways in which context influences decisions, then there is nothing wrong with exploring the possibility of nudging people even in highly charged emotional situations. Defaulting to donation subject to family veto may be more of a comfort to those facing a dreaded choice than being forced to decide what to do in line at the DMV.

Notes

1. For more about the ethics of nudges, see Nagel (2011), Ménard (2010), Lobel and Amir (2009), Bovens (2009), and Rizzo and Whitman (2008). For more about the ethics of nudges, see Nagel (2011), Ménard (2010), Lobel and Amir (2009), Bovens (2009), and Rizzo and Whitman (2008).

2. See also Nelson (2010).

3. Hospitals need to "want" an IHC; that is, they must make the request and provide the necessary facilities for an IHC to become part of the hospital's staff. On the other hand, OPOs require the resources and funding that are necessary to hire, train, and assign IHCs to more hospitals.

4. Consent rates are obtained through calculating the number of consenting donors divided by the number of potential donors. Conversion rates are obtained through calculating the number of actual donors divided by the number of potential donors.

5. A related aspect of our default to donation policy is considering how to improve OPOs. Kieran Healy suggests that there are "three kinds of logistical effectiveness" that directly affect an organization's (such as an OPO's) success in procuring donations. (1) Resources: This is perhaps the most important of all the logistical characteristics. Resources such as money, time, and people are directly related to the amount of success that an OPO will have in procuring organ donations. "A 10 percent increase in spending raises the procurement rate by nearly 0.9 points" (398). Essentially, it is impossible to increase the number of organs given and transplanted if organizations do not have the resources necessary to create a context for giving, which will in turn act as a nudge on potential donors. (2) Scope: This means the range or reach that an OPO has. The larger the scope, the more hospitals and potential donors the OPO will be able to reach out to and affect. It is obvious that scope and resources are intertwined. An OPO could have a lot of resources at its disposal, but at the same time it could focus on a smaller instead of a larger area. (3) Persistence: This is a measure of the amount of effort an OPO puts into finding and interacting with potential donors. In order for an OPO to be as successful as it could be, the organization must be resilient.

References

Abadie, A., and S. Gay. 2006. The impact of presumed consent legislation on cadaveric organ donation: a cross-country study. *Journal of Health Economics* 25(4): 599–620.

Agence Presse-France. 2010. *Spain leads world in organ donations: Minister.* January 11. Available at: http://www.google.com/hostednews/afp/article/ALeqM5gqsAoAuUV9_jYkqw1VX-i2Vp5CEg (accessed May 30, 2011).

Associated Press. 2008. *Pope condemns organ-selling for transplants.* November 7. Available at: http://article.wn.com/view/2008/11/07/Pope_Condemns_Organ-selling_For_Transplants_7 (accessed May 30 2011).

Baily, M. A. 2010. *This is a very bad idea.* nytimes.com. Available at: http://roomfordebate.blogs.nytimes.com/2010/05/02/should-laws-encourage-organ-donation (accessed July 11, 2010).

Bovens, L. 2009. The ethics of nudge. In *Preference change*, ed. T. Yanoff-Grüne and S.O. Hansson, 207–220. New York: Springer.

Childress, J. F. 2001. The failure to give: Reducing barriers to organ donation. *Kennedy Institute of Ethics Journal* 11(1): 1–16.

Chouhan, P., and H. Draper. 2003. Modified mandated choice for organ procurement. *Journal of Medical Ethics* 29: 157–162.

Drake, A. W., S. N. Finkelstein, and H. M. Sapolsky. 1982. *The American blood supply.* Cambridge, MA: MIT Press.

Hamer, C. L., and M. M. Rivlin. 2003. A stronger policy of organ retrieval from cadaveric donors: Some ethical considerations. *Journal of Medical Ethics* 29(3): 196–200.

Hausman, D. M., and B. Welch. 2010. Debate: To nudge or not to nudge. *Journal of Political Philosophy* 18(1): 123–136.

Healy, K. 2004. Altruism as an organizational problem: The case of organ procurement. *American Sociological Review* 69: 387–404.

Healy, K. 2006. *Last best gifts*. Chicago: University of Chicago Press.

Israni, A. K., S. D. Halpern, S. Zink, S. A. Sidhwani, and A. Caplan. 2005. Incentive models to increase living kidney donation: Encouraging without coercing. *American Journal of Transplantation* 5(1): 15–20.

John, P., G. Smith, and G. Stoker. 2009. Nudge nudge, think think: Two strategies for changing civic behaviour. *Political Quarterly* 80:361–370.

Klassen, A. C., and D. K. Klassen. 1996. Who are the donors in organ donation? The family's perspective in mandated choice. *Annals of Internal Medicine* 125: 70–73.

Lobel, O., and O. Amir. 2009. Stumble, predict, nudge: How behavioral economics informs law and policy. *Columbia Law Review* 108: 2098–2138.

Manman, H. 2011. *Organ donor pilot a failure after one year*. BeijingToday.com. Available at: http://www.beijingtoday.com.cn/feature/organ-donor-pilot-a-failure-after-one-year (accessed May 26, 2011).

Ménard, J. 2010. A 'nudge' for public health ethics: Libertarian paternalism as a framework for ethical analysis of public health interventions? *Public Health Ethics* 3(3): 229–238.

Mojaher, S. T. 2011. DMV now requires organ donor answer in California. *Associated Press*. July 24. Available at: http://www.mercurynews.com/breaking-news/ci_18540781.

Nagel, T. 2011. David Brooks' theory of human nature. *New York Times*: http://www.nytimes.com/2011/03/13/books/review/book-review-the-social-animal-by-david-brooks.html

Nelson, J. L. 2010. Donation by default?: Examining feminist reservations about opt-out organ procurement. *International Journal of Feminist Approaches to Bioethics* 3(1): 23–42.

Nytimes.com. 2010. Should laws push for organ donation? ny-times.com. Available at: http://roomforde bate.blogs.nytimes.com/2010/05/02/should-laws-encourage-organ-donation (accessed July 11, 2010).

Phillips, W. G. 2006. My father's life (after death). *Men's Health* 21(10): 163–169, 179.

Postrel, V. 2010. With functioning kidneys for all 2009. Available at: http://www.theatlantic.com/magazine/print/2009/07/with-functioning-kidneys-for-all/7587 (accessed July 11, 2010).

Rizzo, M. J., and D. G. Whitman. 2008. Little brother is watching you: New paternalism on the slippery slopes. *Arizona Law Review* 51: 685–739.

Salim, A., C. Brown, K. Inaba, et al. 2007. Improving consent rates for organ donation: The effect of an in-house coordinator program. *Journal of Trauma-Injury Infection & Critical Care* 62:1411–1415

Satel, S. (ed.). 2009. *When altruism isn't enough: The case for compensating kidney donors*. Washington, DC: AEI Press.

Selinger, E., and K. Powys Whyte. 2010. Competence and trust in choice architecture. *Knowledge, Technology & Policy* 23(3–4): 461–482.

Seniorjournal.com. 2009. *Majority of Americans express interest in organ donations but few register* Available at: http://seniorjournal.com/NEWS/Features/2009/20090413-MajorityOfAmericans.htm

Shafer, T. J., K. D. Davis, S. M. Holtzman, C. T. Van Buren, N. J. Crafts, and R. Durand. 2003. Location of in-house organ procurement organization staff in level I trauma centers increases conversion of potential donors to actual donors. *Transplantation* 75:1330–1335.

Siminoff, L. A., R. M. Arnold, A. L. Caplan, B. A. Virnig, and D.L. Seltzer. 1995. Public policy governing organ and tissue procurement in the United States. Results from the National Organ and Tissue Procurement Study. *Annals of Internal Medicine* 123: 10–17.

Siminoff, L. A., and M. B. Mercer. 2001. Public policy, public opinion, and consent for organ donation. *Cambridge Quarterly of Healthcare Ethics* 10(4): 377–386.

Siminoff, L. A., and C. M. Saunders Sturm. 2000. African-American reluctance to donate: Beliefs and attitudes about organ donation and implications for policy. *Kennedy Institute for Ethics Journal* 10(1): 59–74.

Smith, W. J. 2010. Presumptuous consent. Institute on Religion and Public Life. Available at: http://www .firstthings.com/onthesquare/2010/05/presumptu ous-consent (accessed July 11, 2010).

Spital, A. 1996. Mandated choice for organ donation: Time to give it a try. *Annals of Internal Medicine* 125: 66–99.

Thaler, R., and C. Sunstein. 2008. *Nudge: Improving decisions about health, wealth, and happiness.* New Haven, CT: Yale University Press.

UN/COE. 2009. *Trafficking in organs, tissues and cells and trafficking in human beings for the purpose of the removal of organs.* Strasbourg: Directorate General of Human Rights and Legal Affairs Council of Europe.

Wendler, D., and N. Dickert. 2001. The consent process for cadaveric organ procurement: How does it work? How can it be improved? *Journal of the American Medical Association* 285: 329–33.

WSYR-TV. 2011. Bill would change organ donor application on DMV form. Available at: http://www.9wsyr .com/news/custom/WSYR Links/story/Bill-would -change-organ-donor-application-on-DMV/c8s- J24qvlkWnFLei7896PA.cspx (accessed May 26, 2011).

Zink, S., and S. Wertlieb. 2006. A study of the presumptive approach to consent for organ donation: A new solution to an old problem. *Critical Care Nurse* 26(2): 129–136.

Chapter 23

The Case for "Presumed Consent" in Organ Donation

Ian Kennedy, Robert A. Sells, Abdallah S. Daar, Ronald D. Guttmann, Raymond Hoffenberg, Michael Lock, Janet Radcliffe-Richards, and Nicholas Tilney

Is there a moral case for changing the law regulating organ donation from a system of "contracting in" to "contracting out" or "presumed consent" in those countries that have not yet done so? Contracting in refers to a system in which the law requires that donors and/or relatives must positively indicate their willingness for organs to be removed for transplantation. In a contracting out system, organs may be removed after death unless individuals positively indicate during their lifetimes that they did not wish this to be done, a system also known as presumed consent.

We start with the premise that any measure that increases the supply of organs for transplantation is a good thing. If the contracting out system were to achieve this, the onus would then be on those who oppose it to demonstrate that the benefit that flows from it is outweighed by the harm.

Why Change the Law?

Since 1990 in those countries that have a contracting in system in place the number of cadaver organs available for transplantation has not kept up with demand; indeed the gap is widening.[1,2] Nonetheless, many people believe that the law should not be changed, arguing that a significant improvement in supply could result from public and professional education and measures to simplify the process of donation and retrieval of organs. Although not discounting this possibility, we believe that a contracting out system would achieve the same effect with greater certainty, as has been shown in countries that have changed to this option. Therefore we believe that it is morally unjustified to perpetuate a system that falls short of increasing the availability of organs to people who might benefit from transplantation.

Current Situation

The guiding principles issued by WHO in 1991[3] state that organs may be removed from the body of a dead person if: (a) any consents required by law are obtained; and (b) there is no reason to believe that in the absence of any formal consent given during life the dead person would have objected to such removal.

In countries where transplantation is widely practised, the law permits removal of organs from the cadaver of a person who made known the wish to donate while alive. In practice most people have not made any such formal declaration. In these circumstances the law looks to the relatives for consent. Since most donors will have spent some time in the intensive care unit before death is pronounced, the relatives will be present when the decision is taken to withdraw life support and are then approached. They decide whether organs may be removed and used for transplantation, and their power is in turn laid down by the law.

The laws of different countries fall into five categories. In the absence of a wish expressed by the donor during life, organs may be removed in the following circumstances.

- Only with the consent of the person lawfully in possession of the body and subject to express objection of the deceased or objection of the relatives, if available (UK).[4]
- After the relatives have been informed of the intention to remove organs, but irrespective of their consent (except for that of the nearest relative (Norway)).[5]
- Once it has been ascertained that the relatives do not object (Italy).[5]
- Where the dead person had not expressed an objection, this is confirmed by the relatives and consent is then presumed (Belgium).[5]
- Irrespective of the relatives' views (Austria).[5]

Does Contracting Out Increase the Supply of Organs?

The difference in the rates of organ donation between countries can be explained by several factors, such as the supply of potential donors (which may vary according to the rate of road-traffic accidents or gun laws, for example), religious and cultural responses to death and to the body after death, and practical issues—e.g., the number of intensive-care beds available. Adverse publicity can seriously reduce the supply by reducing the number of potential donors or the consent of relatives. Supply can be increased by energetic educational campaigns,[6, 7, 8] by having more transplant coordinators,[8] by the provision of specialist teams to take over the care of potential donors,[9] and by provision of financial incentives to encourage doctors and institutions to refer patients. All these factors are independent of the nature of the prevailing law. In three western countries there is evidence that changing to a contracting out system resulted in an increase in organs—Spain,[9] Austria,[10] and Belgium[11]—but the change in legislation has not achieved this rise on its own. In Spain, for example, additional measures included the appointment of more co-ordinators and provision of financial incentives. In the case of Belgium there is well documented and convincing evidence that a change in the law from contracting in to contracting out in 1986 led to an increase in organ supply.[11] Staff at the organ- transplantation centre in Antwerp were strongly opposed to the new law and retained a contracting in policy accompanied by enhanced public and professional education; by contrast, at Leuven the new law was adopted. In Antwerp, organ donation rates remained unchanged; in Leuven they rose from 15 to 40 donors per year over a 3-year period. In the whole country organ donation rose by 55% within 5 years despite a concurrent decrease in the number of organs available from road-traffic accidents. Citizens who wish to opt out of the scheme may register their objection at any Town Hall; since 1986 less than 2% of the population have done so. Use of a computerised register has simplified ascertaining the existence of any objection. In Belgium, despite the existence of this law, doctors are encouraged to approach the relatives in all cases and practitioners may decide against removing the organs if in their opinion this would cause undue distress or for any other valid reason.

Less than 10% of families do object compared with 20–30% elsewhere in Europe. Another benefit has been an increase in the number of referrals of cadaver donors from collaborating centres, suggesting that the intensivists have found the new law favourable to donation.[12] It would seem from the Belgian experience that relatives may be reluctant to take a personal decision about the removal of organs, but they find it easier to agree if they are simply confirming the intention of the dead person. If this is so, a contracting out system has a moral benefit of relieving grieving relatives of the burden of deciding about donation at a time of great psychological stress.

A change in the law thus achieves the dual effect of increasing the supply of organs and lessening the distress of relatives. Those who have moral objections to it must produce convincing evidence that the harm that would follow such a change would outweigh these clear benefits.

Possible Moral Objections

The Right of the Individual to Refuse to Donate Organs

This right is allowed for both in principle and in practice by the Belgian model, in which objection can be registered by law and doctors have the discretion to desist if they feel that removal of organs will better reflect the individual's wishes to avoid undue distress to the relatives. It is essential to ensure that simple mechanisms for registering an objection are easily available. In developed countries it should not be difficult to ensure that an opportunity is provided whenever any official business is transacted—e.g., when applying for a passport or driving licence. The safety mechanism of checking the decision with the relatives should minimise the possibility of erroneous interpretation of the dead person's wishes. We conclude that a sensitive, secure, and robust system could be introduced, preceded by a reasonable period of notice and publicity to give time to those who wish to register their objection. Whether this approach recommends itself to developing countries, where other priorities compete, is a separate matter.

The Rights of Relatives

In most legal systems, relatives have no property claim over the body of the deceased. Furthermore, any claim they may seek to assert seems rather weak when set against the claims of the person in need of a transplant. This is not to argue that relatives' interests should be ignored, and indeed the Belgian model takes them into account. This version of the contracting out system, as opposed to one in which the wishes of the relatives are ignored, is consistent with the recommendations of the Conference of European Health Ministers and WHO. The primary role of relatives is thus to corroborate that the dead person did not actually register an objection. They are not put into the position of having to make the decision themselves, but simply to confirm the facts. As a result the refusal rate is much lower.

Possible Counterproductive Consequences of Changing the Law

It may be argued that this change in public policy would invoke such social unease and disquiet that people would turn away from the whole concept of transplantation. This has not been the experience in countries that have changed, where, if anything, the general population and medical professionals are happier with the new law than with the old. In Belgium and Spain an increase in organ supply has been achieved despite a fall in the number of potential donors. Another objection is that the state already has a big enough stake in our lives—e.g., through the tax law, and further incursion into our affairs by assuming possession of our body parts and the right to distribute them to others by law would be a step too far. A study by the King's Fund Institute in 1994[13] concluded that, in the UK, the medical professions, the transplantation community, and the public were split over the ethics of the contracting out law and it would be inappropriate to recommend a change in the law because this might provoke an acrimonious debate that could damage confidence in transplantation technology as a whole. Others may argue that people would feel pressure not to contract out because this would be socially unacceptable. Both arguments are rebutted by the ready acceptance of the law in Belgium and elsewhere, and the immediate benefit it achieved in increasing the supply of organs.

Clearly, from a moral standpoint, the social context in which any law is to operate and any medical action that arises from it must be a significant consideration in determining policy. Before any such law is promulgated, there will have to be an informed public debate and a clear demonstration that it would be morally acceptable to most people. Much of the objection to change would be mitigated by appropriate public education.

We feel that this debate should now take place and, unless there is a majority view against change, the contracting out system of organ donation should be introduced.

References

1. Hauptman JP, O'Connor KJ. Procurement and allocation of solid organs for transplantation. *N Engl J Med* 1997; 336: 422–31.

2. United Kingdom Transplant Special Services Authority. Bristol, UK 1996.

3. WHO, Geneva. 1991. Human Organ Transplantation: a report on developments under the auspices of the WHO (1987–1991). 7.

4. HM Stationery Office. 1961. *The Human Tissue Act.* Section 1 (2) (a) and (b).

5. WHO. *Legislative responses to organ transplantation.* Dordrecht: Kluwer Academic Publishers, 1994: 276–80.

6. Stevens P, Jager KJ, Ryuan M, Blok G, Van Dalen J. *The European Donor Hospital Education Programme.* In: de Charro FT, *et al.* eds. *Systems of Donor Recruitment.* Dordrecht: Kluwer Academic Publishers, Netherlands: 1992, 105–09.

7. Robert A Sells. *The Impact of the European Donor Hospital Education Programme (EDHEP) on Organ Donation rates in North West England: a prospective trial.* (in press).

8. Birkeland SA, Christensen AK, Kosteljanetz M, Svarre HM. Risk of organ donations. *Lancet* 1997; 349: 35.

9. Matesanz R, Miranda B, Felipe C, Naya MT. *Organ procurement in Spain: The National Organisation of Transplants.* In: Touraine JL, *et al,* eds. *Organ shortage: the solutions.* Kluwer Academic Press, Netherlands: 1995, 167–77.

10. Muhlbacher F. *Donor recruitment in Austria.* 1992. In: De Charro FT, *et al,* eds. *Systems of donor procurement.* Dordrecht: Kluwer Academic Publishers, Netherlands, 1992: 65–71.

11. Michelsen P. *Effect of transplantation laws on organ procurement.* In: Touraine JL, *et al,* eds. *Organ shortage: the solutions.* Kluwer Academic Press, Netherlands: 1995, 33–39.

12. Michelsen P. Presumed consent to organ donation: ten years' experience in Belgium. *J R Soc Med* 1996; 89: 663–66.

13. New W, Solomon M. *A question of give and take—improving the supply of donor organs for transplantation. Research report 18.* King's Fund Institute, London; 1994: 25–29.

Chapter 24

AN EXCERPT FROM

A Critical Approach to the Current Understanding of Islamic Scholars on Using Cadaver Organs Without Prior Permission

Sahin Aksoy

Abstract

Chronic organ diseases and the increasing demand for organ transplantation have become an important health care problem within the last few decades. Campaigns and regulations to encourage people to donate organs after their death have not met much success. This article discusses the subject from an Islamic perspective. It begins with some basic information on how Muslims reach legal rulings on a particular issue, and goes on to debate contemporary thinking among Islamic scholars on the ethical legal issues of organ donation and organ transplantation. It is shown that there are two groups of scholars, one allowing organ donation and organ transplantation, the other refusing it in any circumstances. Both groups agree that it is fundamentally wrong to harvest organs from cadavers without the prior permission of the deceased or the relatives. This dogma is reexamined, and it is argued that, under the rule of necessity and the imperative to preserve life, there is enough moral and theological ground to allow the state to harvest organs from the deceased without prior permission.

Introduction

I will not be discussing the reasons for organ failures—reasons like excessive alcohol consumption in liver ailments, or unhealthy diet or lack of exercise in heart diseases. The commonly accepted view in bioethics is that we cannot make moral judgements about the lifestyles of individuals when we provide health care to them. My sole aim in this article is to review current Islamic opinions on organ transplantation and brain death, and offer an alternative to them.

Review and Critique of the Current Majority Consensus

The Exclusion of Any Monetary Transaction or Financial Benefit

The principle that human organs are not an ordinary property or commodity means that they should be donated freely in response to altruistic feelings of brotherhood and love for one's fellow beings. The donation of organs should not be considered as, or ever allowed to become, a legitimate way of trading or otherwise earning a regular living.[1] However, it does not necessarily follow that any financial transaction whatever associated with organ donation must be considered forbidden. Islam is a robust, natural way of life that has always anticipated and allowed exceptions that do not infringe or damage the spirit, purpose and meaning of the 'original message.' For instance, Ibn Quda Amain the 14th century allowed the sale of an organ of a living person. Indeed, permission to re-use the organs of the deceased is based on his ruling.[2] Al-Mahdi, Chairman of the Neurosurgery Department at Ibn Sina Hospital in Kuwait, writing about kidney transplants, concludes that, until we can obtain an adequate supply of organs through voluntary and uncompensated donation, we must countenance the possibility of offering to donors 'material recompense, on condition that no publicity in this respect is made.' He further observes: 'As far as the material recompense is concerned, the Islamic Sheria has actually determined it to be half the blood money. . . . 5,000 Kuwaiti Dinars. By mere coincidence, it is the very sum of money paid by the Health Ministry to procure a kidney from abroad.'[3] Similarly, Muhammad Sayed Tantawi, the Grand Mufti of Egypt and a widely respected authority in Islamic jurisprudence, has said: 'Man's sale of any of his organs is lawfully invalid and prohibited. Such sale is only permissible in the rarest cases decided by reliable doctors when they deem a patient's life contingent upon that sale.'[4] In sum, we may say that the condition—'There should be no monetary transaction or financial benefit from the procedure'—is not absolute and can be waived case by case.

The Problem of 'Brain Death'

One aspect of another condition that needs to be re-examined is that, if the transplantation is from a cadaver, 'the donor should be dead.' As discussed by Bagheri[5] and stated in the 3rd International Conference of Islamic Jurists (Amman 1986), brain death has come to be equated with cardiac and respiratory death.[6] However, this is something new and indicates a double standard. According to Islamic understanding a human life begins when the soul meets with the body, which is claimed to be 120 days after conception.[7] Brain formation or the beginning of electrical activity in the brain which occur well before 120 days are not considered as deciding the beginning of life. But for some reason, after the 1970s (which is, coincidentally, after the first successful cadaveric transplantation) Muslim scholars began to equate brain death with death. Until then, death had traditionally been described and defined by some accompanying signs which are: weakening of vision, limpness of the feet, bending of the nose, whitening of the temples and the stretching of the face and loss of the ability to wrinkle.'[8]

Elsewhere, I have argued that the 120-day period after which human life is thought to be established is based on an expedient interpretation of the texts (intended to enable people to abort foetuses at that late stage), and that the period should instead be 50 days.[9] In the same way, I believe the effort to equate brain death with real death is also an expedient, intended by the authorities to enable organs to be utilised for transplantation. I think shifting the boundaries at either end is suspect as well as unnecessary.

The Dogma of Prior Donor Consent

Another dogma that needs to re-examined and nuanced is the absoluteness attached to the consent of the donor or of the donor's relatives: 'Donation from people who have already died can be used on the basis of their own signed will or authorisation obtained from their relatives post-mortem.'[10] Strictly applied, this condition means that if there is a need for an available organ, that organ cannot be used unless there is a donor card on the person of the deceased person, and/or permission is obtained from the relatives of the deceased. However, strict application of this condition in all circumstances would appear to contradict the important maxim we mentioned earlier, *al-darûrât tubîh al-mahzûrât* (necessities render the prohibited permitted). That maxim means that when there is no other way to save life, forbidden means become permitted; this includes the removal of organs from a cadaver. As I mentioned above, parallel to Harris' controversial suggestion,[11] Ibn Qudâma allowed the re-use of the organs of the deceased six centuries ago.[12] At the First International Conference on Islamic Medicine it was agreed that the donation of body parts is a social obligation, of the kind classified in Islamic law as *fard kifâya* (a collective duty that must be fulfilled by a sufficient number of community members, though not necessarily by all: the commonest example is making proper funeral arrangements for Muslims and doing the funeral prayer). This means the community is under a collective obligation to find the right organs for transplantation in order to preserve the lives and health of its sick members. If a sick person dies while awaiting a transplant, the society as a whole carries some responsibility for that. In this situation, the medical staff in charge of the transplant procedure represent the community as a whole. Once an organ for transplant has been obtained, the community regards itself exempt from seeking further cure for the recipient of the organ.[13] Thus, the condition requiring medical staff to have or obtain the permission of the deceased person and/or his relatives prior to removal of any organ for transplantation cannot be applied in every case. As Shaykh Tantawi said, it is a necessary procedure to seek permission from the inheritors.[14] In case there are not

inheritors, permission should be taken from the appropriate legal authority. Nevertheless, seeking such permission is not a binding condition on competent people, namely reliable doctors, if they believe that the life of a living person is contingent upon the transfer of a human organ from a deceased person. Where there is life-and-death urgency, the medical procedure may be initiated on the famous 'lesser evil' principle, a universal principle whose formulation in Islamic legal thought is: 'The most harmful detriment is removable by the less harmful one.'[15]

Conclusions

Muslims believe Islam to be the final divinely revealed religion, and must therefore expect it to offer solutions to every contemporary issue, provided its principles, ethos and tradition are interpreted with sufficient compassion and imagination. The scarcity of organs for transplantation is an important health care problem in all societies, including Muslim ones. As we have explained above, by applying one of the best-known legal maxims in Islam, namely *al-darûrât tubîh al-mahzûrât* (necessities render the prohibited permitted), the legal-moral difficulties can be negotiated relatively easily. Islam, as a way of life, seeks to balance communitarian and individualistic principles. Islam is individualistic in the sense that it values every individual life as important as the whole world; it is communitarian in that it recognises the need to sacrifice some individual liberties (which in other traditions might be regarded as legal-moral absolutes) for the sake of public benefit. Although Islamic law protects individual rights, public benefit is always prioritised. This is the reason why it is allowed (in the appropriate circumstances, even recommended) to transfer organs from dead bodies without the donors' permission, albeit the ideal procedure is, of course, to obtain permission and consent of the donor and/or relatives. Willingness to countenance the payment of financial compensation to motivate organ donors can also be seen as an example of the robust realism of the Islamic way. It is suggested that if it encourages people to donate their organs and promotes the public benefit there could be some material exchange under the supervision of the state.

Beside these two unorthodox opinions I also tried to emphasise in this article that the brain death criterion is a novel but inappropriate interpretation in contemporary Islamic jurisprudence. Although it is necessary to be open-minded and modern-knowledge-oriented, we should err on the side of caution and not risk the possibility of ending lives prematurely and unjustly.

Notes

This article was given as an oral presentation at the IAB 5th World Congress of Bioethics in London, 21–24 September, 2000.

1. M. al-Qushairi. 1972. *Sahih Muslim bi-Sharh al-Nawawi*. Beirut. Dar al-Fikr: 14:191–200.

2. I. Ghanem. 1982. *Islamic Medical Jurisprudence*. London. Isos Publications: 276

3. M. al-Mahdi. 1989. Donation, sale and unbequeathed possession of human organs. In *The Islamic Vision of Some Medical Practices*. K. al-Mazkur, A. al-Saif, A.R. al-Gindi, and A. Abu-Ghudda, eds. Kuwait. IOMS Publications: 286.

4. M.S. Tantawi. 1989. Judgment on sale or donation of human organs. In *The Islamic Vision of Some Medical Practices*. K. al-Mazkur, A. al-Saif, A.R. al-Gindi, and A. Abu-Ghudda, eds. Kuwait. IOMS Publications: 287–96.

5. A. Bagheri. *The Islamic Views on Brain Death*. Presentation made at Multicultural Ethical Issues in Transplantation Meeting, February 21–22, 1999, Manchester.

6. 3rd Conference of Islamic Jurists. *Fiqh Academy Book of Decrees*. Decree No.5, Amman, October 11–16, 1986.

7. M.A. Albar. 1995. When is the soul inspired? In *Contemporary Topics in Islamic Medicine*. Jeddah. Saudi Publishing and Distributing House: 131–6.

8. V. Rispler-Chaim. Islamic Medical Ethics in the Twentieth Century. *Journal of Medical Ethics* 1989; 5:203–8.

9. S. Aksoy. Can Islamic Texts Help to Resolve the Problem of the Moral Status of the Prenate. *Eubios Journal of Asian and International Bioethics* 1998; 8:76–79.

10. Rispler-Chaim, op. cit.: 36.

11. J. Harris. We should recycle the dead to help the living. *The Independent*, February 19, 1999.

12. I. Ghanem. 1982. *op. cit.*: 276.

13. First International Conference on Islamic Medicine. *Islamic Code of Medical Ethics*. Kuwait. January 1981: 81. In this source it is also mentioned that the Caliph Umar b. al-Khattâb accused the community, one of whose members died of hunger, of killing him, and ordered them to pay *fidya* (ransom). Similarly, the community is held responsible for the death of a person, if the community could not provide blood or organ donation for him/her. A part of the collective responsibility involves the provision of the minimal means of survival for all human beings.

14. Maybe it is more crucial than the will of the deceased since he or she has already gone and cannot benefit or be harmed by the procedure.

15. M.S. Tantawi. 1989. Judgment on sale or donation of human organs. In *The Islamic Vision of Some Medical Practices*. K. al-Mazkur, A. al-Saif, A.R. al-Gindi, and A. Abu-Ghudda, eds. Kuwait. IOMS Publications: 294–5.

Chapter 25

AN EXCERPT FROM

Priority in Organ Allocation to Previously Registered Donors

Public Perceptions of the Fairness and Effectiveness of Priority Systems

Jennifer A. Chandler, Jacquelyn A. Burkell, and Sam D. Shemie

Abstract

A priority system is one in which previously registered donors receive a preference in the allocation of organs for transplant ahead of those who have not registered. Supporters justify these systems on the basis that they are fair and will encourage donor registration. This article reviews existing studies of public reactions to priority systems, as well as studies of the extent to which the moral principle of reciprocity affects decision making in organ donation. The role of reciprocity in the public discourse surrounding the enactment of priority systems in Singapore and Israel is described. One factor that seems to have been relevant in these countries is the existence of a religious minority that is perceived as willing to take an organ but not to donate one. Although this perception may have fueled a resentment of perceived "free-riders," concerns were raised about the social divisiveness of priority systems. In sum, people appear to be sensitive to the principle of reciprocity in the context of organ donation, but this sensitivity does not always translate into support for priority systems. Further research into whether public messaging about organ donation could be modified to encourage registration by appeal to the golden rule would be worthwhile.

Reciprocity or priority systems in organ donation and transplant (also known as solidarity models or preferred status systems) provide priority in the receipt of an organ to transplant recipients who have previously demonstrated their willingness to donate their own organs (as living donors or as registered deceased donors). Proposals vary in the degree of priority provided to registrants, from an extreme of disqualifying non-registrants altogether from receiving a transplant to the use of registration status only to break a tie between patients who are otherwise equivalent. In some systems, the priority reward accrues not just to the registrant but to the family members of registrants should those family members require an organ transplant.

Many assessments of the ethical arguments for and against priority systems have been published since the early days of organ transplants. (1–38) There are 2 central arguments for priority systems. First, priority systems could increase donation rates by offering an incentive for donor registration. Second, such systems address the potential unfairness that a person unwilling to contribute to the pool of scarce lifesaving resources may draw from that pool ahead of a person who is willing to contribute. This second argument is based on the moral principle of reciprocity, also known as the "golden rule" that you should "do to others as you want others to do to you."(39) This principle is widespread among human cultures. (40) These 2 justifications, which are independent of each other, are usually cited in discussions of priority systems.

The counterargument to the proposition that priority systems will increase donation is that the proposed priority incentive is too modest to motivate nondonors. Furthermore, the system might actually decrease registration and donation if those motivated by altruism are repelled by an incentive scheme, or if the system propagates the idea that "free-riding" is prevalent, reducing otherwise positive feelings that people may have toward the organ donation system.

In response to the fairness-based justification for priority systems, opponents argue that it is unfair to discriminate among those in need on the basis of willingness to donate because this unfairly treats all as equally able to donate when in fact people have different and legitimate reasons to find it impossible or difficult to donate their organs (e.g., religion, culture, psychological factors, socioeconomic vulnerability or exclusion). They point out that priority systems may discriminate along problematic and socially divisive lines such as ethnicity or religion and may compound the disadvantage faced already by socially vulnerable minority groups. For example, it may be more difficult for African Americans in the United States to register to donate as a result of historical and current mistrust of the medical system. (41) To treat them as equivalent to those without similar reasons to mistrust the medical system unfairly ignores a relevant difference. (41)

Additional arguments raised against priority systems are that (1) allocation should be based on factors such as need and waiting time

rather than on moral worth as determined by willingness to register, (2) the incentive is coercive, and (3) the system raises various practical problems.

Our research group is currently studying responses of the Canadian public to priority systems. As part of this work, we have searched for existing empirical studies of responses to priority systems, particularly those that address perceptions of fairness or effectiveness. The purpose of this review article is to gather and summarize this literature, and to provide our assessment of the strength of the 2 main justifications for priority systems in light of this literature.

. . .

Discussion

The studies summarized here shed some light on public perceptions of the 2 main justifications for priority systems in organ donation and allocation: (1) that priority systems are fairer because they do not allow someone not willing to donate to receive an organ ahead of someone willing to donate and (2) that priority systems will increase registration (and therefore, donation). In most of the surveys, the respondents' views are not probed in detail, and so it is not clear whether their support or opposition is due to the issues of efficacy or fairness, or both. However, it appears that, on average, the public is split in its support for priority systems.

One interesting dimension that emerges from the focus group study in Israel (38) as well as the review of the Singaporean and Israeli adoption of priority systems is the relevance of identifiable religious or ethnic minorities that are perceived as unwilling to donate. There are suggestions, such as that made by Lavee et al., that priority systems were in part a reaction to a perception that an identifiable minority was free-riding. (48) At the same time, voices in both communities were deeply concerned that priority systems would exacerbate divisions and undermine social cohesion, and were unfair to minorities whose objections were religiously based.

The discussion will address the 2 main justifications in turn, returning to social divisiveness within the discussion on the fairness or unfairness of priority systems.

Do People Think That Priority Systems Will Increase Donor Registration?

When questions about the likely efficacy of priority systems in encouraging registration were put to them, respondents seemed to think a priority system might have some effect on others, and might motivate them as well, although the predicted effects were not huge. Robertson's study is interesting for its demonstration that priming respondents with the idea that they may one day want an organ affects expressed willingness to donate. (33) Whether this effect on expressed willingness to donate would translate into actual registrations is uncertain.

Israel offers an opportunity to test the actual effects of a reciprocity system. A report of the recently enacted reciprocity system is due in 2012. (48) This may offer some basis upon which to judge the efficacy of reciprocity systems, although it may be challenging to do so because the increased awareness of organ donation and transplantation (due to the legal change and associated media campaigns) might also explain any observed increase in registration. (76) Although it is not possible to ascribe the increase in donation among the non–Muslim population of Singapore to the priority system (because presumed consent was enacted at the same time), the priority

penalty applied to Muslims who did not opt in does not appear to have been particularly effective at encouraging them to opt in. (61)

Are Priority Systems Considered Fair?

With respect to the fairness of priority systems, people seem to be deeply divided, with sizeable proportions of respondents finding the system fair, unfair, or morally neutral. The results do demonstrate the strong appeal of the moral principle of reciprocity (the golden rule), but also suggest that, for many people, it does not translate into a willingness to penalize a violator of this norm in the context of the allocation of lifesaving organs as would occur under a priority system.

A review of the experiences in Singapore and Israel, the 2 countries that have enacted priority systems, suggests some possible risks associated with priority systems. In both Israel and Singapore, ethnic and/or religious subpopulations seem to have been identified as a "free-riding" group in the context of organ donation. As outsiders without detailed knowledge of the social and political contexts of those 2 countries, we hesitate to draw conclusions about how and why the priority policies were adopted in those countries, and the extent to which existing social divisions played a role in the politics of the move to priority systems. However, based on a reading of the discourse surrounding the legislative amendments that instituted the priority systems, communal divisions do seem to have been part of the politics of these changes. The concerns about emphasizing differences between social groups that were expressed by some focus group participants in the study conducted by Guttman *et al.*, (38) as well as the observation by authors such as Teo (62) about the risk of damage to communal goodwill and cohesion, underscore the risk of social divisiveness that a priority system can have in a context where a particular minority is identified as unwilling to donate.

In addition to religious objections to donation of the type that were salient in Singapore and Israel, another important aspect of this discussion is that social minority groups may experience exclusion or discrimination that reduces their willingness to donate. As noted above, Goering and Dula (41) have discussed the historical and enduring mistrust of the medical system among the African American community as a factor in willingness to donate. The fairness of a priority system must be assessed in light of these factors. Furthermore, to the extent that ethnic minorities are less willing to donate, a priority system risks reinforcing some of the potential consequences of minority status that might make a person less likely to donate—feelings of exclusion, discrimination, or distrust. Various studies of the attitudes of minority groups to organ donation suggest that reluctance to donate is related to questions of identity and belonging (77) and that greater "acculturation" is significantly associated with more positive attitudes toward organ donation. (78) To the extent that minority groups are less likely to register because they do not feel fully part of the broader community or mistrust that broader community, a policy such as a priority system that emphatically expresses their separateness from the community may just reinforce this feeling.

Conclusion

Regardless of whether policymakers ultimately adopt priority systems or not, the seemingly widespread sensitivity to the golden rule may open up opportunities to vary public messaging in an attempt to increase organ donation registration. There are precedents in other contexts for the use of appeals to reciprocity to encourage donation. For example, the American Red Cross uses an appeal to reciprocity in addition to other arguments in describing the "benefits of donation." Its website suggests that one of the benefits of donation is that "you will help ensure blood is on the shelf when needed—most people don't think they'll ever need blood, but many do." (79) Empirical support for this approach is suggested by findings of a recent meta-analysis of studies of donor motivations and deterrents, which indicated that reciprocity was a commonly cited motivation for blood donation. (80) This reciprocity included donations out of gratitude for the prior receipt of a transfusion as well as donations in order to help ensure an adequate supply in the event the donors one day needed a transfusion. (80)

Some care may be needed in generalizing from blood donation to the organ donation context. As noted earlier, Robertson's survey (33) suggests that people are sensitive to the golden rule in the context of organ donation. Respondents who were asked first about their willingness to take an organ were more likely to express willingness to donate their organs after death than were respondents who were asked the questions in the reverse order. This finding suggests that it may be possible to affect willingness to donate by appealing to feelings of reciprocity. (33) However, if people are primarily driven by reciprocity, a problematic corollary is that the low likelihood that any potential donor will require a transplant would undermine that person's feelings of obligation to donate. This problem is less acute for blood donation, given that the chances of requiring a transfusion one day are higher than the chances of requiring a transplant.

Although people do seem to respond to the

golden rule in the organ donation context, an appeal to it may not be enough to overcome reluctance to donate. (81) Nonetheless, we feel that further research is warranted into whether willingness to donate might be affected by messages that incorporate concepts of reciprocity. In fact, Landry (30) has previously proposed something along these lines. He suggests that potential donors be asked to answer 2 questions: (1) I would want an organ transplant to save my life. Check one: yes or no, (2) In the event of my death, I agree to the donation of my organs. Check one: yes, no, yes with a preference to donate to those who agree to donate their organs. (30)

A message that more explicitly invokes the norm of reciprocity could cover the following points: (1) You or your loved ones may one day need an organ. (2) Would you accept an organ if you need one? (3) Would you want an organ for your loved one who needs one? (4) If you need an organ, should you take an organ ahead of someone who was already registered as a donor if you weren't registered? (5) Why not register now to help others and also to make sure it is fair for you to take an organ later if you need one? Some of these messages may be perceived as heavy-handed or psychologically coercive, and care should be taken to navigate between persuasion and coercion in messaging about organ donation.

Acknowledgments

The authors thank Canadian Blood Services and Health Canada for financial support of their study of public reactions to priority systems in Canada.

References

1. Schwindt R, Vining AR. Proposal for a future delivery market for transplant organs. *J Health Polit Policy Law.* 1986; 11(3): 483–500.

2. Peters DA. A unified approach to organ donor recruitment, organ procurement, and distribution. *J Law Health.* 1988–1989; 3(2):157–187.

3. Capron AM. More blessed to give than to receive? *Transplant Proc.* 1992; 24(5):2185–2187.

4. Kleinman I, Lowy FH. Ethical considerations in living organ donation and a new approach: an advance-directive organ registry. *Arch Intern Med.* 1992; 152(7): 1484–1488.

5. Muyskens J. Should receiving depend upon willingness to give? *Transplant Proc.* 1992; 24(5):2181–2184.

6. Burdick JF, Capron AM, Delmonico FL, Ravenscraft MD, Reckard CR, Shapiro M. Preferred Status for Organ Donors: A Report of the OPTN/UNOS Ethics Committee. http://optn.tranplant.hrsa.gov/resources/bioethics.asp?index= . Accessed April 29, 2012.

7. Gillon R. On giving preference to prior volunteers when allocating organs for transplantation. *J Med Ethics.* 1995; 21(4): 195–196.

8. Jarvis R. Join the club: a modest proposal to increase availability of donor organs. *J Med Ethics.* 1995; 21(4): 199–204.

9. Gubernatis G. Solidarity model as nonmonetary incentive could increase organ donation and justice in organ allocation at the same time. *Transplant Proc.* 1997; 29(8): 3264–3266.

10. Eaton S. The subtle politics of organ donation: a proposal. *J Med Ethics.* 1998; 24(3):166–170.

11. Schwindt R, Vining A. Proposal for a mutual insurance pool for transplant organs. *J Health Polit Policy Law.* 1998; 23(5): 725–741.

12. Daar AS. Altruism and reciprocity in organ donation: compatible or not? *Transplantation.* 2000; 70(4): 704–705.

13. Sells RA. Donation: Will the principle of "do as you would be done by" be enough? *Transplantation.* 2000; 70(4):703–704.

14. Kluge EH. Improving organ retrieval rates: various proposals and their ethical validity. *Health Care Anal.* 2000; 8(3):279–295.

15. Gubernatis G, Kliemt H. A superior approach to organ allocation and donation. *Transplantation.* 2000; 70(4): 699–702.

16. Gubernatis G, Kliemt H. Solidarity model: a way to cope with rationing problems in organ transplantation. *Transpl Int.* 2000; 13(suppl 1):S607–S608.

17. Kolber AJ. A matter of priority: transplanting organs preferentially to registered donors. *Rutgers Law Rev.* 2003; 55(3): 671–740.

18. Blankart CB. Donors without rights—the tragedy of organ transplantation. 2004. http://lvb.wiwi .hu-berlin.de/vwl/oef /dok/docs/donors.pdf. Accessed March 3, 2012.

19. Wigmore SJ, Forsythe JL. Incentives to promote organ donation. *Transplantation.* 2004; 77(1):159–161.

20. Sackner-Bernstein JD, Godin S. Increasing organ transplantation—fairly. *Transplantation.* 2004; 77(1): 157–159.

21. Steinberg D. An "opting-in" paradigm for kidney transplantation. *Am J Bioeth.* 2004; 4(4):4–14.

22. Ravelingien A, Krom A. Earning points for moral behavior: organ allocation based on reciprocity. *Int J Appl Philos.* 2005; 19(1):73–83.

23. Nadel MS, Nadel CA. Using reciprocity to motivate organ donations. *Yale J Health Policy Law Ethics.* 2005; 5(1):293–325.

24. Giles S. An antidote to the emerging two tier organ donation policy in Canada: the Public Cadaveric Organ Donation Program. *J Med Ethics.* 2005; 31(4): 188–191.

25. Chandler JA. Priority systems in the allocation of organs for transplant: should we reward those who have previously agreed to donate? *Health Law J.* 2005; 13: 99–138.

26. Spital A. Should people who commit themselves to organ donation be granted preferred status to receive organ transplants? *Clin Transplant.* 2005; 19(2): 269–272.

27. Undis DJ. Changing organ allocation will increase organ supply. *DePaul Law Rev.* 2005–2006; 55: 889–896.

28. Childress JF, Liverman CT, eds, for the Committee on Increasing Rates of Organ Donation, Board on Health Sciences Policy, Institute of Medicine. *Organ Donation: Opportunities for Action.* Washington DC: National Academies Press; 2006.

29. Bramstedt KA. Is it ethical to prioritize patients for organ allocation according to their values about organ donation? *Prog Transplant.* 2006; 16(2):170–174.

30. Landry DW. Voluntary reciprocal altruism: a novel strategy to encourage deceased organ donation. *Kidney Int.* 2006; 69(6): 957–959.

31. Murphy TF, Veatch RM. Members first: the ethics of donating organs and tissues to groups. *Camb Q Healthc Ethics.* 2006; 15(1):50–59.

32. Siegal G, Bonnie RJ. Closing the organ gap: a reciprocity-based social contract approach. *J Law Med Ethics.* 2006; 34(2):415–423

33. Robertson CT. From free riders to fairness: a cooperative system for organ transplantation. *Jurimetrics.* 2007; 48(1):1–42.

34. Trotter G. Preferred allocation for registered organ donors. *Transplant Rev.* 2008; 22(3):158–162.

35. Gruenbaum BF, Jotkowitz A. The practical, moral, and ethical considerations of the new Israeli law for the allocation of donor organs. *Transplant Proc.* 2010; 42(10):4475–4478.

36. Lifesharers. http://www.lifesharers.org. Accessed April 29, 2012.

37. den Hartogh G. Priority to registered donors on the waiting list for postmortal organs? A critical look at the objections. *J Med Ethics.* 2011; 37(3):149–152.

38. Guttman N, Ashkenazi T, Gesser-Edelsburg A, Seidmann V. Laypeople's ethical concerns about a new Israeli organ transplantation prioritization policy aimed to encourage organ donor registration among the public. *J Health Polit Policy Law.* 2011; 36(4):691–716.

39. Wattles J. *The Golden Rule.* New York, NY: Oxford University Press; 1996.

40. Pfaff DW. *The Neuroscience of Fair Play: Why We (Usually) Follow the Golden Rule.* New York, NY: Dana Press; 2007.

41. Goering S, Dula A. Reasonable people, double jeopardy and justice. *Am J Bioeth.* 2004; 4(4):37–39.

42. Aita K. New organ transplant policies in Japan, including the family-oriented priority donation clause. *Transplantation.* 2011; 91(5):489–491.

43. Kittur DS, Hogan MM, Thukral VK, McGaw LJ, Alexander JW. Incentives for organ donation? The

United Network for Organ Sharing Ad hoc Donations Committee. *Lancet.* 1991; 338(8780):1441–1443.

44. Jasper JD, Nickerson CA, Hershey JC, Asch DA. The public's attitudes toward incentives for organ donation. *Transplant Proc.* 1999; 31(5):2181–2184.

45. Ahlert M, Gubernatis G, Klein R. Common sense in organ allocation. *Analyse Kritik.* 2001; 23: 221–244.

46. Bennett R, Savani S. Factors influencing the willingness to donate body parts for transplantation. *J Health Soc Policy.* 2004; 18(3):61–85.

47. Decker O, Winter M, Brahler E, Beutel M. Between commodification and altruism: gender imbalance and attitudes towards organ donation. A representative survey of the German community. *J Gender Stud.* 2008; 17(3):251–255.

48. Lavee J, Ashkenazi T, Gurman G, Steinberg D. A new law for allocation of donor organs in Israel. *Lancet.* 2010; 375(9720): 1131–1133.

49. Stijnen MMN, Dijker AJM. Reciprocity and need in posthumous organ donation: the mediating role of moral emotions. *Soc Psychol Personal Sci.* 2011; 2(4):387–394.

50. Oz MC, Kherani AR, Rowe A, et al. How to improve organ donation: results of the ISHLT/FACT poll. *J Heart Lung Transplant.* 2003; 22(4):389–410.

51. Siminoff LA, Mercer MB. Public policy, public opinion, and consent for organ donation. *Camb Q Healthc Ethics.* 2001; 10(4):377–386.

52. Batten HL, Prottas JM. Kind strangers: the families of organ donors. *Health Affairs.* 1987; 6(2):35–47.

53. Peters TG, Kittur DS, McGaw LJ, Roy MR, Nelson EW. Organ donors and nondonors: an American dilemma. *Arch Intern Med.* 1996; 156(21):2419–2424.

54. Boulware LE, Troll MU, Wang NY, Powe NR. Public attitudes toward incentives for organ donation: a national study of different racial/ethnic and income groups. *Am J Transplant.* 2006; 6(11):2774–2785.

55. Jasper JD, Nickerson CA, Ubel PA, Asch DA. Altruism, incentives, and organ donation: attitudes of the transplant community. *Med Care.* 2004; 42(4): 378–386.

56. Gandalf Group, for the Trillium Gift of Life Network. Public Opinion Research for a Campaign to Promote Registration. 2009. http://www.giftoflife.on.ca. Accessed April 29, 2012.

57. Schweda M, Schicktanz S. Public ideas and values concerning the commercialization of organ donation in four European countries. *Soc Sci Med.* 2009; 68(6):1129–1136.

58. Schweda M, Wohlke S, Schicktanz S. Understanding public skepticism toward organ donation and its commercialization: the important role of reciprocity. *Transplant Proc.* 2009; 41(6): 2509–2511.

59. Organ Procurement and Transplantation Network. Policy 3.5. Organ Distribution: Allocation of Deceased Kidneys. http://optn.transplant.hrsa.gov/PoliciesandBylaws2/policies/pdfs/policy_7.pdf. Accessed March 3, 2012.

60. United Network for Organ Sharing. Living Donation: Information You Need to Know. 2009. http://www.unos.org/docs/Living_Donation.pdf. Accessed March 3, 2012.

61. Schmidt VH, Lim CH. Organ transplantation in Singapore: history, problems and policies. *Soc Sci Med.* 2004; 59(10): 2173–2182.

62. Teo B. Organs for transplantation: the Singapore experience. *Hastings Cent Rep.* 1991; 21(6):10–13.

63. Iyer TK. Kidneys for transplant—"opting out" law in Singapore. *Forensic Sci Int.* 1987; 35(2–3):131–140.

64. Singapore, Sixth Parliament, 2nd Session. Report of the Select Committee on the Human Organ Transplant Bill (Bill No. 26/86) Presented to Parliament on 22 April 1987. Singapore: Singapore National Printers; 1987.

65. Tan EKB. Keeping God in place: the management of religion in Singapore. In: Lai AE, ed. *Religious Diversity in Singapore.* Singapore: Institute of Southeast Asian Studies; 2008: 55–82.

66. Abu Bakar M. NKF: "Our resources are being drained." *The Straits Times.* September 23, 1993:5.

67. Abu Bakar M. Include Muslims in organ transplant act. *The Straits Times.* September 23, 1993:L4.

68. Nirmala M. Muslims must give kidney issue top priority: Abdullah. *The Straits Times.* January 30, 1994:23.

69. Nirmala M. Don't let prejudices undermine Muslim community's needs. *The Straits Times.* February 20, 1994:16.

70. Ng J. Include us in transplant act: Muslims. *The Straits Times.* January 31, 2003.

71. Gal I. Heart recipient's father: We'll never donate organs. Ynet News. January 29, 2009. http://www.ynetnews.com/articles/0,7340,L-3663653,00.html. Accessed March 3, 2012.

72. Heller A. In Israel, a radical way to boost organ supply: experiment aims to broaden donor pool by enforcing the "Golden Rule." Associated Press. March 14, 2010.

73. http://www.msnbc.msn.com/id/35842049/ns/health-health_care. Accessed March 3, 2012.

74. Freedman S. Saving a life trumps dogma: the principle of saving a life is paramount in Jewish law—so why are ultra-orthodox Jews still opposed to organ donation? *The Guardian.* June 4, 2010. http://www.guardian.co.uk/commentisfree/belief/2010/jun/04/jewish-organ-donation. Accessed March 3, 2012.

75. Israel's organ donation law [transcript]. The World. Public Radio International. January 22, 2010. http://www.theworld.org/2010/01/israels-organ-donation-law. Accessed March 3, 2012.

76. Lynfield B. Israel offers incentive to organ donors: those who donate will go to the top of the queue if they later need a transplant. *The Independent.* December 18, 2009. http://www.independent.co.uk/news/world/middle-east/israel-offers-incentive-to-organ-donors-1844269.html. Accessed March 3, 2012.

77. Rodrigue JR, Cornell DL, Howard RJ. Relationship of exposure to organ donation information to attitudes, beliefs, and donation decisions of next of kin. *Prog Transplant.* 2009; 19(2): 173–179.

78. Morgan M, Mayblin M, Jones R. Ethnicity and registration as a kidney donor: the significance of identity and belonging. *Soc Sci Med.* 2008; 66(1):147–158.

79. Padela AI, Rasheed S, Warren GJ, Choi H, Mathur AK. Factors associated with positive attitudes toward organ donation in Arab Americans. *Clin Transplant.* 2011; 25(5):800–808.

80. American Red Cross. Donating Blood: Benefits of Donation. http://www.redcrossblood.org/donating-blood. Accessed March 4, 2012.

81. Bednall TC, Bove LL. Donating blood: a meta-analytic review of self-reported motivators and deterrents. *Transfus Med Rev.* 2011; 25(4):317–334.

82. Sanner MA. People's attitudes and reactions to organ donation. *Mortality.* 2006; 11(2):133–150.

Chapter 26

The Use of Prisoners as Sources of Organs—An Ethically Dubious Practice

Arthur L. Caplan

Abstract

The movement to try to close the ever-widening gap between demand and supply of organs has recently arrived at the prison gate. While there is enthusiasm for using executed prisoners as sources of organs, there are both practical barriers and moral concerns that make it unlikely that proposals to use prisoners will or should gain traction. Prisoners are generally not healthy enough to be a safe source of organs, execution makes the procurement of viable organs difficult, and organ donation post-execution ties the medical profession too closely to the act of execution.

Strategies for Finding More Organ Donors

The push to find more organs to transplant has led to some very novel ideas. Some cities have decided to send out specially equipped "donor" ambulances to follow regular ambulances. When someone dies outside of a hospital and is pronounced dead by the first ambulance team, a second team can be called in from the trailing donor ambulance, try to get consent from any available family member to attach the corpse to life support, and then transport the body back to a place capable of carrying out procurement. Initially this strategy will only be used when a newly dead person is known to be an organ donor by an advance directive or other means, but the plan is to eventually extend the effort to all newly deceased persons who die outside a hospital, using surrogate consent (New York Organ Donor Network 2010). Still others have proposed routinely offering kidney donation to anyone undergoing elective surgery (Testa et al. 2009). And some procurement teams argue that advance directives regarding termination of life support should never interfere with the possibility of donation (DeVita and Caplan 2007).

The movement to try to close the ever-widening gap between demand and supply of organs by creative strategies has recently arrived at the prison gate. While there is some enthusiasm for using prisoners as sources of organs, there are both practical barriers and moral concerns that make it likely that the use of prisoners will not contribute in any significant way to relieving the problem of organ shortage.

Calls for the Use of Organs from Executed Prisoners

There has been a renewed interest in the use of organs from death-row inmates, as reflected in an editorial in the New York Times written by a death-row inmate, Christian Longo (2011). He wrote that he was in prison in Oregon as a consequence of having killed his wife and three children. He said he had reached the point where he wished not to make any further appeals of his conviction. What he hopes is that after he is put to death he can donate his organs. But prison authorities have rejected his request.

Longo says there are others on death row who want to donate after execution. He has started a movement to insure he and they have the chance to exercise what he claims is his right to donate: "I am seeking nothing but the right to determine what happens to my body once the state has carried out its sentence" (Longo 2011).

Longo has attracted some support for his idea of using executed prisoners as sources of organs (Wood 2011). Longo's idea is not original. Efforts to obtain organs from executed prisoners have attracted attention for many years (Patton 1995; Bartz 2005).

Use of Living Prisoners as Organ Sources in Exchange for Parole or Reduction in Sentence

In January 2011, Mississippi Governor Haley Barbour freed two sisters from life sentences in jail for an $11 armed robbery on the condition that one donate a kidney to the other. Given the offer of parole, Gladys Scott agreed to be a donor for her sister Jamie, who requires dialysis. Barbour was not apparently convinced of the sisters' innocence or meritorious conduct while serving their sentences in prison. He said a key reason for his decision to order the sisters' release was that Jamie Scott's kidney dialysis and treatment was a financial burden on the state of Mississippi (Williams 2011).

In 2007 a state legislator in South Carolina proposed a law to shorten prison sentences in exchange for kidney or bone-marrow donation. State Senator Ralph Anderson proposed bills that would release prisoners 60 days for donating bone marrow and another that would give good-behavior credit of up to 180 days to "any inmate who performs a particularly meritorious or humanitarian act," which Anderson said would include living kidney donation (O'Reilly 2007).

So, do either of these strategies to seek organs from prisoners, dead or living, pass muster either practically or ethically?

Obstacles to Cadaver Donation by Executed Prisoners: Practical and Moral

The Number of Potential Organ Donors Is Very Small

The practice of capital punishment remains ethically controversial. A tiny minority of the world's nations still retain this form of punishment. Some countries that permit capital punishment have not executed any prisoner for many years.

The majority of all executions in the world happen in China, with approximately 5000 per year. Iran, with about 400 per year, is the second highest executioner. No other countries regularly execute more than 100 people per year. The only other countries that regularly execute more than 10 people per year are Iraq, Saudi Arabia, the United States, and Yemen.

As of February 2011 there were 60 federal prisoners in the United States on death row (http://www.deathpenaltyinfo.org/federal-death-row-prisoners). Since the reinstatement of the federal death penalty in 1988, 68 defendants have been sentenced to death. Three have been executed. Six had their death sentence removed.

Thirty-four states permit the death penalty for nonfederal crimes. In 2010, there were 46 executions, down from a peak of 98 in 1999. That number may well decline in the future due to problems raised concerning the manner in which executions are currently conducted.

Many challenges and appeals have been mounted in recent years to execution, protesting the mode of execution used as cruel. This has led to court-ordered stays of all executions in some states. Other states may abandon capital punishment in light of difficulties in obtaining drugs that courts deem necessary for humane execution (Belluck 2011). So the pool of potential candidates may grow even smaller in the future.

Not only are the numbers of potential donors small, but many prisoners would not be eligible to serve as donors due to age, ill health, obesity, or communicable disease. The average time between sentencing and any execution is 10.6 years (Baltimore Sun 2011). This means that executed prisoners are often in their fifties or older, greatly reducing their potential to serve as sources of organs. Inmates engage in drug-related and sexual risk behaviors, and the transmission of HIV, hepatitis, and sexually transmitted diseases occurs at high rates in correctional facilities. The prevalence of HIV and other infectious diseases, whether acquired prior to or during imprisonment, is much higher among inmates than among those in the general community. The burden of disease among inmates is also disproportionately high (Hammett 2006; Kuehn 2010). Those in prison for long periods of time are more likely to become infected with communicable diseases that would either disqualify them as donors or make their organs a high risk for recipients.

Even if one presumes the willingness of all those sentenced to death in the United States to donate, the actual number of executions diminishes the maximum pool of possible donees to roughly 40 to 50 persons per year. That number is declining. Presuming some of those on death row would not be willing to be donors and that others would be medically ineligible due to age or ill health, the use of prisoners as cadaver organ donors cannot yield anything more than a tiny number of organs for those in need.

Ethical opposition to capital punishment is strong and further compromises proposals to use executed prisoners as sources.

Efforts to abolish capital punishment remain vigorous in the United States and around the world. In the United States, fears of false conviction reinforce efforts to do away with the death penalty. The Innocence Project reports 267 post-conviction exonerations in the United States using DNA evidence since 1989. Of these, 17 were prisoners on death row (http://www.innocenceproject.org/Content/Facts_on_PostConviction_DNA_Exonerations.php).

Critics of the practice may see linking organ procurement to execution as increasing the image or social acceptability of capital punishment. The introduction of organ procurement into executions also raises concerns that prosecutors, judges, or juries may be more likely to insist on the death penalty, knowing that lives might be saved.

Opponents of the use of executed prisoners are likely to be very concerned about the impact of legalization in the United States on other nations, since such a move may make it more difficult to condemn controversial international practices involving the execution of persons in order to obtain their organs. Allegations persist of the involuntary and brutal execution and then immediate harvesting of "prisoners" in China (Matas and Kilgour 2010).

Some of those executed may have been

imprisoned for religious or political activities (Matas and Kilgour 2010). Any legitimation of the use of executed prisoners in the United States may make it more difficult to protest cruel and unjust execution practices in other nations.

Yet another moral problem confronting the use of executed prisoners is the role that physicians and health care workers ought play with respect to executions (Caplan 2007). Many maintain that physicians should play no role whatsoever in the process, and some include in this even the pronouncement of death at an execution. This is the position of many national medical associations (American College of Physicians [ACP] 1994; American Medical Association [AMA] 2010; World Medical Association [WMA] 2005). It is not clear whether the professional groups that condemn physician or health care worker involvement with executions would deem it ethical to be involved with organ procurement after an execution has been completed. It is clear that they would not condone any change in the practice of execution in order to achieve procurement (ACP 1994; AMA 2010; WMA 2005).

Putting aside the controversy over the morality of the practice and the permissibility of health care workers involvement with executions, the use of prisoners as cadaver donors is made even more difficult by the complexity, practical and moral, of procurement in the setting of an execution.

Cadaver Donation Would Be Difficult to Achieve Using Executed Prisoners

A large number of methods of execution including electrocution, hanging, and firing squad make organ procurement impossible. However, nearly all executions in the United States are by lethal injection.

Typically, three drugs are used in lethal injection: sodium thiopental is used to induce unconsciousness; pancuronium bromide (Pavulon) is used to cause muscle paralysis and respiratory arrest; and these are followed by potassium chloride to stop the heart. In the past 3 years, two states have used a single-drug execution protocol using only sodium thiopental. The only American company that made this drug stopped manufacturing it due to its use in executions, leading to shortages that have delayed executions.

The primary obstacle to utilizing organs from executed prisoners is that the prisoners do not die on life support. This means that donation must be accomplished using protocols developed from donation after cardiac determination of death without life support. Prisoners would be treated as if they were controlled DCDD (donation after cardiac determination of death) donors. This category refers to patients in intensive care units with nonsurvivable injuries who have treatment withdrawn and a transplant team present to immediately try to retrieve organs after monitored cardiac arrest has occurred.

Hearts cannot be used after a non-life-support death. If the liver, kidneys, or lungs are felt to be suitable for transplantation, the donor in a hospital setting is taken directly to an operating room after cardiac arrest, and, after a waiting period of up to 5 minutes depending on the protocol in place at the hospital, a rapid retrieval operation is performed. The outcomes for kidneys post DCDD procurement seem comparable to those obtained from persons who die on life support. Outcomes for livers and lungs are less certain.

Part of the problem in trying to carry out DCDD recovery from executed prisoners is the extent to which the legal and practical requirements of the execution would diminish the likelihood of successful DCDD procurement. Executions take place in prisons, not hospitals. Most executions involve at least 10 to 15 minutes of examination prior to a final pronouncement of death (http://www.txexecutions.org). If the usual DCDD protocols involving additional waiting time post death to insure death has occurred were to be applied and if, since most prisons lack a facility where DCDD procurement could safely be done, bodies will likely have to be moved to another location, the time involved could well make DCDD procurement impossible. Given these practical challenges, it is likely that only kidneys may be safely used.

This scenario also presumes medical teams would be willing to be involved in the requisite proceedings. The ethics of involvement in monitoring a patient post execution, the use of interventions to preserve organs either prior to, during, or right after the execution, and participating in the movement of the body from the execution chamber to a surgical suite raise issues of complicity with the execution that may violate professional norms. Moreover, the number of physicians and nurses willing to be publicly associated with these activities, given that executions are witnessed events, is likely to prove extraordinarily small. Potential recipients may not be willing to accept organs from executed prisoners, knowing the risks involved (Halpern et al. 2008), or simply out of ethical concerns that they do not want organs from a person executed for terrible crimes.

Could Organ Removal Be Used as the Mode of Execution?

It might be possible to shift the location of executions into hospitals or clinics in order to increase the chance of a successful procurement of more organs. Prisoners might be anesthetized and have their organs removed by a medical team before they are dead. I have dubbed the notion of execution by means of the removal of the heart or other vital organs the "Mayan protocol" after the Mayan practice of human sacrifice by removing a beating heart during certain religious rituals (Wood 2008). It is, however, morally repugnant to involve physicians as executioners or to shift the setting of punishment from prison to hospital. Involvement in causing death in any way is a direct violation of the "dead donor" rule, which has long been maintained as a bright line between death and donation in order to insure public trust and support for cadaver donation (DeVita and Caplan 2007). This principle would even restrict efforts to maximize the likelihood of procurement by the use of drugs and cold perfusion as steps prior to execution.

Donation Undercuts the Morality of Execution

The point of capital punishment is to achieve retribution for terrible crimes. It is also, proponents argue, a deterrent. If either justification is to hold, then is organ donation likely to be compatible with these reasons?

Retribution may be made far more difficult to achieve as families and friends of victims watch as executed perpetrators are lauded in their final days by possible recipients and the media for their altruism in saving lives. Some may find redemption acceptable (Wang and Wang 2010) if it saves lives, but given the horrific nature of the crimes that lead to execution, relatives and friends of victims are not likely to be among them.

Consider Christian Longo, the prisoner behind the movement to permit organ donation post-execution. What were his specific crimes? He killed his wife MaryJane, 34, and children Zachery, 4, Sadie, 3, and Madison,

2. Longo strangled MaryJane and Madison, stuffed their bodies in suitcases, and threw them in a bay. Then he drove Zachery and Sadie to a nearby bridge, tied rocks to their legs, and tossed them into the water to drown. He said he did it because his family was hindering his lifestyle. After the murders he fled to Mexico, where he engaged in a variety of cons and swindles until he was caught. In prison he has made money by writing explicit sex letters to gay men, who pay him for the raw prose (Smith 2011).

Longo now seeks redemption through being an organ donor. If the moral basis for his execution is retribution for his horrific acts, then how is any redemptive gesture on his part consistent with the retributive intent of capital execution (Hill 2009)?

Similarly, the deterrent effect of execution may wane if social good is seen as issuing from the practice. While the needs of those awaiting transplants are real, the aim of the penal system is not to serve medical needs but to achieve justice for those wronged and their families and friends, as well as to deter future crimes. Mitigating the horror of execution by permitting organ donation is not consistent with the deterrent purpose of execution.

Giving the state a motivation to execute beyond retribution or deterrence may be seen as inconsistent with protecting prisoners' rights. Creating the possibility of organ donation may provide an incentive to prisoners or their legal teams to prematurely abandon efforts to appeal death-penalty decisions, particularly if prisoners believe they may be able to expiate their crime and be remembered in a positive manner as a result of donation.

Nor is it true, contrary to Longo's claim (Longo 2011), that being an organ donor is a right. Organ donation is a gift that neither organ procurement agencies nor anyone else is bound to accept. Even freed felons lose their right to vote, to be a party in most lawsuits, to hold public office, and to bear arms, and they suffer restrictions on travel overseas. Why permit prisoners the chance to make posthumous gifts of their bodies if their punishment is in part based on both retribution and their loss of standing within society (Hill 2009)?

The practical and ethical problems facing the use of executed prisoners as donors are overwhelming. Despite ongoing interest in their use, there is absolutely no possibility of this strategy moving forward.

Donations from Living Prisoners

Practical Obstacles

In 2008 there were about one and a half million persons in federal and state prisons and another 785,000 in local jails in the United States at some point during the year (Sabol 2009). This large population might be available to provide kidneys and perhaps portions of liver to those in need of these types of transplants.

There are prisoners willing to consider donation, especially to family members. In the past a few prisoners have done so. And prison officials in many states are willing to consider these requests on a case-by-case basis (http://www.tdcj.state.tx.us/policy/policy-home.htm).

The primary practical problem facing living prisoner donation is the ill health and high rate of infectious disease among prisoners (Hinkle 2002). In the case of the sisters in Mississippi where the governor granted parole on condition of sister-to-sister donation, no donation took place. The would-be donor was too obese to be able to safely donate. The risk factors for prisoners are significant enough that they require special consent requirements to be used in approaching potential recipients to inform them of the dangers of accepting a kidney or lobe of liver from this source (Singer et al. 2008; Halpern et al. 2008; Kucirka et al. 2009).

Ethical Concerns over Use of Living Prisoners

The issue of living donation from prisoners is made morally complex when various incentives or rewards such as parole, reduction in sentence, or the extension of privileges are associated with making an organ available. Federal law prohibits making organs available for "valuable consideration" (NOTA 1984). Arguably, giving a prisoner parole or a reduction in sentence on condition of giving a kidney to another is a form of valuable compensation. That is how various national (UNOS [United Network for Organ Sharing] Ethics Committee 2009) and international groups (Zhiyong 2007) interpret policies that reward prisoners who give up organs for rewards.

In addition to worries about compensation, the question of free choice clouds the issue of prisoner consent (WMA 2005). Many maintain that prisoners cannot consent freely, given the nature of the environment in which they live. The vulnerability of prisoners in terms of coercion and manipulation is explicitly acknowledged in their categorization as a special population for whom informed consent may be compromised in regulations governing prisoner participation in research (National Institutes of Health [NIH] 2011). The ability to comprehend the facts about donation and to make a voluntary choice must be carefully weighed on a case-by-case basis if voluntary consent is to remain a key component for obtaining organs from all living persons.

In most programs for living donors a donor advocate is appointed, a psychological assessment is undertaken, and the donee is made aware that he or she may change his or her mind about donation at any time prior to the actual act. These steps would have to be in place for a vulnerable population such as prisoners, and those carrying them out ought not have a connection to the corrections system, to minimize any possibility of coercion or manipulation.

The arguments against allowing prisoners to donate organs—kidney, liver, or bone marrow—while alive are not as persuasive as the practical and ethical issues raised by cadaver donation from executed prisoners. Still, as the case in Mississippi shows, a decision to commute a sentence conditioned on making an organ available for reasons of cost may well backfire. A high degree of ill health among prisoners, alongside issues around the acceptability of compensation, and the problematic nature of consent by those who are incarcerated make this practice one that needs to be carefully regulated and assessed on a case-by-case basis. Direct promises of reward will have to be replaced by a willingness to consider generous acts as a part of parole decisions without any guarantees. As such, while lives may be saved, living prisoners are not likely to provide a significant source of organs for those in need.

References

American College of Physicians. 1994. *Breach of trust: Physicians participations in executions in the United States.* Available at: http://www.hrw.org/reports/1994 /usdp/index.htm

American Medical Association. 2010. Code of Medical Ethics, Opinion 2.06—Capital punishment. Available at http://www.amaassn.org/ama/pub/physi cian-resources/medical-ethics/code-medical-ethics /opinion206.page

Baltimore Sun. 2011. Death penalty's cruel toll on victims. Available at: http://articles.baltimoresun.com/2011–02–27/news/bs-ed-death-penalty-20110227-1_john-booth-el-capital-punishment-death-row/2

Bartz, C. 2005. Prisoners and organ donation. Available at: http://findarticles.com/p/articles/miqa4100/is200512/ain15957681

Belluck, P. 2011. *What's in a lethal injection cocktail*. Available at: http://www.nytimes.com/2011/04/10/weekinreview/10injection.html?_r=1&ref=todayspaper

Caplan, A. L. 2007. Should physicians participate in capital punishment? *Mayo Clinic Proceedings* 82(9): 1047–1048.

DeVita, M., and A. L. Caplan. 2007. Caring for organs or for patients? Ethical concerns about the Uniform Anatomical Gift Act. *Annals of Internal Medicine* 147:876–879.

Halpern, S., A. Shaked, R. Hasj, and A. L. Caplan. 2008. Informing candidates for solid-organ transplantation about donor risk factors. *New England Journal of Medicine* 358: 2832–2837.

Hammett, T. M. 2006. HIV/AIDS and other infectious diseases among correctional inmates: Transmission, burden, and an appropriate response. *American Journal of Public Health* 96:974–978.

Hill, T., ed. 2009. *The Blackwell guide to Kant's ethics*. Malden, MA: Wiley-Blackwell.

Hinkle, W. 2002. Giving until it hurts: Prisoners are not the answer to the national organ shortage. *Indiana Law Review* 35:593–619.

Kucirka, L. M., R. Namuyinga, C. Hanrahan, R. A. Montgomery, and D. L. Sege. 2009. Formal policies and special informed consent are associated with higher provider utilization of CDC high-risk donor organs. *American Journal of Transplantation* 9:629–635.

Longo, C. 2011. Giving life after death row. Available at: http://www.nytimes.com/2011/03/06/opinion/06longo.html?partner = rss&emc = rss.

Kuehn, B. M. 2010. Inmates with HIV. *Journal of the American Medical Association* 304:1685.

Matas, D., and D. Kilgour. 2010. *Bloody harvest: The killing of Falun Gong for their organs*. Woodstock, Ontario: Seraphim.

National Institutes of Health. 2011. *Research involving vulnerable populations*. Available at: http://grants.nih.gov/grants/policy/hs/prisoners.htm

New York Organ Donor Network. 2010. New York City pilot program expands organ recovery to at-home deaths. Available at: http://www.donatelifeny.org/news-events/news/news-newyork-city-pilot-program-expands-organ-recovery-to-at-homedeaths/#bloom donate.

National Organ Transplant Act. 1984. *Public Law 98–507*. Enacted October 19. Statutes at Large 98: 2339–2348.

Patton, L. 1995. A call for common sense: Organ donation and the executed prisoner. *Virginia Journal of Social Policy & the Law* 3:387–434.

O'Reilly, K. 2007. Prisoner organ donation proposal worrisome. *AMA News*. Available at: http://www.amaassn.org/amednews/2007/04/09/prsb0409.htm

Sabol, W. J., H. C. West, and M. Cooper. 2009. *Bureau of Justice Statistics, Prisoners in 2008*, p.8. Washington, DC: US Department of Justice, NCJ228417. Available at: http://bjs.ojp.usdoj.gov/content/pub/pdf/p08.pdf

Singer, A. L., L. M. Kucirka, R. H. C. Namuyinga, A. K. Subramanian, and D. L. Segev. 2008. The high risk donor: Viral infections in solid organ transplantation. *Current Opinion in Organ Transplantation* 13:400–404.

Smith, W. 2011. Christian Longo's latest con. Available at: http://www.nationalreview.com/corner/261598/christian-longos-latest-con-wesley-j-smith.

Testa, G., P. Angelos, M. Crowley-Matoka, and M. Siegler. 2009. Elective surgical patients as living organ donors: A clinical and ethical innovation. *American Journal of Transplantation* 9(10):2400–2405.

UNOS [United Network for Organ Sharing] Ethics Committee. 2009. Who we are. *UNOS* 7 May 2009. Available at http://www.unos.org/whoWeAre

Wang, M., and X. Wang. 2010. Organ donation by capital prisoners in China. *Journal of Medicine and Philosophy* 35(2):197–212.

Williams, T. 2011. Jailed sisters are released for kidney transplant. *New York Times*. Available at: http://www.nytimes".com/2011/01/08/us/08sisters.html

Wood, G. 2008. *Let's harvest the organs of death-row inmates*. Available at: http://www.good.is/post/lets-harvest-the-organsof-death-row-inmates-777

World Medical Association. 2005. *Resolution on organ donation in China*. http://www.wma.net/en/30publications/10policies/30council/cr5

Zhiyong, C. 2007. *Group pledges restriction on prisoner's organ donation*. Available at: http://tianjin.chinadaily.com.cn/china/2007-10/09/content 6158754.htm

Chapter 27

AN EXCERPT FROM

Presumed Consent to Organ Donation in Three European Countries

Barbara L. Neades

Abstract

United Kingdom Transplant reported that, during 2007–2008, a total of 7655 people were awaiting a transplant; however, only 3235 organs were available via the current 'opt in' approach. To address this shortfall, new UK legislation sought to increase the number of organs available for donation. The Chief Medical Officer for England and Wales supports the adoption of 'presumed consent' legislation, that is, an 'opt out' approach, as used in much of Europe. Little research, however, has explored the impact on bereaved relatives, nurses and medical staff of introducing presumed consent legislation. Adopting a phenomenological approach, this study used responses to an initial questionnaire combined with selected interviews with health care professionals to capture their direct experience of presumed consent legislation in three European countries: Portugal, Norway and Belgium.

Introduction

Published reports have suggested that 65–90% of the UK population is in favour of organ donation (1–3). The Human Tissue Act 2004 (England and Wales) (4) and the Human Tissue (Scotland) Act 2006 (5) are designed to facilitate the donation of parts of the body of a deceased person for the purposes of transplantation, research, education or training, and audit, provided the deceased had authorized this prior to his or her death, either in writing or verbally. In the UK, organ donation is viewed as a voluntary beneficent act undertaken by an individual with the intention of improving the health of another. A fundamental principle of this is the requirement of evidence of individual consent to donation. This 'opt in' system allows people to choose to donate their organs and record their consent to organ donation by completing a donor card or by placing their name on the NHS National Donor Register. Despite these strategies, there continues to be a considerable shortfall in the number of organs available for transplant. In an effort to improve this situation, some European countries have introduced presumed consent legislation (PCL) (6–10). This approach presumes that most individuals are in favour of organ donation and would wish to be donors in the event of their sudden death. Under the terms of this 'opt out' system, if there is no indication of objection to donation, individuals' organs can be procured for transplant.

Perceptions of Organ Donation and Presumed Consent Legislation

The British Medical Association supports moves to introduce this legislation, suggesting that it would increase the number of organs available for transplant (11). The BBC reported that 61% of a survey population were in favour of the introduction of PCL in the UK (12). Others have suggested that it could increase the numbers of organs for donation but create considerable ethical dilemmas for health care professionals (HCPs) and society. These could result in conflict arising between the need to increase organ numbers and the potential harm to the rights of individuals to determine the fate of their body, with further potential harm to bereaved families (13, 14). Public perception of the organ donation system is an important element in any strategy. A report from the House of Lords highlights the public's increasing mistrust of HCPs in this area, citing earlier controversy surrounding the retention of children's organs as an example (15). Debate continues, however, about the benefits and implications of adopting PCL, and a Department of Health task force was established to explore the benefits and challenges of using this approach (3).

Consent to Donation

Controversy exists surrounding the nature of consent that allows organ donation to proceed. Price (16) acknowledged the fundamental ideal that autonomy in health care should be expressed in consent, normally demonstrated by written instructions. Prottas and Batten supported this view, stating that the principles of informed consent and encouraged voluntarism that underpin the act of organ donation are vital and cannot be overlooked (17). Beauchamp and Childress, (18) however, highlighted that another form of consent exists, namely tacit or implicit or implied consent, expressed silently or passively by omission. Price (16) also noted that using presumed consent as a form of consent is unusual, highlighting that silence is not recognized as consent in most other legal contexts. Nursing and medical practice normally require formal written consent from patients for any invasive procedures to be undertaken. This raises the question of whether the lack of an objection to donation can be viewed as consent to or authorization of this procedure by individuals. Other authors have challenged the validity of using tacit or implied consent in organ donation, arguing that implied consent in this situation is consent by default (19–21). They further question if this can actually be regarded as consent, suggesting that it represents an erosion of individuals' right to determine the outcome of their organs after death. They caution that using tacit consent may in due course impact on other rights to autonomous informed decision making and create a 'slippery slope,' with people feeling that they are state owned commodities with little autonomy. Some go further, suggesting that consent provided by default when no evidence of a deceased person's agreement or objection to organ donation exists is ethically unsustainable (22, 23).

Beauchamp and Childress (18) do, however, clarify that this form of consent can be acceptable if it can be demonstrated that the individuals concerned were fully informed of the need to consent or object to an action and also fully aware of the consequences. This suggests that, in order for presumed consent to be valid, evidence of deceased persons' prior knowledge of the law concerning organ donation and the necessary actions in relation to this legislation are required. If there is no evidence that tacit or implied consent exists or that deceased persons were aware of the law and the need to record their consent or objection, then the practice of removing organs under presumed consent perhaps expropriates those organs without any regard to consent. This underlines the need for public education for presumed consent to be valid.

Trust in Health Care Professionals

Public confidence in scientific professionals in the UK is at a low level (15). Any public mistrust in the organ donation system engendered by the introduction of PCL may not only fail to improve the supply of organs for transplant but may also reduce the numbers currently available. This could in turn produce professional and legal consequences for nurses and other HCPs. Few data exist concerning families' knowledge or public understanding of organ donation concepts prior to them being involved in this experience (24). Both Robertson (25) and Koppelman (26) suggested that confusion about definitions of death also results in misunderstandings between HCPs in relation to organ donation practices. The reported public fear that organ harvesting could start prior to people being pronounced dead (27) raises questions about exactly what members of the public understand concerning organ donation.

Impact of Organ Donation on Families

Opinions are divided on the benefits and problems of families being involved in decision making about organ donation. Gore *et al* (28) stressed that the level of support provided by HCPs at the time was very important in facilitating both family members'

understanding of the procedure for diagnosing brain death and their decision to consider a relative as an organ donor. If this level of support is not provided, family objections to organ donation may increase. Haddow (29) supported this view, suggesting that negative beliefs in relation to donation and lack of understanding of organ donation procedures led to mistrust of HCPs and underpinned families' refusal to allow organ donation to proceed. Others warn of potential harm to families if they are asked to make a decision about organ donation very soon after being informed of the sudden death of a relative (30, 31). In recognizing the potential detrimental impact on bereaved families involved in the decision-making process in organ donation, Sque and Payne (32) demonstrated the need for these families to be approached and supported by appropriately trained HCPs when a request for donation is made. At the time of the donation, bereaved families also have to be provided with appropriate information concerning their need to discuss and understand the concepts of brain death and organ donation, and allowed time to come to terms with these. The importance of education programmes to prepare HCPs to undertake this complex role has been highlighted by a number of observers (33–35).

Rationale for the Research Study

Existing literature describes the impact of opt in approaches to organ donation on professionals and families, but little has been published to explore the impact of opt out legislation on the families of deceased persons or on the professionals involved. This lack of data detailing the potential impact of this approach to organ donation was viewed as an important omission in the debate in the UK.

This study therefore sought to capture the experiences of these professionals by identifying the implications for both them and bereaved families of using this legislative framework.

. . .

Discussion

Given the formats of PCL in the three countries included in this study, it could be argued that a form of tacit or implied consent (18) is being adopted to facilitate organ donation. Individuals who have not expressed their views either positively or negatively in relation to donation have therefore done so silently or passively by their omission to register an objection. Organ donation in the UK is based on expressed consent, with recruitment to the organ donation register relying on altruistic behaviour of individuals in society and a public understanding of organ donation. United Kingdom Transplant has reported a considerable proportion of the UK population being in favour of organ donation; (3) however, this does not result in large numbers registering as organ donors. This may be a product of apathy concerning the need for organ donation, lack of knowledge, or public mistrust of the system. A public education strategy aimed at improving knowledge and understanding of concepts such as brain death, combined with knowledge of the appropriate legislation, is therefore required. A national strategy to improve the public's understanding of organ donation and increase the numbers of people placing their names on the register has been implemented (12). These initiatives need to be expanded if a greater awareness of organ donation is to be achieved.

The evidence provided by the participants that families in the countries studied are asked to confirm the view of deceased persons in relation to donation is an interesting finding. In addition to raising questions concerning the validity of families' response as a basis for proceeding to organ donation, this finding demonstrates that there is a dissonance between the legislation and its interpretation by HCPs. It would appear that HCPs do not apply the full tenets of the legislation. Rather, they use the legislation as a guide to practice until the decision to progress to organ donation is verified by families. The role and function of registers of consent or objection as a means of authorization for HCPs to proceed to organ donation therefore require to be considered further.

The application of PCL is often facilitated by the use of registers of objection. Although these may provide a method for competent individuals to record their consent or objection to donation, questions remain about the protection of incapacitated and vulnerable persons from automatically being identified as donors resulting from their inability to record an objection. If PCL were to be applied in the UK, a systematic infrastructure for recording individual objection to organ donation would require to be established. Vulnerable or incapacitated people would have to be protected. This would potentially require a review of all individuals over the age of consent who would be considered exempt, such as persons with severe mental health problems, those with severe learning difficulties or who do not speak English well enough to comprehend the legislation. Such people would have to be identified and considered as automatically exempt from the legislation. Even if these data could be collected, a regular system of updating would be needed to maintain a 'live' register. The organizational and financial implications of establishing such a system would be huge and would need to be explored before a change in legislation could be considered. Practical aspects on how transplant co-ordinators, often but not exclusively nurses in the UK, would appropriately access and use this information also requires to be examined.

The routine involvement of families in decision making in organ donation despite the legislation in place in Portugal, Norway and Belgium had not previously been identified or publicized. This supports the findings of a study in France that found HCPs did not use the full powers of the legislation but allowed families' views to influence their decision to progress to organ donation (42). In Portugal and Norway, objections raised by families veto any agreement to donation recorded previously by the donor. Only in Belgium was a positive decision to donate recorded by the deceased person in life upheld regardless of family opposition.

Thus, despite any intention recorded by the deceased person, it could be said that families are used as a method of proxy authorization or refusal for organ donation. Allowing families to object to organ donation in this manner if the deceased person has indicated a wish to donate poses questions concerning individuals' right to determine what happens to their body after death. The need to respect the wishes of dead persons while also respecting the wishes of their families presented a dilemma for the HCP participants. The view expressed by some participants was that families were able to represent deceased relatives' wishes in relation to organ donation. Without concrete evidence of deceased persons' views, however, this assertion is difficult to support. The role of families in representing their deceased relatives' wishes and the validity of any consent given by families to proceed to organ donation therefore requires to be clarified.

Questions also arise concerning the ra-

tionale behind HCPs seeking families' authorization to proceed to organ donation and in relation to the potential benefits and problems for family involvement. It could be said that seeking the views of families, unless this aspect is required under legislation, cannot establish deceased persons' previously expressed views in relation to organ donation. This practice may instead seek authorization to proceed from families in order to prevent the likelihood of challenges being raised later. The implications of involvement of families in the decision-making process to this degree require to be explored in more detail. Their involvement in the decision making may be less challenging than excluding them from the process, but the benefits and consequences of this require to be researched further.

It appears that, according to the participants, when supporting bereaved families involved in organ donation it is vital that HCPs should not only consider the requirement to care for the donors and obtain the organs for donation, but also reflect upon the welfare of their families. The participant HCPs suggested that there is much to be gained by the families, even at this time of bereavement, by ensuring that they are included in the organ donation decision-making process and supported appropriately during the request to authorize donation.

The development of a trusting relationship between HCPs (who are often nurses) and families is crucial to the success of the donation process. If this does not occur there may be detrimental consequences for families and indeed for the organ donation initiative. The participants in this study indicated that this lack of understanding and fear could result in families involved in organ donation objecting, believing that their relative is not dead and is being inappropriately identified as an organ donor. To address this issue, the participants reported the development and application of detailed communication protocols designed to assist families to understand these concepts, decoupling communication of the diagnosis of brain death from the request for them to agree to organ donation. The adoption of these protocols in support of families throughout the donation process had not previously been reported and clearly demonstrates the importance placed by HCPs on ensuring the physical, psychological, emotional and spiritual well-being of families of potential donors, in addition to obtaining organs for donation.

The respondents reported that, if HCPs are to understand the legislation and its application in practice, there is a requirement for them to receive appropriate education. The data revealed that organ donation presents considerable challenges for HCPs in terms of the ethical dilemmas and emotional challenges it presents. The curricula of both nursing and medical undergraduate programmes in all three countries now include some content relating to the fundamental legal and ethical aspects of organ donation. Education on the principles of organ donation legislation is augmented by the availability of continuing professional development, exploring the bioethical aspects of care and using the European Donor Hospital Education Programme, (41) often facilitated and funded by regional organ donation organizations and supported by central government.

In the UK the curricula for both medical and nursing students contain some fundamental preparation relating to legal and ethical aspects of practice. These programmes however often do not explore the bioethical aspects of organ donation. The question arises, therefore, of whether the UK professional bodies would consider the addition of this topic as a compulsory element of preregistration programmes for nurses and doctors. Additionally, the merits of ensuring that education in this practice area forms part of a mandatory requirement for continuing professional development for HCPs in the UK requires review.

Conclusion

The findings identify a number of key issues that would require careful consideration if PCL were to be adopted in the UK, many of which have been supported by the Department of Health task force (3). Of most importance among these is the need to consider the form of consent that would be acceptable to society to allow organ donation under PCL. The HCPs' responses suggest that in their countries the concept of presumed consent in organ donation is well accepted by the public. The strong objections held by some that a change in the UK legislative approach could have much wider ranging consequences do, however, require to be considered carefully. Exploration of the impact on bereaved relatives identified that the current legislation in the three countries studied demonstrated the variable need for the involvement of families in the organ donation process.

Analysis of the participants' responses in Norway, Portugal and Belgium clearly demonstrated that families are always involved in the decision to accept or reject their deceased relative as an organ donor. In particular, the data suggest that families are not only invited to confirm their deceased relative's views on organ donation but, despite the lack of a requirement to do so from a legislative perspective, they are also asked if they hold any personal objection to the procedure. The involvement of bereaved relatives was viewed by the HCPs as a method of confirming the lack of objection to organ donation by the deceased person and a means of protecting vulnerable or incapacitated people from becoming organ donors by default. If family objections were identified, the organ donation process would be halted because, in the opinion of the participants, families' views must be upheld. The data obtained therefore demonstrated a dissonance between the requirements of the legislation and its application by HCPs, resulting from ethical and professional practice considerations. The involvement of families in the decision-making process to this degree has major implications for both legislators and HCPs involved in the care and support of organ donors and their families. Most important among these considerations was the need to support bereaved relatives during the organ donation decision-making process and develop protocols to facilitate this procedure.

It could be said that the involvement of families in the organ donation decision-making process in these European countries is very similar to the process adopted under existing UK legislation (4, 5). Even when evidence exists that the wishes of a deceased person were in favour of organ donation, in the absence of any positive authorization for organ donation by the deceased person, families can be asked to agree to organ donation. Clearly, family members have a fundamental role in the authorization of organ donation in the European countries surveyed and in the UK, irrespective of whether or not PCL is in force.

The analysis of the participants' responses related to the impact of the application of the legislative framework on the relationship between donor families and HCPs suggests that a trusting relationship can be established between these two groups by the provision of public education in relation to the legislation and the concepts surrounding organ donation.

In particular, information relating to the diagnosis of brain death facilitated transparency in clinical practice and reduced public fears that organ donation is being considered at the expense of patient care. This would indicate that in implementing a change in organ donation legislation and, in addition to providing the public with education regarding legal and administration aspects, there is also a need for public understanding of both the technical aspects of organ donation and eligibility for donor status. Any organ donation strategy developed to support families would also require recognition of religious and cultural sensitivities related to this issue in order to establish trust and facilitate successful organ donation. The involvement of families in the organ donation decision-making process also holds considerable implications for the preparation of HCPs to enable them to approach and adequately support families. The potential role of the 'social nurse' as a successful family advocate in organ donation also requires further study.

References

1. NHS Blood and Transplant. *UK transplant activity report 2007–2008*. Bristol: NHSBT, 2008.

2. Department of Health. *Organs for transplants: a report from the Organ Donation Taskforce*. London: DH, 2008.

3. Department of Health. *The potential impact of an opt out system for organ donation in the UK: an independent report from the Organ Donation Taskforce*. London: DH, 2008.

4. *The Human Tissue Act 2004 (England and Wales)*, chapter 30. Retrieved 21 January, 2009, from: http://www.opsi.gov.uk/ACTS/acts2004/ukpga_20040030_en_1

5. *The Human Tissue (Scotland) Act 2006*. Retrieved 21 January, 2009, from: http://www.opsi.gov.uk/legislation/scotland/acts2006/asp_20060004_en_1

6. New B, Solomon M, Dingwall R, McHale J. *A question of give and take: improving the supply of donor organs for transplantation.* (Kings Fund Institute Research Report.) London: Kings Fund, 1994.

7. Roels, L. Opt out registers for organ donation have existed in Belgium since 1987. *BMJ* 1999; 318: 399.

8. Gimbel RA, Strosberg MA, Lehrman SE, Genfenas E, Taft F. Presumed consent and other predictors of cadaveric organ donation in Europe. *Prog Transplant* 2003; 13:17–23.

9. Abadie A, Gray S. *The impact of presumed consent legislation on cadaveric organ donation: a cross country study.* 2004. (NBER Working Group paper no. 10604.) Retrieved 21 January, 2009, from: http://www.nber.org/papers/w10604

10. Coppen R, Friele RD, Marquet RI, Gevers SKM. Opting-out systems: no guarantee for higher donation rates. *Transplant Int* 2005; 18:1275–79.

11. British Medical Association. *Organ donation in the 21st century: time for a consolidated approach.* London: BMA, 2000.

12. British Broadcasting Corporation. Health donation: opt-in or opt-out, a BBC poll. 2007. Retrieved 21 January, 2009, from: http://news.bbc.co.uk/1/hi/health/7051235.stm

13. Kozlowski LM. Case study in identification and maintenance of an organ donor. *Heart Lung* 1998; 17: 366–71.

14. Riley PL, Coolican MB. Needs of families of organ donors: facing death and life. *Crit Care Nurse* 1999; 19(2):53–55.

15. House of Lords: Report of the Science and Technology Committee. (Lord Jenkins of Roding, chairman.) *The relationship between science and society*, third report. London: House of Lords, 2000.

16. Price D. *Legal and ethical aspects of organ transplantation.* Cambridge: Cambridge University Press, 2002.

17. Prottas JM, Batten HL. The willingness to give: the public and the supply of transplantable organs. *J Health Polit Policy Law* 1991; 16:121–34.

18. Beauchamp TL, Childress JF. *Principles of biomedical ethics*, fifth edition. Oxford: Oxford University Press, 2001.

19. Lamb D. *Organ transplants and ethics.* London: Routledge, 1990.

20. Ellis P. Organ donation and presumed consent [Letter]. *Lancet* 1998; 352:151.

21. Hill DJ, Palmer TC, Evans DW. Presumed consent [Letter]. *BMJ* 1999; 318:1490.

22. Gillon R. On giving preference to prior volunteers when allocating organs for transplant. *J Med Ethics* 1995; 21:195–96.

23. Wilks M. Organ donation and presumed consent. *Lancet* 1998; 352:151.

24. Pellitier M. The organ donor family members' perception of stressful situations during the organ donation experience. *J Adv Nurs* 1992; 17:90–97.

25. Robertson JA. Delimiting the donor: the Dead Donor Rule. *Hastings Cent Rep* 1999; 29(6): 6–14.

26. Koppelman ER. The Dead Donor Rule and concepts of death: severing the ties that bind them. *Am J Bioethics* 2003; 3(1): 1–9.

27. English V, Sommerville A. Presumed consent for transplantation: a dead issue after Alder Hey? *J Med Ethics* 2003; 29:147–52.

28. Gore SM, Cable DJ, Holland AJ. Organ donation from ICUs in England and Wales: two-year confidential audit of deaths in intensive care. *BMJ* 1992; 304:349–55.

29. Haddow G. Donor and non-donor families' accounts of communication and relations with healthcare professionals. *Prog Transplant* 2004; 14:41–48.

30. Garrison RN, Bentley FR, Raque GH. There is an answer to the shortage of organ donors. *Surg Gynecol Obstet* 1991; 173:391–96.

31. Niles PA, Mattice C. The timing factor in the consent process. *J Transpl Coord* 1996; 6:84–87

32. Sque M, Payne S eds. *Organ and tissue donation: an evidence base for practice.* Maidenhead: Open University Press, 2007.

33. Singer P, Rachmani R. Improving attitude and knowledge of healthcare professionals towards organ

donation in Israel: results of 12 European donor hospital education programs. *Transplant Proc* 1997; 29: 3244–45.

34. Randhawa G. Specialist nurse training programme dealing with asking for organ donation. *J Am Nurs* 1998; 28:405–408.

35. Verble M, Worth J. Overcoming families' fears and concerns in donation discussion [Progress in transplantation]. *J Transpl Coord* 2000; 10:155–60.

36. Qualitative Software Research International. *Nvivo computerised data management system*. Victoria, Australia: QSR, 2002.

37. Heidegger M. *Being and time*. (Maquarie J, Robinson E trans.) Oxford: Basil Blackwell, 1962.

38. Assembeia da Republica. (Republic Assembly.) Colheita e transplante de organos e tecidos de origem humana. Lei no 12/93. (Law of Portugal: Collection and transplant of organs and tissues of human origin. No. 12/93.) *Quinta-feria I A Serie* 1960–1963; 94 (in Portuguese).

39. Executive Legal Advisory Body of Belgium. *Koninklijk besluit tot regeling van de waarope de donorof de personen betreffende het wegnemen en transplanteren van organen hun will te kennen geven. (Royal decision concerning regulations pertaining to donors or persons making their wishes known for the removal and transplantation of organs.)* Brussels: Department of Justice Public Health and Environment, 1996 (in Dutch).

40. Royal Norwegian Department of Health and Social Services. *Forskiter om dodsdefinisjonen i relasjon til lov om transplantasjon, sykehusobduksjon og avgivelse av lik M.M. (Act relating to transplantation, hospital autopsies and the donation of bodies.)* Oslo: DHSS, 2004 (in Norwegian).

41. European Transplant Co-ordinators Organisation. *The European Donor Hospital Education Programme (EDHEP)*. Retrieved 21 January, 2009, from: http://www.etco.org/certification_transplant.htm

42. Nowenstein Piery G. Organ procurement rates: does presumed consent legislation really make a difference? *Electronic Law Journals LGD,* 2004; 1. Retrieved 21 January, 2009, from: http://www2.warwick.ac.uk /fac/soc/law/elj/lgd/2004_1/nowenstein/

Chapter 28

AN EXCERPT FROM

Kidney Paired Donation 2011

David Serur and Marian Charlton

Abstract

Patients with incompatible live donors have had to resort to the long wait on the deceased donor list. Now, through kidney paired donation, these incompatible pairs can enter a kidney exchange program where kidneys are "swapped" between incompatible pairs. This review highlights the evolution of kidney paired exchange and reviews the challenges and ethical considerations within a paired exchange system.

Kidney paired donation refers to the exchange or "swap" of kidneys between 2 or more incompatible living donor pairs. This type of exchange is commonly done in the context of ABO incompatibility but can also be used in the case of a positive cross-match.

History

Dr Felix Rapaport of New York first put forth the case for a "living emotionally related international kidney donor exchange registry" in 1986 (4). In Korea in 1991, the first donor exchange program was initiated. This program was in a single center and facilitated 129 transplants in an 11-year period (5). A computer program was not used to match up the pairs.

In 2004, the Netherlands started a paired exchange program. Seven centers were involved using a computer-based match program and a central tissue-typing laboratory. The donor traveled to the recipient hospital. The final cross-matches were performed locally and the transplants were simultaneous. This Dutch program facilitated 128 transplants in 5 years (6).

In the United States, donor exchange programs exist as local or regional consortiums (see below).

US paired exchange programs:
Alliance for Paired Donation
National Kidney Registry
New England Program for Kidney Exchange
Paired Donation Network
Johns Hopkins Paired Exchange Program

The Ohio Solid Organ Transplantation Consortium of 6 Ohio transplant centers was founded in 1984 for non-renal organs. This consortium evolved into 2 different organizations: The Paired Donation Network and the Alliance for Paired Donation. Both programs have accrued about 200 incompatible living pairs from many centers in about 30 states. Both together have been able to facilitate about 115 transplants in several years.

In 2005, the New England Paired Kidney

Exchange was formed. A computerized match run occurs every month or so using pairs from 14 regional centers in New England and 5 centers in New Jersey. Seventy-three transplants have occurred since 2005, most of them initiated by a non-directed altruistic donor (7).

The National Kidney Registry (NKR) began operations in 2008 and has facilitated more than 300 transplants since February 2008. Fifty transplant centers in 20 states enroll incompatible patient pairs into the BestMatch computer program at NKR. Match runs occur twice a week. Recipients and donors both state their preferences such as willingness to travel, the preferred age of the donor, the preferred match with the donor, and cytomegalovirus status. The more stringent the preferences, however, the longer wait time before the preferred transplant is available.

Currently, no national paired donation system exists in the United States, although the United Network for Organ Sharing (UNOS) started a pilot program in 2010. As of February 2011, 130 pairs have been entered into the UNOS program. Only 1 paired exchange has been done so far, resulting in 2 transplants; all matches to date have been closed loops. Plans are being made to initiate chains including non-directed donors in the near future. However, these chains will run no more than 3 deep before ending the chain by transplanting an organ from the deceased waiting list.

Ethics

Some have raised ethical concerns about paired donation. Ross et al, (8) in the *New England Journal of Medicine* in 1997, suggested that in paired donation, the hesitant donor has fewer opportunities to back out. That donor cannot invoke ABO incompatibility as a reason for withdrawal. The donor is under greater stress, as backing out will result in many people not receiving a transplant. Also some may see paired donation as a barter system, a transfer of human organs for valuable consideration. However, in 2007, the US Congress ruled "that criminal penalty does not apply to human organ paired donation"(9). Some have written that paired exchange disadvantages the deceased donor waiting list as non-directed donors (NDDs) are "diverted" into paired exchange as opposed to donating to the patients on the waiting list.(10) But Segev et al. (11) show that an NDD donating to a patient on the waiting list facilitates fewer transplants than a closed or open chain. In a closed chain, the last donor donates to a patient on the waiting list.

Even in an open chain never-ending altruistic donation (NEAD), it is not uncommon for the bridge donor to donate to a patient on the list. In fact, NKR has a program for bridge donors that do not initiate a new chain to donate to children on the list and to the hard-to-match patients on the list who have high levels of panel-reactive antibodies. The effect on the waiting list may not be as detrimental as some have thought.

Bridge Donors

Some are concerned about the effect of a donor from one of the pairs backing out. In a simple 2-way exchange that occurs simultaneously, such a situation is unlikely because the 2 donors are anesthetized at the same time. In more complicated exchanges where there is no strict simultaneity, the risk of a donor backing out is higher. In the case of larger exchanges across different time zones, the theoretical risk is higher still. The NEAD chains use a bridge donor to initiate the next cluster of transplants. The next cluster may not occur in weeks to months, in which time the donor may change his mind or may have life-changing events, such as moving away or illness. In the NKR system, 5 of 32 bridge donors have backed out. The 5 backed out for the following reasons: 2 because of financial hardship and loss of jobs and 3 because their recipient received a transplant (1 of the 3 cited emotional stress as the reason). It is left to the medical professionals to assess the likelihood of a donor backing out. Steps to minimize the risk of a bridge donor backing out are ensuring that the donor has a stable psychosocial environment and that the cluster that he initiates occurs in close time proximity to his own recipient's transplant.

Flying Living Kidneys

An active and busy national paired exchange program needs to rely on the ability to transport living kidneys across state lines, much like the transportation of deceased donor kidneys. Some have expressed concern about the kidney flying instead of the donor flying. Studies by Segev et al. (15) have shown that a cold ischemic time of less than 14 hours does not affect the immediate function of the live kidney transplant. In 200 cases of shipped kidneys in NKR, only 7 cases of delayed graft function. This 3.5% rate of delayed graft function is in keeping with the national average of 3.6% for non-shipped kidneys (16). The 7 cases have all resolved.

It appears that flying live kidneys is a safe option with regards to the functionality of the organ. But what if the organ is lost en route? What if the intended recipient cannot accept that kidney (patient becomes ill or dies while anesthesia is induced)? Some of these dooms-day scenarios have been worked out. The kidney that flies is boxed in the usual orange box with regulatory paperwork similar to a deceased donor flying kidney. A GPS tracking device can be included in the box in the event that the box or the plane is lost. Contents of the kidney box include kidney anatomy data and donor blood tubes so that if the intended recipient cannot accept the kidney then cross-matching can commence with other possible recipients so that the kidney is not wasted.

Financial Aspects

Who pays for the donor surgery in Alabama from which an organ is then shipped to New York to a recipient that the donor has never met? There are no national guidelines on this yet. At our center, the recipient insurance pays donor expenses. In the NKR system, the donor's hospital bills the recipient's hospital for the donor organ recovery. Transportation of the donor organ to the recipient hospital is coordinated by the donor hospital's organ procurement organization, which bills the recipient's hospital for the costs associated with transporting the organ. Whichever financial modality is used, it is clear that there must be cooperation among hospitals for this paired exchange endeavor to work on a large scale.

Summary

In summary, paired exchange is a practical solution for patients who have incompatible live donors. In addition, paired exchange can help patients on the deceased donor list. With an increase in living donor transplants, patients waiting for a deceased donor organ may have a shorter wait time because the waiting list is shortened with every live transplant. Also a bridge donor can elect to donate a kidney to the deceased donor list if initiating the next cluster is not immediately feasible.

(Financial Disclosures: None reported.)

References

1. Rees MA, Kopke JE, Pelletier RP, et al. A non-simultaneous, extended, altruistic-donor chain. *N Eng J Med.* 2009; 360(11):1096–1101.

2. Butt FK, Gritsch HA, Schulam P, et al. Asynchronous, out-of-sequence, transcontinental chain kidney transplantation: a novel concept. *Am J Transplant.* 2009; 9(9): 2180–2185.

3. Segev DL, Gentry SE, Melancon JK, Montgomery, RA. Characterization of waiting times in a simulation of kidney paired donation. *Am J Transplant.* 2005; 5(10): 2448–2455.

4. Rapaport FT. The case for a living emotionally related international kidney donor exchange registry. *Transplant Proc.* 1986; 18(3 suppl 2):5–9.

5. Huh KH, Kim MS, Ju MK, et al. Exchange living-donor kidney transplantation: merits and limitations. *Transplantation.* 2008; 86(3):430–435.

6. de Klerk M, Witvliet MD, Haase-Kromwijk, et al. Hurdles, barriers and successes of a national living donor kidney exchange program. *Transplantation.* 2008; 86(12): 1749–1753.

7. Hanto RL, Reitsma W, Delmonico FL. The development of a successful multiregional kidney paired donation program. *Transplantation.* 2008; 86(12):1744–1748.

8. Ross LF, Rubin DT, Siegler M, et al. Ethics of a paired-kidney-exchange-program. *N Engl J Med.* 1997; 336(24): 1752–1755.

9. H.R. 710: Charlie W. Norwood Living Organ Donation Act. 110th Congress. 2007–2008. http://www.govtrack.us/congress/bill.xpd?bill=h110–710. Accessed April 7, 2011.

10. Woodle ES, Daller JA, Aeder M, et al. Ethical considerations for participation of non-directed living donors in kidney exchange programs. *Am J Transplant.* 2010; 10(6): 1460–1467.

11. Gentry SE, Montgomery RA, Swihart BJ, Segev DL. The roles of dominos and non-simultaneous chains in kidney paired donation. *Am J Transplant.* 2009; 9(6):1330–1336.

12. Optimization. http://optimizedmatch.com./learn_opt.php. Accessed May 4, 2011.

13. Kranenburg LW, Zuidema W, Weimar W, et al. One donor, two transplants: willingness to participate in altruistically unbalanced exchange donation. *Transpl Int.* 2006; 19(12):995–999.

14. Gentry SE, Segev DL, Simmerling M, Montgomery, RA. Expanding kidney paired donation through participation by compatible pairs. *Am J Transplant.* 2007; 7(10): 2361–2370.

15. Segev DL, Veale JL, Berger JC, et al. Transporting live donor kidneys for kidney paired donation: initial national results. *Am J Transplant.* 2011; 11(2):356–360.

16. National Institutes of Health, National Institute of Diabetes and Digestive and Kidney Diseases. *USRDS 2010 Annual Data Report: Atlas of Chronic Kidney Disease and End-Stage Renal Disease in the United States.* Bethesda, MD: National Institutes of Health, National Institute of Diabetes and Digestive and Kidney Diseases; 2010:318.

Chapter 29

AN EXCERPT FROM

Kidney Paired Donation

C. Bradley Wallis, Kannan P. Samy, Alvin E. Roth,
Michael A. Rees

Abstract

Kidney paired donation (KPD) was first suggested in 1986, but it was not until 2000
when the first paired donation transplant was
performed in the USA. In the past decade,
KPD has become the fastest growing source
of transplantable kidneys, overcoming the
barrier faced by living donors deemed incompatible with their intended recipients. This review provides a basic overview of the concepts
and challenges faced by KPD as we prepare
for a national pilot program with the United
Network for Organ Sharing. Several different
algorithms have been creatively implemented
in the USA and elsewhere to transplant paired
donors, each method uniquely contributing to
the success of KPD. As the paired donor pool
grows, the problem of determining allocation
strategies that maximize equity and utility will
become increasingly important as the transplant community seeks to balance quality and
quantity in choosing the best matches. Financ-
ing for paired donation is a major issue, as phi-
lanthropy alone cannot support the emerging
national system. We also discuss the advent of
altruistic or non-directed donors in KPD, and
the important role of chains in addition to exchanges. This review is designed to provide insight into the challenges that face the emerging

national KPD system in the USA, now 5 years
into its development.

Introduction

Kidney transplantation has been established as the best treatment for patients
suffering from end stage renal disease (ESRD).
Patients fortunate enough to receive a kidney
transplant, on average, live 10 years longer
than those who remain on dialysis [1], and it is
now clear that a living donor kidney transplant
is better than a kidney from a deceased donor.
The average deceased donor kidney transplant will function for 8.6 years, while a living
donor kidney provides an average of >16 years
of dialysis-free survival [2]. Sadly, the demand
for a kidney transplant far exceeds the supply
that can be met by deceased donors, so much
so that roughly 19 patients die each day in the
USA, while waiting for a kidney donation [3].
Unfortunately, all too often, a willing living
donor is deemed incompatible due to blood
type or unacceptable donor-specific antibodies. Kidney paired donation (KPD) provides
a solution to this dilemma by pairing two incompatible pairs together to facilitate an exchange between the willing donors' kidneys.

. . .

Allocation in Paired Donation

Two driving factors have fueled KPD innovation over the years: maximizing the number of incompatible pairs that can be served and finding the best possible matches between participants. Maximizing the quantity of KPD exchanges is a straightforward concept: larger pool sizes and successful matching equals more transplants. Determining the quality of matches is more complex as it requires allocation decisions that, until the advent of paired donation, are typically limited to the realm of deceased donor kidneys. In KPD, living donors do not choose their recipients; the matching algorithm must do this. For this reason, the entity that controls allocation of KPD kidneys must carefully consider allocation principles as there are many different perspectives as to what defines the best match. According to the National Organ Transplant Act, donated organs are to be allocated equitably among transplant patients [53]. The United Network for Organ Sharing (UNOS) defines 'equitable' as a balance between utility and justice [54]. KPD fosters utility by creating viable transplants out of a pool of donors who are unable to give their loved one a kidney. Justice is less intuitive. Justice requires balancing the perspectives of recipients, donors, transplant centers and society as a whole, which tend to vary greatly, in terms of the proper allocation of living organs [46, 55]. The recent inability of UNOS to gain consensus on life years from transplant (LYFT) as a new strategy for allocating deceased donor organs emphasizes the controversial nature of determining quality in organ allocation [56].

Whereas living donor kidneys historically have been allocated by the living donor themselves, or in the case of non-directed donors by the local transplant center, a paradigm shift is required if KPD is to expand between many centers on a regional or national scale. Not only does KPD require consensus regarding the allocation of living donor kidneys but the new allocation system will also need to consider the desire of local transplant programs to maximize the number of transplants for patients at their center. Take the following example: one transplant center has two pairs that can simply participate in a two-way exchange. However, if these two pairs are put into a national pool, they may get matched to two other pairs from other transplant centers, so that a child and a highly sensitized patient are transplanted, allowing four people to be transplanted instead of two [57]. The risk for the center enrolling these two pairs into the national system is that only one patient of their two might get matched, while their other patient is left untransplanted. In this sense, they are not advocating the best for 'their' two patients. Thus, as more transplant centers are drawn into cooperation with one another, it is likely that effective matching protocols will have to give centers appropriate incentives to submit all of their incompatible patient–donor pairs to the kidney exchange pool, and not just those for whom they cannot arrange exchanges internally [57]. If centers are doing some internal exchanges without making those pairs available to the national pool, that means those exchanges, de facto, had higher priority than, for example, children at other centers. One can imagine, based on the stark differences between these competing allocation philosophies, how challenging it will be to achieve a national consensus on how to quantify quality so that transplant programs will accept the allocation approach and agree to put all their pairs into a single pool, thus offering all patients the best opportunity through KPD.

While it may appear that efforts to increase the quality of transplants would do so at the expense of higher quantity matches and vice versa, there are many strategies that seek to improve both. The simplest way quantity and quality of KPD matching is improved is through increasing pool size. In simulations of paired donation pools and calculations of outcomes, the number of potential matches will exponentially increase as the paired donor pool increases [21,44,47,58]. While there has been no determination of a 'critical mass' or a volume of enrolled incompatible pairs that would begin a cascade of transplants, some have suggested that a pool size of at least 100 pairs is necessary for sustainable matching [59]. Naturally, as more incompatible pairs are added to a KPD registry, more transplants are made possible and the likelihood that hard-to-match and highly sensitized pairs will find suitable donors increases, as illustrated in the previous example [58]. This fundamental concept has inspired programs to create national pools in spite of substantial logistical obstacles that invariably stand in the way [10,21,22,60]. Other methods to improve quality and quantity involve utilizing specific computer algorithms and allocation protocols. Originally, the process of finding a match among a pool of incompatible pairs followed a 'first-accept' scheme, which entails matching pairs without considering the impact of that choice on all the other possible choices. This algorithm would remove easy-to-match pairs, hurting the remaining hard-to-match pairs by concentrating them in the pool [61]. Most programs today have adopted an 'optimization' algorithm, which searches for every possible match in the available pool and then analyzes which option will generate both the highest quantity of matches and the best quality of matches [8,14,60,62,63]. Match quality

is ensured by establishing a list of specific allocation criteria that helps guide the computer in coordinating its match run. This set of criteria goes beyond blood type compatibility and human leukocyte antigen (HLA) sensitization to include factors such as age, travel distance, wait-time on dialysis and any number of additional parameters that facilitate the best possible outcomes.

Although specific-allocation criteria may differ, most programs agree that there is a delicate balance between assigning too few criteria, which leads to poor matching and outcomes and assigning too complex criteria, which can limit matching, particularly in smaller pools [47]. The most successful programs are able to straddle this line and therefore maximize KPD outcomes. Our program, the Alliance for Paired Donation (APD), is overseen by a Scientific Operations Committee (SOC) composed of representatives from each participating transplant program and led by an executive committee from 10 of these programs. Our SOC regularly reevaluates the matching algorithm to ensure that the optimized matches reflect desired priorities. The upcoming UNOS KPD pilot program has likewise sought to achieve a consensus on allocation—a process that has taken >5 years to develop. Experience and careful study of the different allocation approaches currently in practice should yield critical insights to create an optimal algorithm for increasing the quantity and quality of paired donation transplants achieved [64].

As stated previously, a three-way exchange not only enables more transplants than a two-way but also allows higher quality matching since pairs no longer require a reciprocal match [20–22,62,63]. Altruistic donors provide a similar advantage. By initiating chains with an altruistic donor, both domino-paired donation (DPD) and never-ending altruistic donation (NEAD) chains, like three-way exchanges, bypass the need for reciprocal matching, providing higher quality matches to participants and allowing more pairs to profit [49–51]. Additionally, DPD and NEAD chains permit better matching just by including altruistic donors alone, which typically represent the blood type frequencies of the general population. This means that there is a high probability that any given altruistic donor will be blood type O and will therefore be able to match with a hard-to-match O recipient to initiate a chain. All of these advantages give altruistic donor chains an unmistakable edge in the effort to maximize quality and quantity.

Ethical Issues in Paired Donation

As with any new approach in transplantation, there have been ethical concerns since the beginning of KPD. A new issue arising with paired donation is the involvement of separate unrelated patients participating in an exchange; this raises the question of maintaining anonymity between exchanging pairs [6]. While some KPD programs allow full contact between participating pairs, others prevent contact until after the procedure and still others discourage meeting altogether [12, 16,23,43,50,62,65,68,69,75,76]. Those that support anonymity argue that there is a risk of anger or frustration with poor transplant outcomes [16, 76], that it might affect the decision to participate in the exchange, or that loss of anonymity might promote unethical or unlawful interactions such as coercion or bartering [23]. In our experience with the APD, anonymity has been the decision of the participating transplant centers. At the authors' home transplant center, patients are offered

the choice and only 1 pair in 25 has chosen to remain anonymous. All the other recipients and donors met prior to the transplant procedure and in every case, the meetings have been a positive experience. Others have also allowed donor–recipient pairs to meet with positive responses [23, 43], whereas many of the arguments supporting anonymity have been based on speculation and do not correlate with studies evaluating patient desires [77]. Thus, anonymity between KPD participants is an area that requires data to help guide future policy development.

Until recently, KPD transplants were performed simultaneously in order to prevent donor reneging [11,43,62,69,75,78]. Domino chain donations are also done simultaneously for the same reasons [32, 79]. A NEAD chain, on the other hand, has the potential for 'bridge' donor reneging, but this controversial risk of inequity has been justified by a belief that non-simultaneous chains would provide better utility [49,62,64,77–79]. Experience will need to determine whether risking donor reneging by non-simultaneous chains results in utility gains and sufficiently low renege rates in order to continue its practice.

Coercion has been a concern for living donation since its beginning, and some argue that KPD places donors under even greater pressure to donate because it eliminates incompatibility as an excuse to avoid donation [6, 76]. In addition, since NEAD chains create a situation where bridge donors' incompatible recipients have already received transplants, some argue that this inappropriately limits the donor's ability to withdraw and by its very nature is coercive [80]. Further ethical concerns include privacy, confidentiality, exploitation and commercialization [80]. Danovitch et al. [81] argue that the benefits of NEAD chains outweigh the hypothetical concerns about the unintended consequences of such a policy. Again, experience will distill those concerns with merit and clarify the best way forward.

Discussion

While there are many other issues that could be explored in the evolving field of KPD, this review has summarized different matching strategies and some of the barriers to developing a national program in the USA. It is therefore worth noting that UNOS initiated a KPD pilot program in the fall of 2010 [67]. In this pilot, four coordinating centers have been chosen: the APD, the Johns Hopkins Program, the New England Program for Kidney Exchange and a UCLA-led consortium. Through these coordinating centers, >75 transplant programs will participate in a pilot that has been under development for >5 years. However, the limitations of the pilot emphasize the challenges—highlighted in this review—that hinder movement from the UNOS pilot to a national program. The initial UNOS pilot does not allow for chains, but is limited to two- and three-way exchanges. There is no strategy in place to pay for incompatible donor evaluations, the expenses of the coordination centers, or for donor or kidney shipping. There is no web-based data entry portal and there is no provision for a centralized laboratory to perform screening crossmatches. Another limitation is that the matching algorithm does not provide assurances to transplant centers that encourage them to enroll all of their pairs instead of performing internal exchanges utilizing their easy-to-match pairs.

This list of deficiencies is not meant as a criticism but as an example of the difficulty of building consensus. UNOS as an organization is dependent on achieving consensus. As

such, it is less able to innovate and this review makes clear that KPD remains a rapidly evolving field. Furthermore, while a contractor for the federal government, UNOS does not control the allocation of federal funding that is required to support a national KPD program. For these reasons, KPD is likely to remain in the hands of smaller regional programs that have the advantage of driving innovation, but the disadvantage of limited pool size that by definition will not provide the greatest number of opportunities for patients with incompatible, but willing living donors. Nonetheless, the UNOS KPD Pilot Program represents the nascent beginning of a national KPD program in the USA that promises hope to the growing number of patients suffering from ESRD.

Editors' Note: All figures and diagrams have been omitted.

Acknowledgments: This work was supported in part by Health Resources and Services Administration contract 234–2005–37011C and National Science Foundation Grant 0616733. The content is the responsibility of the authors alone and does not necessarily reflect the views or policies of the Department of Health and Human Services nor does mention of trade names, commercial products, or organizations imply endorsement by the U.S. Government.

Conflict of interest statement: None declared.

References

1. Wolfe RA, Ashby VB, Milford EL et al. Comparison of mortality in all patients on dialysis, patients on dialysis awaiting transplantation, and recipients of a first cadaveric transplant. *N Engl J Med* 1999; 341:1725–1730.

2. SRTR. 2008 *Annual Report of the U.S. Organ Procurement and Transplantation Network and the Scientific Registry of Transplant Recipients: Transplant Data*

1998–2007. Rockville, MD:Health Resources and Services Administration, Healthcare Systems Bureau, Division of Transplantation, 2008.

3. UNOS. www.optn.org. (Accessed February 1, 2011).

4. Rapaport FT. The case for a living emotionally related international kidney donor exchange registry. *Transplant Proc* 1986; 18:5–9.

5. Kwak JY, Kwon OJ, Lee KS et al. Exchange-donor program in renal transplantation: a single-center experience. *Transplant Proc* 1999; 31:344–345.

6. Thiel G, Vogelbach P, Gurke L et al. Crossover renal transplantation: hurdles to be cleared! *Transplant Proc* 2001; 33:811–816.

7. Zarsadias P, Monaco AP, Morrissey PE. A pioneering paired kidney exchange. *Student BMJ* 2010; 18:c1562.

8. de Klerk M, Keizer KM, Claas FH et al. The Dutch national living donor kidney exchange program. *Am J Transplant* 2005; 5:2302–2305.

9. Terasaki PI, Gjertson DW, Cecka JM. Paired kidney exchange is not a solution to ABO incompatibility. *Transplantation* 1998; 65:291.

10. Montgomery RA, Cooper M, Kraus E et al. Renal transplantation at the Johns Hopkins Comprehensive Transplant Center. *Clin Transpl* 2003:199–213.

11. Delmonico FL. Exchanging kidneys–advances in living-donor transplantation. *N Engl J Med* 2004; 350: 1812–1814.

12. Delmonico FL, Morrissey PE, Lipkowitz GS et al. Donor kidney exchanges. *Am J Transplant* 2004; 4:1628–1634.

13. Goody AJ. Donor exchange for renal transplantation. *N Engl J Med* 2004; 351:935–937; author reply—7.

14. Montgomery RA, Zachary AA, Ratner LE et al. Clinical results from transplanting incompatible live kidney donor/recipient pairs using kidney paired donation. *JAMA* 2005; 294:1655–1663.

15. Norman DJ. Kidney paired donation: a single-center study of feasibility and outcomes. *Nat Clin Pract Nephrol* 2006; 2:302–303.

16. Park K, Moon JI, Kim SI, Kim YS. Exchange donor program in kidney transplantation. *Transplantation* 1999; 67:336–338.

17. Roth AE, Sonmez T, Unver MU. Kidney Exchange. *Quart J Econ* 2004; 119:457–488.

18. Roth AE, Sönmez T, Unver MU. Pairwise kidney exchange. *J Econ Theory* 2004; 125:151–188.

19. Woodle ES, Goldfarb D, Aeder M et al. Establishment of a nationalized, multiregional Paired Donation Network. *Clin Transpl* 2005; 247–258.

20. Montgomery RA, Katznelson S, Bry WI et al. Successful three-way kidney paired donation with cross-country live donor allograft transport. *Am J Transplant* 2008; 8: 2163–2168.

21. Roth AE, Sönmez T, Unver MU. Efficient Kidney Exchange: Coincidence of Wants in Markets with Compatibility-Based Preferences. *Am Econ Rev* 2007; 97:828–851.

22. Saidman SL, Roth AE, Sonmez T et al. Increasing the opportunity of live kidney donation by matching for two- and three-way exchanges. *Transplantation* 2006; 81:773–782.

23. Lucan M. Five years of single-center experience with paired kidney exchange transplantation. *Transplant Proc* 2007; 39:1371–1375.

24. Roth AE, Sonmez T, Unver MU, Delmonico FL, Saidman SL. Utilizing list exchange and non-directed donation through 'chain' paired kidney donations. *Am J Transplant* 2006; 6:2694–2705.

25. Gentry SE, Segev DL, Montgomery RA. A comparison of populations served by kidney paired donation and list paired donation. *Am J Transplant* 2005; 5:1914–1921.

26. den Hartogh G. Trading with the waiting-list: the justice of living donor list exchange. *Bioethics* 2010; 24: 190–198.

27. Axelrod DA, McCullough KP, Brewer ED et al. Kidney and pancreas transplantation in the United States, 1999–2008: the changing face of living donation. *Am J Transplant* 2010; 10:987–1002.

28. Gentry SE, Segev DL, Simmerling M et al. Expanding kidney paired donation through partici-

pation by compatible pairs. *Am J Transplant* 2007; 7:2361–2370.

29. Ratner LE, Rana A, Ratner ER et al. The altruistic unbalanced paired kidney exchange: proof of concept and survey of potential donor and recipient attitudes. *Transplantation* 2010; 89:15–22.

30. Roth AE, Sonmez T, Unver MU. Kidney paired donation with compatible pairs. *Am J Transplant* 2008; 8:463.

31. Roth AE, Sonmez T., Utku Unver M. A Kindey Exchange Clearinghouse in New England. *American Economic Review, Papers and Proceedings* 2005; 95:376–380.

32. Mahendran AO, Veitch PS. Paired exchange programmes can expand the live kidney donor pool. *Br J Surg* 2007; 94:657–664.

33. Montgomery RA. Renal transplantation across HLA and ABO antibody barriers: integrating paired donation into desensitization protocols. *Am J Transplant* 2010; 10:449–457.

34. Montgomery RA, Simpkins CE, Segev DL. New options for patients with donor incompatibilities. *Transplantation* 2006; 82:164–165.

35. Warren DS, Montgomery RA. Incompatible kidney transplantation: lessons from a decade of desensitization and paired kidney exchange. *Immunol Res* 2010; 47:257–264.

36. Gloor JM, Lager DJ, Moore SB et al. ABO-incompatible kidney transplantation using both A2 and non-A2 living donors. *Transplantation* 2003; 75: 971–977.

37. Jordan SC, Quartel AW, Czer LS et al. Posttransplant therapy using high-dose human immunoglobulin (intravenous gammaglobulin) to control acute humoral rejection in renal and cardiac allograft recipients and potential mechanism of action. *Transplantation* 1998; 66:800–805.

38. Tanabe K, Takahashi K, Sonda K et al. Long-term results of ABO incompatible living kidney transplantation: a single-center experience. *Transplantation* 1998; 65:224–228.

39. Wilpert J, Fischer KG, Pisarski P et al. Long-term outcome of ABO incompatible living donor kidney transplantation based on antigen-specific desensitization. An observational comparative analysis. *Nephrol Dial Transplant* 2010; 25:3778–3786.

40. Gloor JM, Winters JL, Cornell LD et al. Baseline donor-specific antibody levels and outcomes in positive cross-match kidney transplantation. *Am J Transplant* 2010; 10:582–589.

41. Haririan A, Nogueira J, Kukuruga D et al. Positive cross-match living donor kidney transplantation: longer-term outcomes. *Am J Transplant* 2009; 9:536–542.

42. Montgomery RA. Renal transplantation across HLA and ABO antibody barriers: integrating paired donation into desensitization protocols. *Am J Transplant* 2010; 10:449–457.

43. Gilbert JC, Brigham L, Batty DS Jr. et al. The non-directed living donor program: a model for cooperative donation, recovery and allocation of living donor kidneys. *Am J Transplant* 2005; 5:167–174.

44. Johnson RJ, Allen JE, Fuggle SV et al. Early experience of paired living kidney donation in the United Kingdom. *Transplantation* 2008; 86:1672–1677.

45. Adams PL, Cohen DJ, Danovitch GM et al. The non-directed live-kidney donor: ethical considerations and practice guidelines: A National Conference Report. *Transplantation* 2002; 74:582–589.

46. Montgomery RA, Gentry SE, Marks WH et al. Domino paired kidney donation: a strategy to make best use of live non-directed donation. *Lancet* 2006; 368: 419–421.

47. Ferrari P, de Klerk M. Paired kidney donations to expand the living donor pool. *J Nephrol* 2009; 22: 699–707.

48. Ferrari P, Woodroffe C, Christiansen FT. Paired kidney donations to expand the living donor pool: the Western Australian experience. *Med J Aust* 2009; 190: 700–703.

49. Rees MA, Kopke JE, Pelletier RP et al. A non-simultaneous, extended, altruistic-donor chain. *N Engl J Med* 2009; 360:1096–1101.

50. Butt FK, Gritsch HA, Schulam P et al. Asynchronous, out-of-sequence, transcontinental chain kid-

ney transplantation: a novel concept. *Am J Transplant* 2009; 9: 2180–2185.

51. Rees MA, Bargnesi D, Samy K et al. Altruistic donation through the Alliance for Paired Donation. *Clin Transpl* 2009; 235–246.

52. AP. 13-way Kidney Transplant Sets Record. Washington, DC: *The Washington Times*, 2009.

53. The National Organ Transplant Act 42. In: *98th Congress ed*; 1984:42 U.S.C. Sec. 273.

54. General principles for allocating human organs and tissues. *Transplant Proc* 1992; 24:2227–2235.

55. Marks W. Towards understanding living non-directed donation. *Symposium on Living Non-Directed Donation*. Seattle:WA, 2004.

56. Wolfe RA, McCullough KP, Schaubel DE et al. Calculating life years from transplant (LYFT):methods for kidney and kidney-pancreas candidates. *Am J Transplant* 2008; 8:997–1011.

57. Roth AE. What have we learned from market design? *Econ J* 2007; 118:285–310.

58. Basu G, Daniel D, Rajagopal A et al. A model for human leukocyte antigen-matched donor-swap transplantation in India. *Transplantation* 2008; 85:687–692.

59. Bingaman AW, Wright FH, Murphey CL. Kidney paired donation in live-donor kidney transplantation. *N Engl J Med* 2010; 363:1091–1092.

60. Zenios SA. Optimal Control of a Paired-Kidney Exchange Program. *Manage Sci* 2002; 48:328–342.

61. Segev DL, Gentry SE, Melancon JK et al. Characterization of waiting times in a simulation of kidney paired donation. *Am J Transplant* 2005; 5:2448–2455.

62. Hanto RL, Reitsma W, Delmonico FL. The development of a successful multiregional kidney paired donation program. *Transplantation* 2008; 86:1744–1748.

63. Kaplan I, Houp JA, Montgomery RA et al. A computer match program for paired and unconventional kidney exchanges. *Am J Transplant* 2005; 5:2306–2308.

64. Ashlagi I GD, Roth AE, Rees MA. Nonsimultaneous Chains and Dominos in Kidney Paired Donation–Revisited. *Am J Transplant* 2011; 11:1–11.

65. Gohh RY, Morrissey PE, Madras PN et al. Controversies in organ donation: the altruistic living donor. *Nephrol Dial Transplant* 2001; 16:619–621.

66. Goldfarb DA. Kidney paired donation and optimizing the use of live donor organs. *J Urol* 2005; 174:1911–1912.

67. Pondrom S. The AJT Report: news and issues that affect organ and tissue transplantation. *Am J Transplant* 2009; 9:1699–1700.

68. Ratner LE, Ratner ER, Kelly J et al. Altruistic unbalanced paired kidney exchange at Columbia University/New York-Presbyterian hospital: rationale and practical considerations. *Clin Transpl* 2008:107–112.

69. de Klerk M, Weimar W. Ingredients for a successful living donor kidney exchange program. *Transplantation* 2008; 86:511–512.

70. de Klerk M, Witvliet MD, Haase-Kromwijk BJ et al. Hurdles, barriers, and successes of a national living donor kidney exchange program. *Transplantation* 2008; 86:1749–1753.

71. Simpkins CE, Montgomery RA, Hawxby AM et al. Cold ischemia time and allograft outcomes in live donor renal transplantation: is live donor organ transport feasible? *Am J Transplant* 2007; 7:99–107.

72. Terasaki PI, Cecka JM, Gjertson DW et al. High survival rates of kidney transplants from spousal and living unrelated donors. *N Engl J Med* 1995; 333:333–336.

73. Waki K, Terasaki PI. Paired kidney donation by shipment of living donor kidneys. *Clin Transplant* 2007; 21:186–191.

74. Segev DL, Veale JL, Berger JC et al. Transporting Live Donor Kidneys for Kidney Paired Donation: Initial National Results. *Am J Transplant* 2011; 11:356–360.

75. Chapman JR, Allen RD. Paired kidney exchange: how far and how wide? *Transplantation* 2008; 85:673–674.

76. Ross LF, Rubin DT, Siegler M et al. Ethics of a paired-kidney-exchange program. *N Engl J Med* 1997; 336:1752–1755.

77. Hizo-Abes P, Young A, Reese PP et al. Attitudes to sharing personal health information in living kidney donation. *Clin J Am Soc Nephrol* 2010; 5:717–722.

78. Ross LF. The ethical limits in expanding living donor transplantation. *Kennedy Inst Ethics J* 2006; 16:151–172.

79. Gentry SE, Montgomery RA, Swihart BJ et al. The roles of dominos and non-simultaneous chains in kidney paired donation. *Am J Transplant* 2009; 9:1330–1336.

80. Woodle ES, Daller JA, Aeder M et al. Ethical considerations for participation of non-directed living donors in kidney exchange programs. *Am J Transplant* 2010; 10:1460–1467.

81. Danovitch G, Veale J, Hippen B. Living donor kidney donation in the United States: quo vadis? *Am J Transplant* 2010; 10: 1345–1346.

Chapter 30

Some High Risk Kidneys Safe for Transplant

Kristina Fiore

ATLANTA—Patients who received kidneys from deceased donors considered to be at high risk for transmission of infectious disease fared well more than 2 years after transplant, researchers reported here.

In a single-center study, 87% of transplanted patients whose donor kidneys were considered high-risk had good kidney function and no trace of infection over nearly 2.5 years of follow-up, Moya Gallagher, RN, of Columbia University Medical Center, and colleagues reported at Kidney Week here.

Using these organs offers "an opportunity for shortening wait times . . . while antibody and PCR testing functioned well at 2 years of follow-up with no evidence of infectious seroconversion, providing good outcomes and an extremely low level of risk for transmission of infections," Gallagher said in a statement.

She noted that for most deceased organ donors, their medical history is obtained second or third hand and may not be reliable.

"Therefore," she said, "we believe that the current dichotomized classification is misleading and does a disservice to those patients on the waiting list."

Roslyn Mannon, MD, of the Comprehensive Transplant Institute at the University of Alabama at Birmingham, who was not involved in the study, called it an "excellent abstract," noting that "patients die daily on the kidney list, waiting for a deceased [donor's] organ."

"With the limited availability of organs for the waiting list population, we cannot be discarding kidneys without a good reason," Mannon told *MedPage Today* in an email.

About 10% of deceased donor kidneys are classified as high-risk for infection with HIV or with hepatitis B or C (HBV or HCV) based on CDC criteria. But technology has improved and the researchers said it's unlikely that infection would not be detected by modern nucleic acid testing for these diseases.

Indeed, Mannon said, many centers perform careful screening on donor organs and inform recipients of the potential risks. They also follow them closely, and "by and large, they have done well."

To assess how patients who are given these potentially high-risk organs fare, Gallagher and colleagues studied 170 patients who had received kidneys that met CDC's criteria for being high risk at their center since 2004.

All of these patients had pre-transplant screening for HIV, HCV, HBV, and were also screened by antibody and polymerase chain reaction (PCR) testing—to look for DNA evidence of these diseases—at 6, 12, and 24 weeks after transplant. All patients were on standard immunosuppression when they received their transplants.

The donors did indeed have high-risk characteristics, including a history of injection drug use (57%), high-risk sexual behavior (26%), incarceration (12%), being men who had sex with men (7%), and receiving multiple blood transfusions (5%).

Most of these transplanted kidneys had been imported from other centers (78%), Gallagher noted, suggesting those centers refused to use those organs, likely because of their high-risk status.

But the researchers found that after two and a half years, 87% of kidney transplants in these patients were functioning well, with a mean creatinine of 1.62 mg/dL, and there was no evidence of any of the infectious diseases that had been absent on initial screening.

Gallagher concluded that these findings suggest the relative safety of so-called "high-risk" deceased donor organs, and that the CDC criteria should perhaps classify these organs as "identified risk" instead.

Primary source: American Society of Nephrology

Source reference: Gallagher MB, et al "CDC high-risk designation for deceased kidney donors is a misnomer" ASN 2013; Abstract 2603.

Part V

Gaming the System

Arthur L. Caplan

One of the hardest moral challenges an ethicist working in the field of transplantation ethics can face is the question from someone waiting for a transplant—what can I do to get a better shot at an organ? Those desperate to live or to find some way for their loved one to receive a scarce transplant want to know if they can somehow "game the system." They want to know if there is anything that can be done to push their name or their loved one's name up the waiting list or to find an organ by other-than-routine means.

This part reviews the realities and the ethics of gaming the system. There are in fact ways that people can and do use to increase their odds of receiving a transplant. The first three chapters in the part discuss transplant tourism wherein those in need travel to other nations where doctors are willing, for a considerable fee, to obtain organs for them and to give them priority in receiving organs even over the fellow citizens of the doctors. Transplant tourism often involves paying a poor person for an organ, usually a kidney. Then that person, once in agreement, is either brought to a transplant center where a patient is waiting or goes to a transplant center to meet a would-be patient who has also traveled there. The sellers of organs are almost always very poor, leading

to the likelihood that they will be exploited in the course of this transaction. Middlemen and surgeons tend to take in the profits, while the seller goes home with little and often no follow-up care should it be needed postsurgery. This type of trafficking in body parts has elicited much condemnation from various groups and governments, but it is estimated that close to a quarter of all kidneys transplanted worldwide come from black market sales from the very poor to the wealthy.

Worse, in some nations such as China and Cambodia prisoners are executed on demand for organs to be sold for those rich enough to get to China to receive them. This murder-for-hire practice again has drawn much criticism, but many of the rich around the world who are unwilling to wait for an organ accept them, knowing they came from those killed for parts.

There are other ways in which the rich can gain advantage over the poor in the competition for scarce organs. Some like the entrepreneur Steve Jobs had enough money to multiple-list himself at many US transplant centers when he needed a liver. Since organs are distributed partly on the basis of geography, being able to list at more than one center confers an edge on access for those who can afford to pay each program to evaluate them and fly quickly to a center if an organ becomes available.

Another way to game the system is to launch campaigns on social media or the mainstream media or both to try to find a willing living donor. This has happened many times in the United States and other nations where those wealthy enough or savvy enough to utilize public-relations help can obtain access to a kidney or even an organ from a deceased donor by being the loudest voice in the room.

The motives of those seeking to game the system are very understandable—self-interest leads each of us to want to live and to help those we love continue to live. But transplant tourism, multiple-listing, and social media campaigns are not equitable ways of distributing scarce life-saving transplants.

Chapter 31

The Declaration of Istanbul on Organ Trafficking and Transplant Tourism

Participants in the International Summit on Transplant Tourism and Organ Trafficking

Convened by the Transplantation Society and International Society of Nephrology in Istanbul, Turkey, April 30–May 2, 2008

Preamble

Organ transplantation, one of the medical miracles of the twentieth century, has prolonged and improved the lives of hundreds of thousands of patients worldwide. The many great scientific and clinical advances of dedicated health professionals, as well as countless acts of generosity by organ donors and their families, have made transplantation not only a life-saving therapy but a shining symbol of human solidarity. Yet these accomplishments have been tarnished by numerous reports of trafficking in human beings who are used as sources of organs and of patient-tourists from rich countries who travel abroad to purchase organs from poor people. In 2004, the World Health Organization, called on member states "to take measures to protect the poorest and vulnerable groups from transplant tourism and the sale of tissues and organs, including attention to the wider problem of international trafficking in human tissues and organs" (1).

To address the urgent and growing problems of organ sales, transplant tourism and trafficking in organ donors in the context of the global shortage of organs, a Summit Meeting of more than 150 representatives of scientific and medical bodies from around the world, government officials, social scientists, and ethicists, was held in Istanbul from April 30 to May 2, 2008. Preparatory work for the meeting was undertaken by a Steering Committee convened by The Transplantation Society (TTS) and the International Society of Nephrology (ISN) in Dubai in December 2007. That committee's draft declaration was widely circulated and then revised in light of the comments received. At the Summit, the revised draft was reviewed by working groups and finalized in plenary deliberations.

This Declaration represents the consensus of the Summit participants. All countries need a legal and professional framework to govern organ donation and transplantation activities, as well as a transparent regulatory oversight system that ensures donor and recipient safety and the enforcement of standards and prohibitions on unethical practices.

Unethical practices are, in part, an undesirable consequence of the global shortage of organs for transplantation. Thus, each country should strive both to ensure that programs to prevent organ failure are implemented and to provide organs to meet the transplant needs of its residents from donors within its own population or through regional cooperation. The therapeutic potential of deceased organ donation should be maximized not only for kidneys but also for other organs, appropriate to the transplantation needs of each country. Efforts to initiate or enhance deceased donor transplantation are essential to minimize the burden on living donors. Educational programs are useful in addressing the barriers, misconceptions and mistrust that currently impede the development of sufficient deceased donor transplantation; successful transplant programs also depend on the existence of the relevant health system infrastructure.

Access to healthcare is a human right but often not a reality. The provision of care for living donors before, during and after surgery—as described in the reports of the international forums organized by TTS in Amsterdam and Vancouver (2–4)—is no less essential than taking care of the transplant recipient. A positive outcome for a recipient can never justify harm to a live donor; on the contrary, for a transplant with a live donor to be regarded as a success means that both the recipient and the donor have done well.

This Declaration builds on the principles of the Universal Declaration of Human Rights (5). The broad representation at the Istanbul Summit reflects the importance of international collaboration and global consensus to improve donation and transplantation practices. The Declaration will be submitted to relevant professional organizations and to the health authorities of all countries for consideration. The legacy of transplantation must not be the impoverished victims of organ trafficking and transplant tourism but rather a celebration of the gift of health by one individual to another.

Definitions

Organ trafficking is the recruitment, transport, transfer, harboring or receipt of living or deceased persons or their organs by means of the threat or use of force or other forms of coercion, of abduction, of fraud, of deception, of the abuse of power or of a position of vulnerability, or of the giving to, or the receiving by, a third party of payments or benefits to achieve the transfer of control over the potential donor, for the purpose of exploitation by the removal of organs for transplantation (6).

Transplant commercialism is a policy or practice in which an organ is treated as a commodity, including by being bought or sold or used for material gain.

Travel for transplantation is the movement of organs, donors, recipients or transplant professionals across jurisdictional borders for transplantation purposes. Travel for transplantation becomes *transplant tourism* if it involves organ trafficking and/or transplant commercialism or if the resources (organs, professionals and transplant centers) devoted to providing transplants to patients from outside a country undermine the country's ability to provide transplant services for its own population.

Principles

1. National governments, working in collaboration with international and nongovernmental organizations, should develop and implement comprehensive programs for the screening, prevention and treatment of organ failure, which include:
   a. The advancement of clinical and basic science research;
   b. Effective programs, based on international guidelines, to treat and maintain patients with end-stage diseases, such as dialysis programs

for renal patients, to minimize morbidity and mortality, alongside transplant programs for such diseases;

   c. Organ transplantation as the preferred treatment for organ failure for medically suitable recipients.

2. Legislation should be developed and implemented by each country or jurisdiction to govern the recovery of organs from deceased and living donors and the practice of transplantation, consistent with international standards.

   a. Policies and procedures should be developed and implemented to maximize the number of organs available for transplantation, consistent with these principles;

   b. The practice of donation and transplantation requires oversight and accountability by health authorities in each country to ensure transparency and safety;

   c. Oversight requires a national or regional registry to record deceased and living donor transplants;

   d. Key components of effective programs include public education and awareness, health professional education and training, and defined responsibilities and accountabilities for all stakeholders in the national organ donation and transplant system.

3. Organs for transplantation should be equitably allocated within countries or jurisdictions to suitable recipients without regard to gender, ethnicity, religion, or social or financial status.

   a. Financial considerations or material gain of any party must not influence the application of relevant allocation rules.

4. The primary objective of transplant policies and programs should be optimal short- and long-term medical care to promote the health of both donors and recipients.

   a. Financial considerations or material gain of any party must not override primary consideration for the health and well-being of donors and recipients.

5. Jurisdictions, countries and regions should strive to achieve self-sufficiency in organ donation by providing a sufficient number of organs for residents in need from within the country or through regional cooperation.

   a. Collaboration between countries is not inconsistent with national self-sufficiency as long as the collaboration protects the vulnerable, promotes equality between donor and recipient populations, and does not violate these principles;

   b. Treatment of patients from outside the country or jurisdiction is only acceptable if it does not undermine a country's ability to provide transplant services for its own population.

6. Organ trafficking and transplant tourism violate the principles of equity, justice and respect for human dignity and should be prohibited. Because transplant commercialism targets impoverished and otherwise vulnerable donors, it leads inexorably to inequity and injustice and should be prohibited. In Resolution 44.25, the World Health Assembly called on countries to prevent the purchase and sale of human organs for transplantation.

   a. Prohibitions on these practices should include a ban on all types of advertising (including electronic and print media), soliciting, or brokering for the purpose of transplant commercialism, organ trafficking, or transplant tourism.

b. Such prohibitions should also include penalties for acts—such as medically screening donors or organs, or transplanting organs—that aid, encourage, or use the products of, organ trafficking or transplant tourism.

c. Practices that induce vulnerable individuals or groups (such as illiterate and impoverished persons, undocumented immigrants, prisoners, and political or economic refugees) to become living donors are incompatible with the aim of combating organ trafficking, transplant tourism and transplant commercialism.

PROPOSALS

Consistent with these principles, participants in the Istanbul Summit suggest the following strategies to increase the donor pool and to prevent organ trafficking, transplant commercialism and transplant tourism and to encourage legitimate, life-saving transplantation programs:

TO RESPOND TO THE NEED TO INCREASE DECEASED DONATION:

1. Governments, in collaboration with health care institutions, professionals, and non-governmental organizations should take appropriate actions to increase deceased organ donation. Measures should be taken to remove obstacles and disincentives to deceased organ donation.

2. In countries without established deceased organ donation or transplantation, national legislation should be enacted that would initiate deceased organ donation and create transplantation infrastructure, so as to fulfill each country's deceased donor potential.

3. In all countries in which deceased organ donation has been initiated, the therapeutic potential of deceased organ donation and transplantation should be maximized.

4. Countries with well-established deceased donor transplant programs are encouraged to share information, expertise and technology with countries seeking to improve their organ donation efforts.

TO ENSURE THE PROTECTION AND SAFETY OF LIVING DONORS AND APPROPRIATE RECOGNITION FOR THEIR HEROIC ACT WHILE COMBATING TRANSPLANT TOURISM, ORGAN TRAFFICKING AND TRANSPLANT COMMERCIALISM:

1. The act of donation should be regarded as heroic and honored as such by representatives of the government and civil society organizations.

2. The determination of the medical and psychosocial suitability of the living donor should be guided by the recommendations of the Amsterdam and Vancouver Forums (2–4).

a. Mechanisms for informed consent should incorporate provisions for evaluating the donor's understanding, including assessment of the psychological impact of the process;

b. All donors should undergo psychosocial evaluation by mental health professionals during screening.

3. The care of organ donors, including

those who have been victims of organ trafficking, transplant commercialism, and transplant tourism, is a critical responsibility of all jurisdictions that sanctioned organ transplants utilizing such practices.

4. Systems and structures should ensure standardization, transparency and accountability of support for donation.

   a. Mechanisms for transparency of process and follow-up should be established;

   b. Informed consent should be obtained both for donation and for follow-up processes.

5. Provision of care includes medical and psychosocial care at the time of donation and for any short- and long-term consequences related to organ donation.

   a. In jurisdictions and countries that lack universal health insurance, the provision of disability, life, and health insurance related to the donation event is a necessary requirement in providing care for the donor;

   b. In those jurisdictions that have universal health insurance, governmental services should ensure donors have access to appropriate medical care related to the donation event;

   c. Health and/or life insurance coverage and employment opportunities of persons who donate organs should not be compromised;

   d. All donors should be offered psychosocial services as a standard component of follow-up;

   e. In the event of organ failure in the donor, the donor should receive:

      i. Supportive medical care,

including dialysis for those with renal failure, and

      ii. Priority for access to transplantation, integrated into existing allocation rules as they apply to either living or deceased organ transplantation.

6. Comprehensive reimbursement of the actual, documented costs of donating an organ does not constitute a payment for an organ, but is rather part of the legitimate costs of treating the recipient.

   a. Such cost-reimbursement would usually be made by the party responsible for the costs of treating the transplant recipient (such as a government health department or a health insurer);

   b. Relevant costs and expenses should be calculated and administered using transparent methodology, consistent with national norms;

   c. Reimbursement of approved costs should be made directly to the party supplying the service (such as to the hospital that provided the donor's medical care);

   d. Reimbursement of the donor's lost income and out-of-pockets expenses should be administered by the agency handling the transplant rather than paid directly from the recipient to the donor.

7. Legitimate expenses that may be reimbursed when documented include:

   a. the cost of any medical and psychological evaluations of potential living donors who are excluded from donation (*e.g.*, because of medical or immunologic issues discovered during the evaluation process);

b. costs incurred in arranging and effecting the pre-, peri- and post-operative phases of the donation process (*e.g.*, long-distance telephone calls, travel, accommodation and subsistence expenses);

c. medical expenses incurred for post-discharge care of the donor;

d. lost income in relation to donation (consistent with national norms).

References

1. World Health Assembly Resolution 57.18, Human organ and tissue transplantation, 22 May 2004, http://www.who.int/gb/ebwha/pdf_files/WHA57/A57_R18-en.pdf.

2. The Ethics Committee of the Transplantation Society (2004). The Consensus Statement of the Amsterdam Forum on the Care of the Live Kidney Donor. *Transplantation* 78(4):491–92.

3. Barr ML, Belghiti J, Villamil FG, Pomfret EA, Sutherland DS, Gruessner RW, Langnas AN & Delmonico FL (2006). A Report of the Vancouver Forum on the Care of the Life Organ Donor: Lung, Liver, Pancreas, and Intenstine Data and Medical Guidelines. *Transplantation* 81(10):1373–85.

4. Pruett TL, Tibell A, Alabdulkareem A, Bhandari M, Cronon DC, Dew MA, Dib-Kuri A, Gutmann T, Matas A, McMurdo L, Rahmel A, Rizvi SAH, Wright L & Delmonico FL (2006). The Ethics Statement of the Vancouver Forum on the Live Lung, Liver, Pancreas, and Intestine Donor. *Transplantation* 81(10):1386–87.

5. Universal Declaration of Human Rights, adopted by the UN General Assembly on December 10, 1948, http://www.un.org/Overview/rights.html.

6. Based on Article 3a of the Protocol to Prevent, Suppress and Punish Trafficking in Persons, Especially Women and Children, Supplementing the United Nations Convention Against Transnational Organized Crime, http://www.uncjin.org/Documents/Conventions/dcatoc/final_documents_2/convention_%20traff_eng.pdf.

The Participants in the International Summit on Transplant Tourism and Organ Trafficking and the manner in which they were chosen and the meeting was organized were as follows:

Process and Participant Selection

Steering Committee

The Steering Committee was selected by an Organizing Committee consisting of Mona Alrukhami, Jeremy Chapman, Francis Delmonico, Mohamed Sayegh, Faissal Shaheen, and Annika Tibell.

The Steering Committee was composed of leadership from The Transplantation Society, including its President-elect and the Chair of its Ethics Committee, and the International Society of Nephrology, including its Vice President and individuals holding Council positions. The Steering Committee had representation from each of the continental regions of the globe with transplantation programs.

The mission of the Steering Committee was to draft a Declaration for consideration by a diverse group of participants at the Istanbul Summit. The Steering Committee also had the responsibility to develop the list of participants to be invited to the Summit meeting.

Istanbul Participant Selection:

Participants at the Istanbul Summit were selected by the Steering Committee according to the following considerations:

- The country liaisons of The Transplantation Society representing virtually all countries with transplantation programs;
- Representatives from international societies and the Vatican;
- Individuals holding leadership positions in nephrology and transplantation;
- Stakeholders in the public policy aspect

of organ transplantation; and

- Ethicists, anthropologists, sociologists, andlegal scholars well-recognized for their writings regarding transplantation policy and practice.

No person or group was polled with respect to their opinion, practice, or philosophy prior to the Steering Committee selection of the Istanbul Summit. After the proposed group of participants was prepared and reviewed by the Steering Committee, they were sent a letter of invitation to the Istanbul Summit, which included the following components:

- the mission of the Steering Committee to draft a Declaration for all Istanbul participants' consideration;
- the agenda and work group format of the Summit;
- the procedure for the selection of participants;
- the work group topics;
- an invitation to the participants to indicate their work group preferences;
- the intent to communicate a draft and other materials before the Summit convened;
- the Summit goals to assemble a final Declaration that could achieve consensus and would address the issues of organ trafficking, transplant tourism and commercialism, and provide principles of practice and recommended alternatives to address the shortage of organs;
- an acknowledgment of the funding provided by Astellas Pharmaceuticals for the Summit;
- provision of hotel accommodations and travel for all invited participants.

Of approximately 170 persons invited, 160 agreed to participate and 152 were able to attend the Summit in Istanbul on April 30–May 2, 2008. Because work on the Declaration at the Summit was to be carried out by dividing the draft document into separate parts, Summit invitees were assigned to a work group topic based on their response concerning the particular topics on which they wished to focus their attention before and during the Summit.

Preparation of the Declaration

The draft Declaration prepared by the Steering Committee was furnished to all participants with ample time for appraisal and response prior to the Summit. The comments and suggestions received in advance were reviewed by the Steering Committee and given to leaders of the appropriate work group at the Summit. (Work group leaders were selected and assigned from the Steering Committee.)

The Summit meeting was formatted so that breakout sessions of the work groups could consider the written responses received from participants prior to the Summit as well as comments from each of the work group participants. The work groups elaborated these ideas as proposed additions to and revisions of the draft. When the Summit reconvened in plenary session, the Chairs of each work group presented the outcome of their breakout session to all Summit participants for discussion. During this process of review, the wording of each section of the Declaration was displayed on a screen before the plenary participants and was modified in light of their comments until consensus was reached on each point.

The content of the Declaration is derived from the consensus that was reached by the participants at the Summit in the plenary sessions which took place on May 1 and 2, 2008. A formatting group was assembled immediately after the Summit to address punctuation, grammatical and related concerns and to record the Declaration in its finished form.

Participants in the Istanbul Summit

Last Name First Name Country

Abboud Omar Sudan
*Abbud-Filho Mario Brazil
Abdramanov Kaldarbek Kyrgyzstan
Abdulla Sadiq Bahrain
Abraham Georgi India
Abueva Amihan V. Philippines
Aderibigbe Ademola Nigeria
*Al-Mousawi Mustafa Kuwait
Alberu Josefina Mexico
Allen Richard D.M. Australia
Almazan-Gomez Lynn C. Philippines
Alnono Ibrahim Yemen
*Alobaidli Ali Abdulkareem United Arab Emirates
*Alrukhaimi Mona United Arab Emirates
Álvarez Inés Uruguay
Assad Lina Saudi Arabia
Assounga Alain G. South Africa
Baez Yenny Colombia
*Bagheri Alireza Iran
*Bakr Mohamed Adel Egypt
Bamgboye Ebun Nigeria
*Barbari Antoine Lebanon
Belghiti Jacques France
Ben Abdallah Taieb Tunisia
Ben Ammar Mohamed Salah Tunisia
Bos Michael The Netherlands
Britz Russell South Africa
Budiani Debra USA
*Capron Alexander USA
Castro Cristina R. Brazil
*Chapman Jeremy Australia
Chen Zhonghua Klaus People's Republic of China
Codreanu Igor Moldova

Cole Edward Canada
Cozzi Emanuele Italy
*Danovitch Gabriel USA
Davids Razeen South Africa
De Broe Marc Belgium
*De Castro Leonardo Philippines
*Delmonico Francis L. USA
Derani Rania Syria
Dittmer Ian New Zealand
Domínguez-Gil Beatriz Spain
Duro-Garcia Valter Brazil
Ehtuish Ehtuish Libya
El-Shoubaki Hatem Qatar
Epstein Miran United Kingdom
*Fazel Iraj Iran
Fernandez Zincke Eduardo Belgium
Garcia-Gallont Rudolf Guatemala
Ghods Ahad J. Iran
Gill John Canada
Glotz Denis France
Gopalakrishnan Ganesh India
Gracida Carmen Mexico
Grinyo Josep Spain
Ha Jongwon South Korea
*Haberal Mehmet A. Turkey
Hakim Nadey United Kingdom
Harmon William USA
Hasegawa Tomonori Japan
Hassan Ahmed Adel Egypt
Hickey David Ireland
Hiesse Christian France
Hongji Yang People's Republic of China
Humar Ines Croatia
Hurtado Abdias Peru
Ismail Moustafa Wesam Egypt
Ivanovski Ninoslav Macedonia
*Jha Vivekanand India
Kahn Delawir South Africa
Kamel Refaat Egypt
Kirpalani Ashok India
Kirste Guenter Germany
*Kobayashi Eiji Japan

Koller Jan   Slovakia
Kranenburg Leonieke   The Netherlands
*Lameire Norbert   Belgium
Laouabdia-Sellami Karim   France
Lei Ruipeng   People's Republic of China
*Levin Adeera   Canada
Lloveras Josep   Spain
Lõhmus Aleksander   Estonia
Luciolli Esmeralda   France
Lundin Susanne   Sweden
Lye Wai Choong   Singapore
Lynch Stephen   Australia
*Maïga Mahamane   Mali
Mamzer Bruneel Marie-France   France
Maric Nicole   Austria
*Martin Dominique   Australia
*Masri Marwan   Lebanon
Matamoros Maria A.   Costa Rica
Matas Arthur   USA
McNeil Adrian   United Kingdom
Meiser Bruno   Germany
Meši Enisa   Bosnia
Moazam Farhat   Pakistan
Mohsin Nabil   Oman
Mor Eytan   Israel
Morales Jorge   Chile
Munn Stephen   New Zealand
Murphy Mark   Ireland
*Naicker Saraladevi   South Africa
Naqvi S.A. Anwar   Pakistan
*Noël Luc   WHO
Obrador Gregorio   Mexico
Oliveros Yolanda   Philippines
Ona Enrique   Philippines
Oosterlee Arie   The Netherlands
Oyen Ole   Norway
Padilla Benita   Philippines
Pratschke Johann   Germany
Rahamimov Ruth   Israel
Rahmel Axel   The Netherlands
Reznik Oleg   Russia
*Rizvi S. Adibul Hasan   Pakistan

Roberts Lesley Ann   Trinidad and Tobago
*Rodriguez-Iturbe Bernardo   Venezuela
Rowinski Wojciech   Poland
Saeed Bassam   Syria
Sarkissian Ashot   Armenia
*Sayegh Mohamed H.   USA
Scheper-Hughes Nancy   USA
Sever Mehmet Sukru   Turkey
*Shaheen Faissal A.   Saudi Arabia
Sharma Dhananjaya   India
Shinozaki Naoshi   Japan
Simforoosh Nasser   Iran
Singh Harjit   Malaysia
Sok Hean Thong   Cambodia
Somerville Margaret   Canada
Stadtler Maria   USA
*Stephan Antoine   Lebanon
Suárez Juliette   Cuba
Suaudeau Msgr. Jacques   Italy
Sumethkul Vasant   Thailand
Takahara Shiro   Japan
Thiel Gilbert T.   Switzerland
*Tibell Annika   Sweden
Tomadze Gia   Georgia
*Tong Matthew Kwok-Lung   Hong Kong
Tsai Daniel Fu-Chang   Taiwan
Uriarte Remedios   Philippines
Vanrenterghem Yves F.C.   Belgium
*Vathsala A.   Singapore
Weimar Willem   The Netherlands
Wikler Daniel   USA
Young Kimberly   Canada
Yuldashev Ulugbek   Uzbekistan
Zhao Minggang   People's Republic of China

* = Members of the Steering Committee.
(William Couser, USA, was also a member of the Steering Committee but was unable to attend the Summit.)

Chapter 32

The Hazards of Transplant Tourism

Francis L. Delmonico

In the November issue of the CJASN, Jagbir Gill et al. present a University of California Los Angeles (UCLA) series of 33 patients that underwent kidney transplantation in a foreign country and returned to the United States for post-transplant care. "Transplant tourists" are traveling to established destinations to obtain readily accessible organs for transplantation, available from the poor of that destination country who sell mostly kidneys, but in some instances, a lobe of the liver or a cornea. These practices have been well known for more than a decade. In 2004, the World Health Assembly (WHA) issued a resolution urging member states "to take measures to protect the poorest and vulnerable groups from transplant tourism and the sale of tissues and organs, including attention to the wider problem of international trafficking in human tissues and organs."

Although the WHA 2004 resolution was unambiguous in its objection to trafficking and transplant tourism, a comprehensive description of these unethical practices was still needed. To address the concerns of the WHA, a Summit Meeting of more than 150 international representatives of scientific and medical bodies, government officials, social scientists, and ethicists was held in Istanbul, Turkey from April 30 to May 2, 2008. The result of these deliberations was the Istanbul Declaration on Organ Trafficking and Transplant Tourism.

Gill describes the transplant tourist as a resident of the United States who underwent transplantation outside the United States and then returned for follow-up care. The UCLA group makes no conclusion regarding the ethical propriety of this practice, disclaiming social circumstances that may have propelled these patients to travel for transplantation. The Istanbul Declaration, however, distinguishes travel for transplantation from transplant tourism by means of the following: "travel for transplantation is the movement of organs, donors, recipients or transplant professionals across jurisdictional borders for transplantation purposes. Travel for transplantation becomes transplant tourism if it involves organ trafficking and/or transplant commercialism or if the resources (organs, professionals and transplant centers) devoted to providing transplants to patients from outside a country undermine the country's ability to provide transplant services for its own population." The practical basis for concern arises when the destination country places its own resident patient population at disadvantage for gaining access to the list because lucrative arrangements for patients from the client countries simultaneously claim an allocation priority. Meanwhile, in the client country, readily available access to organs (in the destination country) prevents deceased-donor programs from gaining widespread support.

Nevertheless, not all recipient travel for transplantation in a foreign country is unethical. The Istanbul Declaration provides additional guidance that travel for transplantation may be ethical if the following conditions are fulfilled:

For Live Donors

If the recipient has a dual citizenship and wishes to undergo transplantation from a live donor that is a family member in a country of citizenship that is not their residence;

if the donor and recipient are genetically related and wish to undergo transplantation in a country not of their residence.

For Deceased Donors

If official regulated bilateral or multilateral organ sharing programs based on a reciprocated organ sharing programs exist between or among countries or jurisdictions.

Gill reports that 17 (52%) of the 33 UCLA tourist patients had infections, with nine requiring hospitalization. The 1-year graft survival was 89% for tourists and 98% for the matched UCLA cohort. The comparative outcome of the tourist patients is a compelling revelation of the hazards of undergoing transplantation in a foreign country. These data are important to transplant physicians who advise their patients not to undertake such risks without some acceptance of the fate that comes with an unpredictable transplant experience. Donor transmitted infection may not be surprising if the kidney is obtained from an executed prisoner in China, where tuberculosis and hepatitis are more prevalent, rather than a deceased donor in the United States.

Notwithstanding these UCLA data, the transplant physician ultimately has to care for the transplant tourist, despite the appropriate admonition to such a patient. The transplant physician has an obligation to care for patients and not judge them. Nevertheless, the Israeli Ministry of Health has recently developed a more practical approach: if it is illegal to undergo transplantation in a foreign country (for example, now in the Philippines), then insurance companies should not condone or provide support for such an illegal activity. This approach would not solve the conundrum of care for the physician, but it would be a substantial deterrent for transplant tourists who seek to undergo the procedure in a foreign country.

The UCLA data and the Istanbul Declaration represent a concerted effort to establish a national self-sufficiency in every country with transplantation practices. Client countries should no longer presume that donor organs from the poor will be preferentially available to their rich patient population because of their affluence and ability to travel. The data from this UCLA report should also be a stark reminder that transplantation care requires an expertise best provided by a transplant center that is devoted to the patient's interest, not to the patient's resources.

See related article, "Transplant Tourism in the United States: A Single-Center Experience," on pages 1820–1828 of the November 2008 issue of CJASN.

Chapter 33

Transplant Tourism in China
A Tale of Two Transplants

Rosamond Rhodes and Thomas Schiano

Abstract

The use of organs obtained from executed prisoners in China has recently been condemned by every major transplant organization. The government of the People's Republic of China has also recently made it illegal to provide transplant organs from executed prisoners to foreign transplant tourists. Nevertheless, the extreme shortage of transplant organs in the U.S. continues to make organ transplantation in China an appealing option for some patients with end-stage disease. Their choice of traveling to China for an organ leaves U.S. transplant programs with decisions about how to respond to the needs of patients who return after transplantation. By discussing two cases that raised this dilemma, we argue for upholding medicine's commitments to traditional principles of beneficence and nonjudgmental regard in sorting out the policies that a transplant program should adopt. We also explain how position statements that aim for the high ground of moral purity fail to give appropriate weight to the needs and suffering of present and future patients in the U.S. and in China.

Introduction

Organ transplantation raises numerous ethical issues. The most serious issues involve questions about who is to provide the organs and how the limited number should be allocated among the many patients who need them. Generally, an ethically justified allocation requires attending to the morally relevant factors and ignoring irrelevant factors. Beyond that general framework, it requires justice in treating similar cases similarly. That said, when we come to allocating scarce transplant organs and scarce medical resources, we are left with the difficulty of determining which factors are relevant, which should be ignored, and what makes cases morally similar.

These critical issues for transplantation become especially complicated when transplant tourism is involved and transplant centers have to sort out which, if any, medical care or additional transplant organs they should provide for returning transplant tourists (Boschert 2007). The circumstances of transplant tourism vary significantly, and much can be said about each of the different circumstances. Certainly, a great deal can also be said about the background institutional arrangements, cultural attitudes, and personal choices that lead patients to become transplant tourists.

Yet, in what follows, we focus narrowly on the issues of professional responsibility and the duties of transplant centers and discuss the matter by explaining our response to two cases that we encountered. Our analysis weaves together several relevant considerations and thereby requires us to piece them together and follow out several separate threads.

A Case from Long Ago

About a dozen years ago, a young girl with kidney failure needed a kidney transplant to survive. No one in her family was willing to donate a kidney to a female child, and, given the waiting time for a transplant organ, she was not expected to get one from the deceased donor list in time to save her.[1]

The family was wealthy and well-connected at home in China. Even though the family members were not willing to go so far as to donate a kidney, they did love their daughter. Short of donating an organ, they wanted to do whatever they could to save her life. After consulting with doctors in China, they offered to pay all the expenses for a transplant team from our program to go to China and perform the surgery. They explained that the team could dictate its own schedule and that everything would be done at the team's convenience. They also wanted the team from our center to teach Chinese transplant surgeons the fine points of performing a kidney transplant to a child from an adult donor, because, at the time, the Chinese surgeons did not know how it was done.

Our kidney transplant program declined the invitation. Little information on the practices in China was then available. Without any significant investigation, we were convinced that the transplant organ would be taken without consent from an executed Chinese prisoner. We were convinced that we were, therefore, justified in refusing to participate. We reasoned that using executed prisoners as organ donors would lay the Chinese judicial process open to corruption by providing perverse incentives to increase the number of executions. Because it would surely be wrong to do anything to encourage executions or anything that would contribute to the corruption of the judicial process, we concluded that we should refuse to collaborate in any way.

In the end, no deceased donor organ became available for the little girl. In spite of the program's best efforts to save her, she died shortly after we declined her parents' offer.

Concurring Opinions from the Transplant Community

While we could find no professional recommendations to guide our decision way back then, in the past couple of years professional societies have begun to publish their advice and guidelines on how to proceed.[2] In April 2007 the International Society for Heart and Lung Transplant (ISHLT) issued a statement on accepting organs from prisoners that echoes our thinking in the case of the little Chinese girl. The ISHLT Statement on Transplant Ethics argues that the practice:

- Contravenes the principles of voluntary donation.
- Provides perverse incentives to increase number of executions.
- Lays the judicial process open to corruption.

The ISHLT therefore concludes that members should discourage patients from seeking transplant in countries where there is no external scrutiny and assurance of ethical standards and declares that members should not participate in, or support, the transplantation of organs from prisoners. The statement goes on to hold out sanctions against those who would fail to comply with their position. It states, "Members found to have contravened this principle may have their rights and privileges as members suspended or revoked." In conformance with its stand, this society now requires a personal declaration that the author adheres to these principles to accompany all submissions to *The Journal of Heart and Lung Transplantation*.

It should be noted that the Declaration of Istanbul on Organ Trafficking and Transplant Tourism has condemned transplant tourism and related practices. This declaration was endorsed by the American Society of Nephrology (ASN), one of the organizations sponsoring the Istanbul meeting. In the same vein, the United Network for Organ Sharing (UNOS) Board of Directors issued a Statement on Transplant Tourism on June 27, 2007. In it, this board too condemns transplant tourism. Interestingly, both the declaration and the statement stop short of offering further direction to transplant programs. The statement "recommends that emergent care be provided to such recipients," but it goes no further. It also includes a specious exemption from the duty to provide non-emergent care for those "physicians who raise a conscientious objection."[3]

Similarly, the American Association for the Study of Liver Diseases (AASLD) and the International Liver Transplant Society (ILTS) have recently endorsed the same line of argument and created policies to uphold similar standards. They have taken positions against exploitation of donors and recovery of organs from executed prisoners, and they have gone farther, to also condemn the use of paid living donors. They have also stated that original publications should explicitly exclude the use of executed prisoners or paid donors. In addition, in March 2008, NATCO, The Organization for Transplant Professionals, adopted a similar stance. Citing its Code of Ethics, which requires "all transplant personnel . . . [to] maintain the highest standard of professional conduct and act to protect the health and safety of organ donors and recipients," it concludes, without argument, that "Organ tourism is not in harmony with these goals, thus NATCO condemns the practice." While holding that "Patients who participate in organ tourism should not be abandoned," but allowing physicians to opt out of their treatment, NATCO goes on to impose sanctions against those "who knowingly participate in organ tourism" and to exclude publications and presentations that include data from studies which violate their principles.

The United States Today

That said, a Scientific Registry of Transplant Recipients (SRTR) analysis published in August 2007 identified 173 wait-list removals, including 158 patients waiting for a kidney transplant, as having been transplanted at foreign centers. The authors of this analysis estimate that an additional 200–335 patients had received transplants abroad, for a total of 373–408 transplant patients, with about 75% occurring between 2004 and 2006. Furthermore, it is estimated that more than 40% of these transplant tourists reside in New York and California. All of this amounts to saying that our rare and unusual situation from years ago is no longer either rare or unusual (Merion 2008).

The transplant tourism phenomenon is not all that surprising, given the marked scarcity of transplant organs in the United States. As of June 7, 2009, there were 101,943 waitlist candidates on the UNOS list, with a new patient added to the list approximately every 14 min. In 2008, there were fewer than 8,000 organ donors and fewer than 22,000 transplanted organs. That means patients do die while waiting for a transplant organ from a deceased donor. For example, 15% of patients die on the liver transplant waiting lists annually. This shortage of transplant organs also involves enormous morbidity and financial costs associated with treating organ failure when no transplant organ is available.

Several factors account for the growing transplant lists and the increasing shortfall of transplant organs. Ever-improving patient and graft survival increases the number of patients who opt for transplantation as a treatment for their end-stage organ failure. In addition, the success of the technology has made transplantation a viable treatment for more conditions. Furthermore, patients who were previously excluded from transplantation are now transplant candidates (e.g., some patients who are HIV+, some patients with liver cancer). And, because transplant organs do not always last indefinitely, some patients come to need re-transplantation.

In the United States, listing for transplant, organ procurement, and organ allocation are all strictly regulated by UNOS. Different rules govern the allocation of each type of organ, but in all cases, prioritization is based on the medical criteria of:

- Urgency.
- Need.
- Tissue match/organ compatibility.
- Time on the list.

Patients who need a transplant organ have few options for improving their chance of receiving one. Patients who need a kidney or a liver transplant could receive one from a living donor. Yet only about 10% of patients who need a kidney or liver have a suitable live donor, and for those who do, live donation involves attendant risks for the donor that have to be taken into account. Patients with the wherewithal to do so have the option of multi-institutional listing, which can increase the chance of a patient from a region with a long waiting list to receive an organ at a center in a region with a shorter waiting list. Often multi-institutional listing is not feasible because of geography, health insurance, or lack of financial resources. Using extended criteria donors is another option for increasing a patient's chance for getting a transplant organ. These organs, from less than optimal donors, could save a recipient's life, but they also offer poorer patient/graft survival than the organs that would otherwise be used in transplantation.

Last Year's Case

A 45 year old lawyer was found to have hepatitis B virus, cirrhosis, and liver cancer. He was listed for liver transplantation. After he had waited on the list for a year, friends suggested that he go to China where he could obtain a liver transplant for a fee. Our patient investigated the option, made the necessary arrangements, and informed his doctors at our transplant center that he was going to China to receive a liver transplant.

Three months later the patient returned to our program requesting follow-up care. He explained that he had received a liver transplant in China, but, when questioned, claimed that he knew nothing about the source of the transplant organ.

Two months later, the patient developed

sepsis due to bile-duct problems and hepatic artery thrombosis. These serious problems were probably iatrogenic, related to injury during the transplant surgery. At this point, he was very ill, and re-transplantation was his only treatment option. There was no potential live organ donor.

Opinions on the liver transplant team were divided on the issue of whether he should be listed for a liver transplant. Some argued that he should not be listed for another liver transplant. Others held that as our patient we must list him. Others were unsure how to proceed. The matter was referred to the Ethics Committee of the Medical Board for advice.

An Ethics Committee meeting was promptly convened. At our institution the Ethics Committee has 25 members appointed by the Medical Board. It includes a member from the hospital administration, a bioethicist, someone from the community, someone from the legal department, a nurse, a patient representative, a social worker, and physicians from an array of clinical departments, many at the level of department chair, vice-chair, or division chief. All members of the liver transplant team who were interested in attending were invited to participate in the meeting, and many did.

After hearing all of the accounts presented by team members, and after raising and discussing whatever questions participants wanted to air, we were left with the sense that there was a good chance that the original transplant organ came from an executed Chinese prisoner. Nevertheless, the Ethics Committee members, as well as those from the transplant team who participated in the conversation, were convinced of the importance of our abiding by central principles of medical ethics.

In this case, we recognized the professional responsibility to adhere to medicine's distinctive moral obligations. A central tenet of medical ethics, with roots way back in the Hippocratic tradition, is the commitment to nonjudgmental regard. This professional responsibility requires health professionals to render care to patients who need it without being influenced by any judgment as to the patient's worthiness. After all, enemy soldiers, prisoners, and even Tony Soprano are entitled to good medical care delivered with compassion and respect. And our patient had not directly caused harm to anyone. In fact, his receiving a transplant organ in China had initially advantaged all of the patients behind him on the waiting list by removing someone ahead of them. We understood that our professional commitment to nonjudgmental regard required us to avoid disparaging this patient, or his choice for transplant tourism, in any way.

We also recognized that doctors have a positive duty of beneficence, that is, a professional obligation to promote the good of patients. Furthermore, as we saw it, doctors actually have a fiduciary responsibility to their patients, which amounts to using the knowledge, powers, and privileges entrusted to them for the good of patients, even when that requires physicians to put the good of patients before their own.

Based on our recognition of these profession-defining responsibilities, the Ethics Committee concluded that the transplant team should treat their transplant tourist as any other patient with a similar need. The committee therefore recommended that the patient should be listed for re-transplantation and treated as any other patient with similarly urgent needs would be. By the end of the meeting, the committee's recommendation was unanimous, and there was no opposition from any member of the transplant team.

The patient was listed for re-transplantation. While he waited on the list, his condition deteriorated and he required multiple hospitalizations. When a transplant organ became available, transplantation was performed. Unfortunately, there was primary non-function of the transplanted organ, and the patient required another transplant. Because of his critical condition, he was quickly allocated another organ and he received a third liver transplant. After a 3-month hospitalization the patient was discharged. He continues to do well.

Some Background Information on Transplant Tourism

Multiple reports have documented trafficking in human organs worldwide. For example, in December 2003 an international kidney transplant trafficking ring was busted. It was revealed that organ transplant recipients had paid $100,000 to the ring for a kidney transplant, while living donors had received only $800. It was also reported that a kidney could be had for $1,000 to $10,000 (Delmonico 2002) and a liver transplant from an executed prisoner in the People's Republic of China (PRC) could be had for $94,000 (BBC 2006). These revelations were followed by international condemnation of paid living donor transplantation in India, Pakistan, the Philippines, China, and South Africa. The denunciation and legal sanctions have driven some of these transplant tourism activities underground. It is assumed, however, that they continue, but without government oversight or regulation (Rakela 2007).

Transplant tourism has been associated with significant problems for those who sell their organs. The money that they are promised is paltry, and they are frequently swindled out of some of the procurement fee. The surgery used to procure the organs and the post-transplant care are often substandard. After-care that should be provided is typically not made available (Budiani-Saberi 2008).

According to most studies, patients who receive organs as transplant tourists also experience significant problems.[4] They too are frequently victims of shoddy surgical techniques. In addition, their transplants are compromised by poor organ matching, unhealthy donors, and post-transplant infection. Typically, organ recipients do not receive adequate patient education either pre- or post-transplant, and there is poor communication throughout because of language barriers. They are discharged from the facility prematurely and encouraged to travel prematurely, and their immunosuppression is inadequate. And when they return to their home transplant center they have inadequate records of what was done or no records at all. All of these problems compromise their health, their lives, and their transplant organs (Bramstedt 2007; Canales 2006; Chugh 2000; Higgins 2003; Inston 2005; Ivanovski 1997; Kennedy 2005; Prasad 2006; Sevcr 1994; Sever 2001).

Combined, the practices associated with transplant tourism could translate into problems for the entire transplant community. Health professionals who work in transplantation worry that the transplant tourism industry could undermine our reliance on altruism for organ donation, undermine society's trust in transplant programs, and ultimately have a negative impact on future organ donation.

Liver Transplantation in the People's Republic of China

The People's Republic of China has a population of more than 1.3 billion, and 20–30%

of the population is infected with hepatitis B virus (HBV). HBV often leads to liver disease, and complications of liver disease are a leading cause of death in the PRC (Rakela 2007).

It is estimated that about 1.5 million people in the PRC need organ transplantation, whereas only about 10,000 organs are available for transplantation each year. Modernization and the improved standard of living in China have led to an increased demand for organ transplantation, including liver transplantation as treatment for end-stage liver disease. Although the technical developments that make liver transplantation possible have advanced, in China there is still little regulation or oversight of organ transplantation and no national organ registry or network has been developed.

Because of the prevailing religious traditions, China, like most other Asian countries, has no "brain death" law. For that reason, almost all organ transplants in most Asian countries come from living donors. Yet, in the PRC, approximately 95% of liver transplants come from deceased donors. In 2005, approximately 3,500 liver transplants were performed in China. The country now has about 10 well-established centers that perform the vast majority of the liver transplants. There are also more than 200 additional centers with developing programs that perform a small number of liver transplants. The official reported survival in Chinese programs is close to the reported survival in the United States, 85% for one-year survival and 70% for 5-year survival. (Huang 2007)

The obvious implication of these data is that approximately 3,325 transplanted livers come from executed prisoners in the PRC. On its face, this looks like a tremendously high number of executed prisoners. A comparison with the execution rate in the state of Texas, however, puts the number in perspective.

Executions carried out in Texas in each year of this millennium:

Year	2000	2001	2002	2003	2004	2005	2006	2007	2008
#	40	17	33	24	23	19	24	22	18

Texas Department of Criminal Justice, http://www.tdcj.state.tx.us/stat/executedoffenders.htm
Additional data
20,851,820 = Texas population in 2000
24,324,976 = Texas population in 2008
U.S. Census Bureau, http://quickfacts.census.gov/qfd/states/48000.html
U.S. Census Bureau, http://www.census.gov/census2000/states/tx.html

Adjusting for population, a comparable rate of execution in 2000 would have yielded approximately 2,476 executed prisoners in the PRC, about 75% of the number of prisoners whose organs are used there in liver transplantation. Comparing an average of the 3 years of this millennium with the highest number of executions in Texas with the population size of the PRC would yield approximately 1,733 executions, about 52% of the executed prisoners whose livers were used for transplantation in 2008. Although we have scant information about the legal processes in the PRC, or the kinds of crimes that are punishable with death, or the proportion of executed prisoners whose organs are used in transplantation, in light of the comparison with Texas, what is being done in the PRC does not seem on an order of magnitude so egregious as to merit the sanctions and policies imposed by the majority of transplant organizations.[5]

Commercialization of organ transplantation in the People's Republic of China benefits wealthy patients. The use of executed prisoners as a source of deceased donor organs is publicly accepted, and Vice-Minister of Health Huang has publicly acknowledged that the majority of deceased donors are prisoners who were subjected to capital punishment (BBC 04/19/2006). He has claimed that the donors or their families give consent for the use of the organs in transplantation. There is no documented remuneration to families. In the past, executions have been carried out by gunshot to the head after the administration of medications to promote organ perfusion. It is claimed that transplant surgeons are not at all involved in the execution process (Huang 2007).

The Non-Issue of Informed Consent

Huang appears to be responding to the many critics who complain about the lack of informed consent in the use of organs from executed prisoners. This is an odd complaint in view of the fact that by dint of being prisoners, individuals are, typically, deprived of numerous rights. Without their consent, others make decisions about where they live, when they wake, when they sleep, what they eat, what they do, if and when they die, and how. Prisoners are not allowed to refuse medical treatment or food. Prisoners who try to refuse have treatment or food forced upon them. Traditionally, the state can even decide on the disposition of a prisoner's corpse. Claiming that informed consent is ethically required for the disposition of the organs of an executed prisoner requires an argument to show why

this particular decision is, or should be, an exception to state authority. We have not found any in the literature.

Furthermore, in one form or another, presumed consent for organ procurement is now an accepted practice in numerous countries, including Austria, Belgium, France, Italy, Spain, Sweden, and the United Kingdom. Policies of presumed consent reflect two concepts, (1) that individual consent for organ donation is not ethically necessary, and (2) that it is good to conserve scarce resources and to avoid wasting them. The procurement of organs from executed prisoners in the PRC reflects these same reasons. As long as the transplant community withholds criticism and sanctions from countries that employ presumed consent, their opposition to the transplant practices in the PRC on the basis of lack of informed consent appears to lack grounds.

Sophocles' play *Antigone* provides a relevant example. After the death of Oedipus, his two sons, Polyneices and Etiocles, are to share the throne of Thebes. When Etiocles usurps complete control, Polyneices, accompanied by six foreign princes, descends on Thebes. The two brothers kill each other in battle, leaving Creon, their uncle, on the throne. Creon orders that Polyneices should not be allowed funeral rites because he attacked his own kingdom. Antigone, the sister of Polyneices, is then torn between her political duty to obey Creon, her sovereign, and her personal duties to her brother and her gods (Sophocles, 1998).

Two points should be noted: (1) Antigone does not dispute Creon's political authority over the disposition of her brother's corpse. In other words, there is a long history of accepting the legitimacy of political power over decisions about the disposition of dead bodies, particularly the corpses of those who have violated the law of the land. (2) Antigone's dilemma illustrates how duties can have different sources and conflict with one another for that reason. In her case, she faces a conflict between personal morality and political responsibility. In this paper, we argue that professional responsibility provides a third source of duty.

Mount Sinai Transplant Program's Experience with Transplant Tourism

Patients in our program who have been transplant tourists learned about the option from abroad by word of mouth. In the period from 2004 to 2009, nine of our patients had liver transplantation in the PRC. Six of these patients were known to our program prior to their transplants. Eight of the nine patients had HBV, and seven of the nine had hepatocellular carcinoma. For the past year, the official policy in the PRC has excluded foreigners from organ transplant candidacy. Nevertheless, one patient returned from the PRC after recently receiving a liver transplant there.

One of these patients required re-transplantation, and three developed biliary problems. Three patients had worsening of liver disease due to the substandard care that they received abroad. One patient died of liver failure. In addition, as far as we know, five of our patients had a kidney transplant in either China or India. Three of these transplanted kidneys failed. These results corroborate the reports that U.S. patients who receive kidney or liver transplants in China or India receive substandard care.

The Distinctive Ethics of Medicine

Our cases, taken together with the background information already given here, allow us to foresee questions that any major U.S. transplant program will have to confront. To determine what should have been done in our two cases, and to answer the questions that loom on the horizon, requires us to take a stand on a critical core issue of medical ethics. Are the ethics of medicine an extrapolation from common morality, or does the ethical practice of medicine rest on distinctive justifications, distinctive principles, and distinctive moral virtues? In other words, could the answers to questions posed from different perspectives be different?

Consider these three questions with respect to our first case: (1) How should these parents of a little girl in kidney failure respond? (2) How should our government respond to questionable legal practices surrounding the death penalty in another country? (3) How should the physicians in a transplant center respond? To us, these are very different questions and different kinds of considerations are relevant to each answer. The first is a personal question, and personal commitments and values are relevant factors. The second is a political question. Goals and reasons that are broadly shared by the members of our society as well as previous commitments by our government are relevant to the answer. The third is a question about professional responsibility. Personal commitments and political stands are not relevant. It has to be answered from the perspective of the duties of the profession.

The point of distinguishing these three questions is to show that the ethics of medicine are significantly different from the ethics of everyday life in dramatic and important ways, and that clinicians need a clear understanding of the special responsibilities of medicine (Rhodes 2007) To clarify this point, consider the following profession-endorsed principles that should be used to guide medical behavior, specifically, three principles of medical ethics that are germane to our cases and questions about transplant tourism.

Fiduciary Responsibility and Beneficence

People appreciate their susceptibility to injury and disease. So, with respect to medical need, they would want attention from skilled and knowledgeable practitioners who could cure disease, alleviate symptoms, restore function, ease suffering, and save lives. These realizations create a broadly accepted consensus that the distinctive knowledge, skills, powers, and privileges that society allows to doctors must be used for the good of patients and society. This is the core of medicine's fiduciary responsibility and commitment to beneficence. These two principles require doctors to act as trusted agents of their patients' welfare and to put their patients' good before their own.

While ordinary morality allows people to distance themselves from the unpalatable choices of others, that luxury is incompatible with the practice of medicine. Medicine's fiduciary responsibility and commitment to beneficence require physicians to use their knowledge and skills to promote their patients' good. Respect for autonomy in this sense requires physicians to accept their patients' views of the good and their patients' ranking of values.

Nonjudgmental Regard

Great wits are often especially adept at identifying flaws in others and making them the butts of jokes and the objects of derision. In times of war, people feel free to hate the enemy. And, frequently, we think that others should be held accountable for their own misfortune. Yet, when it comes to medical care, we want doctors to attend to our loved one's needs regardless of whether or not they were somehow at fault for their current medical

predicament and regardless of their worth in the eyes of others. In fact, we expect physicians to provide excellent medical care to people with whom they might not otherwise associate, to prisoners with medical needs, and to wounded enemy soldiers.

Transplant Tourism in China

Because we never know how unworthy we or our loved ones may appear in the eyes of others, or where or how disheveled one of us is likely to be when we happen to need medical attention, we expect doctors to promote the good of those with medical needs without first judging their worth. Physicians, therefore, have to be nonjudgmental in their allocation of caring concern and medical attention, and they have to try hard to avoid feeling frustrated by patient noncompliance or angered by patient deception, disrespect, or demands.

Ethical Issues for a U.S. Transplant Program

The Ethics Committee that considered our second case responded to the questions, "Should a transplant program provide ongoing treatment to patients who have secured transplant organs under ethically questionable circumstances?" and "Should patients who have received a transplant under questionable circumstances be eligible for re-transplantation if the need arises?" Committee members drew their responses from the professional commitments of medicine. The core commitments to nonjudgmental regard, beneficence, and fiduciary responsibility dictated that it was a medical responsibility to provide care for patients who needed it, and to treat patients based on their need, regardless of what they might have done or how they secured their transplanted organ.

Other questions are, however, on the horizon. We have already noted that some patients who have returned to our program after transplantation abroad had good results, and others had poor results, apparently related to poor medical care. When future patients announce their intention to go abroad for an organ transplant, should a U.S. program steer them away from institutions that seem to provide shoddy care? To the extent that the information is available, should a U.S. program offer information on the quality of foreign transplant programs as guidance for their patients? Again, medicine's commitment to serving patients, that is, the commitments to nonjudgmental regard, beneficence, and fiduciary responsibility, all point to a duty to inform. And knowing that foreign programs typically provide inadequate patient education and inadequate records suggests that a U.S. program should offer its patients the education that they will need, along with forms to elicit and communicate relevant information to the home institution about the organ donor, the surgery, and the postsurgical treatment.

Taking this line of thought a step further will lead programs to consider the lot of their patients who can be expected to die for lack of a transplant organ, given the current organ shortage. Should patients be informed about the possibility of transplant tourism when they would not be eligible for a transplant in the United States or when they are likely to die before reaching the top of the transplant list? Again, the medical responsibility to put a patient's well-being before one's own, the commitment to beneficence, and physicians' fiduciary responsibility all dictate that the information should be provided.

Then, we have to consider all of the thousands of Chinese patients in need of transplantation and the inferior standard of care that has been documented in the returning transplant tourists. This leads us to ask, "Should we provide training in transplant medicine and surgery to visiting physicians from countries known to obtain organs through ethically questionable means and to cater to transplant tourists?" Or, should we go farther and provide on-site training in transplant medicine and surgery at foreign centers that engage in this work? Once more, the commitments to beneficence and the welfare of all patients, including organ failure patients in distant lands with questionable legal practices, dictate that medical expertise should be shared when patients stand to benefit.

Given the tremendous number of Chinese patients who need transplantation, the ability of many wealthy Chinese patients to pay for their deceased donor transplants, and the relatively small number of U.S. patients who travel to the PRC for an organ transplant, it is hard to imagine that the position of U.S. transplant programs could have any impact at all on the policies surrounding the Chinese legal system or the use of organs from executed prisoners in transplantation. For that reason, the positions by transplant societies that oppose interaction of medical professionals with the Chinese transplant community are likely to provide no benefit to anyone. Extrapolating from the experience of the transplant tourists who have returned to our program after receiving an organ transplant in the PRC, there is a significant need for improving transplantation techniques and the care of transplant patients in China. Interaction with the Chinese transplant community could, therefore, provide significant benefit to future Chinese patients whose medical care could be improved significantly by the training and communication that come from interaction with the international community of transplant medicine.

A Concurring Opinion from the Transplant Community

The Transplantation Society has published a "Policy on Interaction with China" that aligns with our position in some respects. The Transplantation Society maintains that health professionals from China should be accepted as registrants at meetings. Lecturing and sharing expertise in China in order to promote ongoing dialogue and education are condoned. And training physicians from China is condoned as long as they comply with the society's Policy and Ethics statements (TTS/Transplantation 2007; 84: 292–294). Similarly, other groups of transplant surgeons have reached conclusions that are in line with ours (Sever 2001, 1482).

A Moral Quandary

Clearly, we reached different conclusions in our two cases. Clearly, the professional transplant societies have reached similarly different conclusions. Clearly, both of the conclusions that point in opposite directions cannot be right. Yet it is also obvious that a good deal of thoughtful attention went into developing the contradictory positions on both sides. It is, therefore, instructive to account for these diametrically opposed views.

A careful examination of the reasons underlying each position explains the radical difference and also suggests a way of understanding the disagreement. From what they say in justifying their stands, we can see that the discussants were asking different questions, and different questions get different answers. In our first case, we considered the personal question, "What should I do?," and the political question, "What should our country's public policy be?" We wanted to know if we would have dirty hands or guilty consciences by involving ourselves in the questionable legal practices and executions of Chinese convicts and the shady practice of taking their organs for paid transplants. We were also concerned about the possibility of corrupting the political justice system in China that might be inclined to hand out death sentences for trivial crimes if there was a profit to be made. (Chang and Thompkins 2002; David 1999) These are legitimate questions for individuals to consider and matters that our political leaders should address in molding our public policies and our relations with other countries of the international community. These also seem to be the concerns that motivated the positions of the International Society for Heart and Lung Transplant, the American Association for the Study of Liver Diseases, NATCO, and the International Liver Transplant Society.

For medical professionals and bioethicists who see the ethics of medicine as merely the extension of common morality to medical issues, those considerations would be the end of the discussion. But, as we have explained, there is another view of medical ethics as the distinctive responsibilities of medical professionals (Pellegrino 1979; 1987; 2002). According to persuasive arguments from proponents of such views, the commitments of medicine are different from common morality, and even when the principles of medical ethics and common morality appear to be similar, the justification for the principles is very different. Those who acknowledge the distinctiveness of medical ethics, the special knowledge, powers, and privileges that society allows to the medical professions, and the trust and reliance that members of society extend to the members of the profession appreciate that the standards of medical professionalism should hold sway in guiding the behavior of medical professionals and determining their policies.

In light of this distinction, it is easy to see that the decision we reached in our second case was a response to the professional question, "What should the patient's doctors do?" We wanted to know what our professional responsibilities entailed and what we owed to our patient. Regardless of how uncomfortable the situation made us feel, we saw concern for our own dirty hands or guilty consciences as self-serving and contrary to our professional fiduciary responsibility of acting as his trusted agents in promoting our patient's welfare.

The Transplantation Society has also viewed the issue from the perspective of professional responsibility. As a professional society it apparently looked to the well-being of all of the hundreds of thousands of prospective Chinese patients, and also the few hundred U.S. patients, who might suffer or benefit because of their stance. The society seems to have looked back to the Hippocratic tradition of sharing knowledge and training with colleagues so that patients can receive the high-quality care that they trust doctors to provide. And the society held to the professional commitment of nonjudgmental regard and showing respect to all, colleagues and patients alike.

Like transplantation, ethics is not as simple as it may seem. Since the beginning of the recent bioethics movement in the mid-1960s, and the rise to prominence of the Beauchamp and Childress four principles approach (i.e., respect for autonomy, beneficence, nonmaleficence, justice), the simple view that common morality was the tool for resolving all ethical dilemmas has ruled. But, looking back to the Hippocratic tradition, we find an understanding of medicine as a higher calling based on principles that are different from and more demanding than common morality. And moral philosophers, including the prominent 20th century philosopher John

Rawls, have recognized that "there are parts of the social world that have their own ethics" (Rawls 1997, 372). These insights point out the need for starting moral deliberation with the identification of the appropriate perspective for answering the question that is being asked. In considering what to do, one first has to sort out what sort of question is at issue. The kinds of factors that could be very significant in answering personal questions (e.g., How will doing this affect my child or my career?) could be totally irrelevant in answering a political question (i.e., What should the law of the land be?) or a professional question (i.e., What do the commitments of the profession require?). In crafting policy to guide the medical profession, those responsible need to be aware that they are answering professional questions. That focus determines the kinds of reasons that will be relevant in their deliberation. Personal feelings and political agendas have to be set aside and the ethics of the profession must be allowed to rule.

Acknowledgments: We are grateful for the research assistance of Shira Bender, Lauren Flicker, and Laura Goodman. We are also grateful for the comments and questions from audience members when we delivered presentations as we developed this paper: Symposium on Science, Technology and Values, Stevens Institute of Technology, Hoboken, NJ, April 25, 2008; Dilemmas and Struggles in Transplantation Conference, Northwestern University Feinberg School of Medicine, Chicago, April 5, 2008; Bioethics Retreat, Lake George, NY, July 14, 2007; David Thomasma Memorial International Bioethics Retreat, St. Catherine's College, Cambridge University, June 20, 2007. Some of the issues discussed in this paper are also addressed in Thomas D. Schiano and Rosamond Rhodes, The dilemma and reality of transplant tourism: An ethical perspective for liver transplant programs. Liver Transplantation (in press).

Notes

1. Although a great deal could be said about this family's attitude toward a female child, such a discussion is beyond the scope of this paper. Our focus is on the ethical responsibility of medical professionals, and we are not discussing the matters of personal morality that would be relevant to a critique of the parents' choices.

2. Similar statements have been published by international organizations that are not organizations of the medical profession, for example: Council of Europe, *Additional Protocol to the Convention on Human Rights and Biomedicine, on Transplantation of Organs and Tissues of Human Origin*, Strasbourg, 24 January 2002; *Recommendation 1611: Trafficking in organs in Europe, 2003*; and 57th World Health Assembly, *Human Organ and Tissue Transplantation*, WHA57.18, October 2000.

3. A discussion of physician claims to an exemption from the duty to provide care based on conscientious objection goes beyond the scope of this discussion. It is relevant to note that conscientious objectors, such as pacifists and Dr. Martin Luther King, impose no burden on others and accept the consequences of abiding by their principles. When health professionals refuse to provide patient care, they expect patients or colleagues to bear the burden of their comfort. Rhodes has discussed these points elsewhere (2006a; 2006b; 2006c).

4. The study by Morad and Lim (2000) reports comparably good outcomes in terms of patient and graft survival for their patients who received a kidney transplant from a living related donor (LRD) as compared with patients who received commercial live donor (CLD) transplants in India or commercial cadaveric donor (CCD) transplants in China.

5. Although we in no way endorse the death penalty, prisoners are executed in many countries, including many states in the United States; see http://www.infoplease.com/ipa/A0777460.html. Presently, acceptance of the death penalty does not place a country beyond the pale in terms of international relations. That is why we advocate toleration and adherence with the ethics of the profession, instead of shunning and ostracization. As John Rawls explains in *The Law of Peoples*, "Provided a non-liberal society's basic institutions meet specified conditions of political right and justice and lead its people to honor a reasonable and just law for the Society of Peoples, a liberal people is to tolerate and accept that society" (Rawls 2001, 59–60).

References

American Society of Transplantation. 2007. *Position statement on transplant tourism.* March 2. Available at http://www.a-st.org/files/pdf/publicpolicy/keyposition/PositionStatementTransplantTourism.pdf

BBC News. 2006. *China 'selling' prisoners' organs.* April 19. Available at http://news.bbc.co.uk/2/hi/asia-pacific/4921116.stm

BBC News. 2006. *Organ sales 'thriving' in China.* September 27. Available at http://news.bbc.co.uk/2/hi/5386720.stm

Boschert S. 2007. 'Transplant tourists' pose ethical dilemmas for U.S. physicians. *GI & Hepatology News* June: 11.

Bramstedt, K. A., and J. Xu. 2007. Checklist: Passport, plane ticket, organ transplant. *American Journal of Transplantation* 2007(7):1698–1701.

Budiani-Saberi, D. A., and F. L. Delmonico. 2008. Organ trafficking and transplant tourism: A commentary on the global realities. *American Journal of Transplantation* 8(5):925–929.

Canales, M. T., B. L. Kasiske, and M. E. Rosenberg. 2006. Transplant tourism: Outcomes of United States residents who undergo kidney transplantation overseas. *Transplantation* 82(12): 1658–1661.

Chang, T. F. H., and D.E. Thompkins. 2002. Corporations go to prisons: The expansion of corporate power in the correctional industry. *Labor Studies Journal* 2002:27–45.

Chugh, K. S., and V. Jha. 2000. Problems and outcomes of living unrelated donor transplants in the developing countries. *Kidney International* 57: S131.

Council of Europe. 2002. *Additional protocol to the convention on human rights and biomedicine* (Oviedo Convention) *on transplantation of organs and tissues of human origin*. Strasbourg, 24 January. Available at http://conventions.coe.int/Treaty/EN/Treaties/html/164.htm

Council of Europe. 2003. *Recommendation 1611: Trafficking in organs in Europe.* Available at http://assembly.coe.int/Main.asp?link=/Documents/AdoptedText/ta03/EREC1611.htm

David, M. 1999. *Prisoners of the American dream: Politics and economy in the history of the U.S. working class.* New York: Verso.

Delmonico, F. L., R. Arnold, N. Scheper-Hughes, L. A. Siminoff, J. Kahn, and S. J. Younger. 2002. Sounding board: Ethical incentives—not payment—for organ donation. *New England Journal of Medicine* 346: 2002–2005.

Higgins, R., N. West, S. Fletcher, A. Stein, F. Lam, and H. Kashi. 2003. Kidney transplantation in patients travelling from the UK to India or Pakistan. *Nephrology Dialysis Transplantation* 18(4):851–852.

Huang, J. 2007. Ethical and legislative perspectives on liver transplantation in the People's Republic of China. *Liver Transplantation* 13:193–196.

Inston, N. G., D. Gill, A. Al-Hakim, and A. R. Ready. 2005. Living paid organ transplantation results in unacceptably high recipient morbidity and mortality. *Transplant Proceedings* 37(2): 560–562.

International Society for Heart and Lung Transplant. 2007. *Statement on transplant ethics*, approved April 2007. Available at https://www.dafoh.org/ISHLT—Statement on Tran.php

Ivanovski, N., L. Stojkovski, K. Cakalaroski, G. Masin, S. Djikova, and M. Polenakovic. 1997. Renal transplantation from paid, unrelated donors in India—It is not only unethical, it is also medically unsafe. Letter. *Nephrology Dialysis Transplantation* 12(9): 2028–2029.

Kennedy, S. E., Y. Shen, J. A. Charlesworth, J. D.

Mackie, J. D.Mahony, J. J. P.Kelly, and B. A. Pussell. 2005. Outcome of overseas commercial kidney transplantation: An Australian perspective. *Medical Journal of Australia* 182(5):224–227.

Merion, R. M., A. D. Barnes, M. J. Lin, V. B. Ashby, V.McBride, E. Ortiz-Rios, J. C.Welch, G. N. Levine, F. K. Port, and J. Burdick. 2008. Transplants in foreign countries among patients removed from the U.S. transplant waiting list. [2007 SRTR report on the state of transplantation.] *American Journal of Transplantation* 8(part 2):988–996.

Morad, Z., and T. O. Lim. 2000. Outcome of overseas kidney transplantation in Malaysia. *Transplantation Proceedings* 32:1950–1951.

NATCO, The Organization for Transplant Professionals. 2008. *Position statement: Organ tourism*. March.

Pellegrino, E. D. 1979. Toward a reconstruction of medical morality: The primacy of the act of profession and the fact of illness. *Journal of Medicine and Philosophy* 4:32–56.

Pellegrino, E. D. 1987. Physician's duty to treat: Altruism, self-interest and medical ethics. *Journal of the American Medical Association* 258(October 9):1939–1940.

Pellegrino, E. D. 2002. Professionalism, profession and the virtues of the good physician. *Mount Sinai Journal of Medicine* 69(6):378–384.

Prasad, G. V., A. Shukla, M. Huang, R. J. D'A Honey, and J. S. Zaltzman. 2006. Outcomes of commercial renal transplantation: A Canadian experience. *Transplantation* 82(9):1130–1135.

Rakela, J., and J. J. Fung. 2007. Liver transplantation in China. *Liver Transplantation* 13:182.

Rawls, J. 1993. *Political liberalism.* New York: Columbia University Press.

Rawls, J. 2001. *The law of peoples.* Cambridge, MA: Harvard University Press.

Rhodes, R. 2006a. The ethical standard of care. *American Journal of Bioethics* 6(2):76–78.

Rhodes, R. 2006b. The priority of professional ethics over personal morality. *British Medical Journal*, Rapid Response to Julian Savulescu, Conscientious objection in medicine, *BMJ* 2006; 332:294–297. 9 February 2006. Available at http://bmj.bmjjour nals.com/cgi/eletters/332/7536/294#127934

Rhodes, R. 2006c. The professional obligation of physicians in times of hazard and need: A response to the opinion of the AMA Council on Ethical and Judicial Affairs. *Cambridge Quarterly of Healthcare Ethics* 15(4):424–428.

Rhodes, R. 2007. The professional responsibilities of medicine. In *The Blackwell guide to medical ethics*, ed. R. Rhodes, L. Francis, and A. Silvers, 71–87. Boston: Blackwell.

Sever, M. S., R. Kazancioglu, A. Yildiz, A. Turkmen, T. Ecder, S. M. Kayacan, V. Celik, S. Sahin, A. E. Aydin, U. Eldegez, and E. Ark. 2001. Outcome of living unrelated (commercial) renal transplantation. *Kidney International* 60:1477–1483.

Sever, M. S., T. Ecder, A. E. Aydin, A. Trkmen, I. Kih- caslan, V. Uysal, H. Eraksoy, S. Calangu, M. Carin, and U. Eldegez. 1994. Living unrelated (paid) kidney transplantation in Third-World countries: High

risk of complications besides the ethical problem. *Nephrology Dialysis Transplantation* 9:350–354.

Sophocles. 1998. *Antigone*. Oxford: Oxford University Press.

Steering Committee of the Istanbul Summit. 2008. *The declaration of Istanbul on organ trafficking and transplant tourism*, Meeting convened by the Transplantation Society and International Society of Nephrology, Istanbul, Turkey, April 30 through May 2.

The Transplantation Society. 2007. Policy on interaction with China. *Transplantation* 84:292–294.

UNESCO. 2005. *Universal declaration on bioethics and human rights,* 19 October. Available at http://portal .unesco.org/shs/en/ev.php-URLID=1883&URLD O=DOTOPIC&URLSECTION=201.html

57th World Health Assembly. 2000. *Human organ and tissue transplantation*, WHA57.18. October. Available at http://afrolib.afro.who.int/RC/RC%2054%20 Doc-En/AFR.RC54.6%20Ways%20and%20means %20of%20implementing%20resolutions-5a.pdf

Chapter 34

AN EXCERPT FROM

Multiple Listing in Kidney Transplantation

Mohammad Sanaei Ardekani and Janis M. Orlowski

Abstract

The increasing number of patients with end-stage renal disease and the expanding waiting lists for various solid-organ transplants, particularly kidney transplants, has compelled prospective transplant recipients and their care teams to explore novel ways to accelerate this process, initiating the practice of multiple listing. Multiple listing is defined as being listed for an organ transplant at more than 1 transplant center. Current policy allows patients to be listed at more than 1 transplant center in 1 or more organ procurement organization. Multiple listing can be beneficial for different groups of transplant candidates. Current data support a beneficial effect for the patient on multiple waiting lists, most notably portending a survival advantage for transplant recipients. The kidney transplant list has the most patients who are multiple listed (4.7%), followed by the liver transplant list at 3.8%. The main potential downside of multiple listing is its effect on patients not on multiple lists, as well as the cost accrued to achieve multiple listings. With the newly clarified policy of the United Network for Organ Sharing, a pivotal role for nephrologists in educating patients about the option of multiple listing becomes more apparent. In this article, current practices and policies regarding multiple listing are reviewed and opinions and ethics relating to the practice are discussed.

Conclusion

Current data support an advantageous role of multiple listing for a wide variety of patients on the transplant waiting list. Recent data show the association of a beneficial effect of multiple listing on patient and transplant survival. The concerns of inequities in access for those unable to be on multiple lists have not been shown statistically, but must be reviewed again in light of the recent review by Merion et al, (15) which shows an advantage to those with higher socioeconomic status. Benefits for those willing and able to multiple list and in particular the likelihood of obtaining a transplant remain high. Transplant center variation in practice and regional variation in donor types may broaden the opportunity for transplant in those who are multiple listed.

Whether this is an individual's right to aggressively pursue access to transplant has been debated. Concerns regarding access equity remain, but have not been shown in simulated studies. There has been no significant change in the percentage of multiple-listed patients on the US waiting list.

Box 1. Current and Future Considerations in Multiple Listing

- Education provided by transplant centers to transplant candidates regarding the importance of waiting time transfer and waiting list–donor ratio characteristics may be important to an individual's decision-making process
- Multiple listing is especially beneficial for medically urgent cases and highly sensitized patients
- Transplant centers and treating nephrologists have a role in informing patients about the likely negligible beneficial effect of being on multiple waiting lists within the same organ procurement organization area
- Data from the postban era in New York State explicitly show no significant changes in waiting time and access rate. With current data, we know that single-state–driven banning strategies may not be the solution to expanding equity
- The United Network for Organ Sharing Kidney Committee presently is redesigning the kidney organ allocation system. The publicly released draft proposal does not address multiple listing (www.unos.org)

The main concern regarding multiple listing is its disadvantageous impact on patients not on multiple lists. Multiple listing increases waiting time for patients on the waiting list in the second organ procurement organization (OPO), but at the same time decreases the waiting time on the first OPO. Concerns have been raised regarding the increase in cost to maintain multiple listings.

There also was concern that if an individual from outside a given OPO network receives a procured organ, it may endanger the organ donation rate. An OPTN poll showed that only 25% of responders wanted the organ to be allocated to the area where the donor lived; (21) thus, this concern may not be substantiated.

To establish balance between equity and autonomy of access to kidney transplant as a life saving treatment, expanding geographic coverage of OPOs (the harvested organ will become available to a larger number of patients, especially in neighboring OPOs), and educating patients entering the transplant waiting list may be considered initial steps (Box 1). Multiple listing of ten is motivated by geographic disparities in waitlist time. Lack of public awareness of multiple listing can be addressed by new UNOS strategies. New policy language and clarifications from March 2009 will certainly be helpful to overcome the previous ambiguity of policy.

Support: None.

Financial Disclosure: The authors declare that they have no relevant financial interests.

References

1. US Renal Data System. USRDS 2008 Annual Data Report: Atlas of End-Stage Renal Disease in the United States. Bethesda, MD: National Institutes of Health, National Institute of Diabetes and Digestive and Kidney Diseases; 2008.

2. Suthanthiran M, Strom TB. Renal transplantation. *N Engl J Med.* 1994; 331(6):365–376.

3. Wolfe RA, Ashby VB, Milford EL, et al. Comparison of mortality in all patients on dialysis, patients on dialysis awaiting transplantation, and recipients of a first cadaveric transplant. *N Engl J Med.* 1999; 341(23): 1725–1730.

4. Ojo AO, Port FK, Wolfe RA, Mauger EA, Williams L, Berling DP. Comparative mortality risks of chronic dialysis and cadaveric transplantation in black end-stage renal disease patients. *Am J Kidney Dis.* 1994; 24(I):59–64.

5. Port FK, Wolfe RA, Mauger EA, Berling DP, Jiang K. Comparison of survival probabilities for dialysis patients vs cadaveric renal transplant recipients. *JAMA.* 1993; 270(11):1339–1343.

6. Schnuelle P, Lorenz D, Trede M, Van Der Woude FJ. Impact of renal cadaveric transplantation on survival in end-stage renal failure: evidence for reduced mortality risk compared with hemodialysis during long-term follow-up. *J Am Soc Nephrol.* 1998; 9(II):2135–2141.

7. Evans RW, Manninen DL, Garrison LP Jr, et al.

The quality of life of patients with end-stage renal disease. *N Engl J Med.* 1985; 312(9):553–559.

8. Cohen DJ, St. Martin L, Christensen LL, Bloom RD, Sung RS. Kidney and pancreas transplantation in the United States, 1995–2004. *Am J Transplant.* 2006; 6(5 pt 2):1153–1169.

9. Abecassis M, Bartlett ST, Collins AJ , et al. Kidney transplantation as primary therapy for end-stage renal disease: a National Kidney Foundation/Kidney Disease Outcomes Quality Initiative (NKF/KDOQT™) conference. *Clin J Am Soc Nephrol.* 2008; 3(2):471–480.

10. Delmonico FL, McBride MA. Analysis of the wait list and deaths among candidates waiting for a kidney transplant. *Transplantation.* 2008; 86(12):1678–1683.

11. Meier-Kriesche HU, Port FK, Ojo AO, et al. Effect of waiting time on renal transplant outcome. *Kidney Int.* 2000; 58(3):1311–1317.

12. United Network for Organ Sharing. www.unos .org.

13. Sanfilippo FP, Vaughn WK, Peters TG, et al. Factors affecting the waiting time of cadaveric kidney transplant candidates in the United States. *JAMA.* 1992; 267(2):247–252.

14. White A, Ozminkowski RJ, Hassol A, Dennis JM, Murphy M. The relationship between multiple listing and cadaveric kidney transplantation and the effects of a multiple listing ban. *Transplant Rev.* 1997; 11(2): 76–83.

15. Merion RM, Guidinger MK, Newmann JM, Ellison MD, Port FK, Wolfe RA. Prevalence and outcomes of multiple-listing for cadaveric kidney and liver transplantation. *Am J Transplant.* 2004; 4(1):94–100.

16. UNOS, OPTN/UNOS Patient Affairs Committee. Report to the Board of Directors. Houston, TX; 2009.

17. UNOS. Organ Distribution Policies, section 3.2.2 (3.2.2 Multiple Listings Permitted). http://www .unos.org/PoliciesandBylaws2/policies/pdfs/policy_4 .pdf. Accessed Feb-ruary 9, 2010.

18. Kumar V, Julian BA, Deierhoi MH, Curtis JJ. Secondary listing for deceased-donor kidney transplantation does not increase likelihood of engraftment at a large transplant center. *Am J Transplant.* 2009; 9(7): 1671–1673.

19. White AJ, Ozminkowski RJ, Hassol A, Dennis JM, Murphy M. The effects of New York State's ban on multiple listing for cadaveric kidney transplantation. *Health Serv Res.* 1998; 33(2 pt 1):205–222.

20. Winkelmayer WC, Weinstein MC, Mittleman MA, Glynn RJ, Pliskin JS. Health economic evaluations: the special case of end-stage renal disease treatment. *Med Decis Making.* 2002; 22(5):417–430.

21. Ankeny RA. Recasting the debate on multiple listing for transplantation through consideration of both principles and practice. *Camb Q Healthc Ethics.* 1999; 8(3):330–339.

Chapter 35

Can Any System of Rationing Withstand the Plea of a Ten-Year-Old Girl?

Arthur L. Caplan and Jennifer deSante

Is rationing possible in health care? Obviously, many health systems do ration based on the patient's ability to pay, accept long queues to delay access to services, limit benefit coverage, or restrict the choices patients and doctors can make among tests or treatments. These strategies are often disconnected from information about what interventions are effective. And they are almost never transparent.

Can tough rationing decisions in the face of scarcity be made fairly and transparently using the best available data? Many believe the answer has to be yes if escalating health care costs are to be constrained (1, 2). A highly publicized (3) controversy concerning eligibility for a lung transplant for a ten-year-old girl challenged whether hard choices can be made about the distribution of life-saving resources on the basis of objective criteria and not emotional pleas or publicity campaigns.

In the United States and in Western Europe, deciding who gets scarce organs for transplant has relied on rule-based, medically determined rationing (4). Determining who receives a transplant based on medically predetermined rules has, for many decades, been a paradigm for making tough rationing decisions in healthcare.

Ten-year-old Sarah Murnaghan, from Newtown Square, Pennsylvania, was born with severe cystic fibrosis. She had been on the transplant waiting list with priority one status since December 2011. In December 2012, she was started on continuous, noninvasive respiratory therapy at home. Two months later, her disease worsened. She was admitted to Children's Hospital of Philadelphia (CHOP) where she had received care since the age of one (3). As the months progressed, her lungs began to fail and she was eventually intubated.

While she had been on the waiting list for a lung transplant no organ deemed suitable by her transplant team had become available (3). When no acceptable donor organ became available, her parents told members of the media that they had only recently learned that Sarah was not eligible to receive adult lungs from cadaver donors (3). From her original listing in 2011, Sarah had been listed for both lung and lobar transplantation. However, given her age, she was not given a lung allocation score (LAS), the system under which adult organs are allocated, that would compete for adult lungs.

The United Network for Organ Sharing (UNOS), a medical group that is charged by Congress with rationing the supply of donated cadaver organs (5), had implemented a lung allocation policy in 2005. Adult organs went to adults first based on lung allocation score, regional location, blood type, and size. Children under twelve would have the best outcomes with organs from donors under twelve years old. Further, the medical conditions of children under twelve are different enough from adults that it was thought to be difficult to calculate an accurate LAS (6). An update to the pediatric lung policy in 2010 put two tiers in place for children. Lungs from pediatric donors went to two groups. Adolescent donors (ages 12–17) were prioritized to adolescent recipients, then to children under twelve and then to adults. Lungs from donors under twelve went first to candidates under twelve, then to adolescents, then to adults (7). Those over the age of twelve were given an allocation score by UNOS based on how urgently they needed a transplant and the severity of their medical condition (4). The rationale was that there was some data on the efficacy of adult lungs in adult recipients and little experience or data on outcomes of partial lobes of lung given to children, especially those under the age of twelve (8, 9, 10). In fact, the only long-term outcomes for partial lobar transplants in patients of any age are studies with fewer than ten patients (8, 11).

Child lung donors are rare. And some child lung transplant programs, unlike adult programs, are conservative as to the cadaver organs they will accept. In 2011 in the United States, there were just nineteen transplants for children under eighteen (12). More than seventeen hundred were given to adults in that same year (4). Of the over four hundred donors a year under twelve years old, less than 10 percent of them provide lungs, compared to more than 35 percent of the over four hundred adolescent donors a year. The scarcity is not because of a lack of donors but because of the constrictions of geography. Proximity to the recipient is critical given the short

ischemic time of lungs. Therefore, nearly 30 percent of lungs from donors under twelve are transplanted into adults.

Sarah's parents were determined to give their daughter the best chance at life they could. They launched a publicity campaign to get her priority access to lungs obtained from the adult cadaver donor list despite the UNOS rationing rule. The campaign drew wide attention in the media in the United States and, interestingly, in other nations, especially the UK (13). Representatives requested that President Obama's Secretary of Health and Human Services, Kathleen Sebelius, void the ban on adult lungs for children under twelve. Lou Barletta (R-PA) noted that "with the stroke of a pen [the Secretary] could have granted Sarah a waiver" that would give her a chance to live (14).

What the congressman did not note was that if Sarah was given greater priority on all waiting lists and received lungs, someone else might not. Nor did he note that Sarah at age ten might push aside another child of twelve or thirteen. Nor that the odds of success for adult lung transplant in any recipient were poor, with overall survival at six years less than 50 percent along with a high risk of acute lung failure (15). Nor did he note the additional surgical difficulties of a lobar lung transplant, which Sarah would require to allow adult lungs to fit into her body. Nor the fact that lobar transplants are very rare in pediatric lung centers and a few surgeons in the country are willing to perform this procedure. When Sebelius, deferring to medical expertise about the optimal use of scarce donor lungs (16), refused to overrule the UNOS policy, the family sought the assistance of a prominent Philadelphia law firm, Pepper Hamilton.

With Sarah dying, an emergency hearing on a lawsuit challenging the rule excluding Sarah was held in Philadelphia before Federal

Judge Michael Baylson. On June 5, 2013, Baylson ordered Sebelius to allow Sarah to be moved to the adult lung transplant list (17). Another child at the CHOP, not as sick as Sarah, was added to the adult list as well (18). These appeals led to an emergency meeting of a key UNOS committee that upheld the existing rationing rule but granted an appeals path that was used to create an exception for Sarah and the other patient.

On June 12, 2013, Sarah received a transplant of partial lungs from an adult donor. They failed (19). Sarah was placed immediately on VA-ECMO and relisted that evening. She received a second partial set three days later on June 15 (19). This set of lungs was infected with pneumonia, but the infected segment was removed prior to transplantation (20). It is not clear whether they would have been deemed suitable for any other person waiting on the adult list. Sarah continued to have many more challenges after this second transplant, including infection, a tracheostomy, and surgery on her diaphragm, but she was discharged home and "was taken off oxygen, although she still gets support from a machine that helps her to breathe" (21).

Never in the history of rationing by UNOS has a federal judge intervened to void the medically determined rules for rationing any organ. People in need have engaged in publicity campaigns to try to motivate designated cadaver or living organ donation but never to challenge UNOS rationing rules. Until Sarah's case, patients waiting on transplant lists had found little fault with the rules that UNOS had made public for guiding the distribution of scarce, life-saving organs. And with the exception of a UNOS proposal to share organs more widely rather than locally, Congress had found no reason to challenge the allocation rules either.

There is no avoiding the issue of rationing regarding organ transplantation. The question is not *whether* there should be rationing of scarce, life-saving resources, but *how* the scarce resources should be rationed. And as Sarah's case shows, there are actually two critical questions about the ethics of rationing in health care: who do we want making rationing decisions and on what basis? Further, do we want our healthcare resources distributed by federal judges, members of Congress or those who can mount media campaigns? If not, then who ought to decide?

We would argue that rationing of healthcare should not be the job of federal judges, attorneys, or public relations firms. These groups lack the requisite expertise for deciding who can and cannot benefit from access to medical resources or for undertaking the research requisite for creating rules sensitive to data on need or outcomes. While there should be avenues available to consider and eliminate possibly groundless forms of discrimination in access to organs, rule-making about rationing is best left primarily in the hands of those who can bring expertise to bear to determine need and other critical factors that shape successful transplant outcomes.

Nor should it be the sole responsibility of doctors at the bedside to ration scarce medical resources. Physicians have a fiduciary responsibility to their patients, which requires them to act in the best interest of that particular patient even at the cost of denying resources to others. Families want to know that their doctor is making decisions with only them, their child or their family member in mind. When at a patient's bedside, a physician is advocating for what is best for that patient, even albeit marginally best, regardless of outside factors and limitations.

Still the number of organs is greatly outstripped by need. A body such as UNOS, which has members with expertise in all areas of transplantation, patient and public representation, is the appropriate organization to set the rules for rationing. UNOS has developed a system of prioritizing distribution of organs to those on waiting lists based on medical need, chances of a successful transplant, physical location, and immunologic compatibility. This process is revised and updated when new information becomes available.

All rules are and should be available for public comment so that the system is seen as both just and fair by those in need and the general public who supplies cadaver organs for transplant. UNOS has sought to be transparent in this way. There should also be an internal review process allowing challenges of existing rules.

Sarah's parents had every right to advocate for their child as best they saw fit, including involving the media and taking legal action. Sarah's doctors were correct in supporting every realistic opportunity and option for Sarah's care. But in transplant, as in many areas of health care, rationing decisions must be made. For almost three decades, Americans have allowed the United Network for Organ Sharing to make these rationing decisions in transplantation. In the Murnaghan case, a federal judge for the first time overrode UNOS when he ordered Sarah and another young patient to be added to the adult list for lungs. He argued that the UNOS rule was "arbitrary," capricious, and based on inadequate evidence (17). If this is true, then the intervention by the judge was morally and legally correct. But this ruling is not a precedent for rethinking who should decide or on what basis rationing ought to proceed. The evidence-based UNOS system has done a good job of allocating scarce organs without favor or politics for decades.

Sarah Murnaghan's parents (and lawyers), in deciding to fight for Sarah's chance at life, threaten to topple one of the few transparent rationing schemes that has secured public and governmental support. Instead they have substituted a favoring of a competition that privileges those who can command publicity and legal firepower.

More rationing is in our future. Those who would turn to evidence-based rules as the path to distributing scarce resources like cadaver organs need to be alert to the possibility that data and expert opinion may be overwhelmed by the plight of a particular patient. Rationing schemes do need to protect against invidious discrimination. They may even need to build in some special consideration for children and infants simply because they are persons with very limited lives (22). But they also need to be sufficiently transparent and grounded in reasonable rules able to withstand the emotional tsunami that a dramatic case can cause.

References

1. Aaron, H.J. Health care rationing: Inevitable but impossible? *Georgetown Law Journal*, 2008; 96(2): 539–558.

2. Webb, D.J. Value-based medicine pricing: NICE work? *Lancet* 377, 2011:1552–53.

3. Levs, J., et al. "Dying Girl's Plight Sparks Fight over Organ Transplants." *CNN. Cable News Network*, 29 May 2013. Web: 04 Sept. 2013. http://edition.cnn.com/2013/05/29/health/pennsylvania-girl-lungs.

4. United Network of Organ Sharing. *Questions and Answers for Transplant Candidates about Lung Allocation Policy*. 2010. Web: http://www.unos.org/docs/Lung_Patient.pdf.

5. "OPTN: Organ Procurement and Transplantation Network." *OPTN: Organ Procurement and Transplantation Network*. OPTN, Web: 04 Sept. 2013. http://optn.transplant.hrsa.gov/policiesAndBylaws/nota.asp.

6. Kadin, K., and W.D. Hanto. "Rational Lung Transplants-Procedural Fairness in Allocation and Appeals." *New England Journal of Medicine*. August 2013; 369(7): 599–601.

7. *Http://optn.transplant.hrsa.gov*. Rep. no. Policy 10: Allocation of Lungs. OPTN, Aug. 2013. Web. http://optn.transplant.hrsa.gov/ContentDocuments/OPTN_Policies_PC_08-2013.pdf#nameddest=Policy10.

8. Keating, D., et al. "Long-term outcomes of cadaveric lobar lung transplantation: helping to maximize resources." *J Heart Lung Transplant*. April 2010; 29(4):439–44.

9. Benden, C., et al. "Size-reduced lung transplantation in children—an option worth to consider!" *Pediatric Transplantation*. 2010; 14:529–533.

10. Marasco, S.F., et al. "Cadaveric Lobar Lung Transplantation: Technical Aspects." *Ann Thorac Surg*. 2012; 93:1836–42.

11. Mohite, P.N., et al. "Living related donor lobar lung transplantation recipients surviving well over a decade: still an option in times of advanced donor management." *J Cardiothoracic Surg*. March 7, 2013; 8:37.

12. Department of Health & Human Services. "2011 Annual Data Report." *SRTR. Scientific Registry of Transplant Recipients*. Web: 04 Sept. 2013. http://srtr.transplant.hrsa.gov/annual_reports/2011/default.aspx.

13. Warren, L., and A. Sanders. "'Sarah Has Been Left to Die': Parents of 10-year-old Girl with Cystic Fibrosis in Need of Lung Donation Plead with Public to Help save Their Daughter." *Daily Mail Online*, 2 June 2013. Web: 04 Sept. 2013, http://www.dailymail.co.uk/news/article-2334957/Sarah-Murnaghan-parents-10-year-old-cystic-fibrosis-sufferer-need-lung-donation-plead-public-help-save-daughter.html.

14. Hoffman, B. "Rep. Barletta: Sebelius Could Easily Have Interceded in Sick Girl's Case." *Newsmax*. 6 June 2013. Web: 04 Sept. 2013, http://www.newsmax.com/US/barletta-sebelius-sick-girl/2013/06/06/id/508548.

15. "What Are the Risks of Lung Transplant?" NIH: NHLBI, 1 May 2011. Web: 04 Sept. 2013, http://www.nhlbi.nih.gov/health/health-topics/topics/lungtxp/risks.html.

16. Letter to Secretary Sebelius from OPTN Board of Directors. May 30, 2013.

17. Baylson, M.M., U.S.D.J. *Janet and Francis Murnaghan v. United States Department Of Health & Human Services*. Rep. no. CIVIL ACTION 13-3083. United States District Court, June 2013. Web: 4 Sept. 2013, http://www.paed.uscourts.gov/documents/opinions/13D0484P.pdf.

18. Jaslow, R. "Children Added to Adult Lung Transplant List amid Outcry a Dilemma for Doctors." *CBS News*. CBS Interactive, 7 June 2013. Web: 04 Sept. 2013, http://www.cbsnews.com/8301-204_162-57588287/children-added-to-adult-lung-transplant-list-amid-outcry-a-dilemma-for-doctors/.

19. "Pennsylvania Girl Underwent Two Lung Transplants, Family Reveals." *CNN*. Cable News Network, 30 June 2013. Web: 04 Sept. 2013, http://edition.cnn.com/2013/06/28/health/pennsylvania-girl-transplant.

20. Loviglio, J. "Sarah Murnaghan Now Has Pneumonia in One Lung." *NBC News*. 8 July 2013. Web: 04 Sept. 2013, http://www.nbcnews.com/health/sarah-murnaghan-now-has-pneumonia-one-lung-6C10570533.

21. Dale, M. "Sarah Murnaghan Discharged From Hospital, Returns Home After Lung Transplants." *Huffington Post*, 27 August 2013, www.huffingtonpost.com/2013/08/27sarah-murnaghan-discharged_n_3823126.html.

22. Reese, P.R., and A.L. Caplan. "Better off Living—The Ethics of the New UNOS Proposal for Allocating Kidneys for Transplantation." *Clinical Journal of the American Society of Nephrology*. 2011; 9:2310–12.

Contributors

Sahin Aksoy, MD, PhD, is a professor and chair of the Department of Medical Ethics and History of Medicine at Harran University Sanliurfa, Turkey. He is on the board of the *Journal of Medical Ethics*, with the *British Medical Journal*, and has contributed to a significant number of bioethical publications.

Mohammad Sanaei Ardekani, MD, is an Iranian specialist in nephrology. He currently practices medicine at the Washington Hospital Center, in Washington, DC, and he works with the Kidney and Hypertension Specialists group in Virginia.

David A. Asch, MD, MBA, currently works with the Philadelphia Veterans Affairs Medical Center and the University of Pennsylvania School of Medicine. A well-published researcher, Asch received his AB in philosophy from Harvard University, his MD from Cornell University, and his MBA from the Wharton School at the University of Pennsylvania. His research expertise includes clinical economics, medical decision making, and bioethics health policy surveys.

James L. Bernat, MD, the Louis and Ruth Frank Professor of Neuroscience at Dartmouth Medical School, earned a BA from the University of Massachusetts and an MD from Cornell University Medical College. He

trained in internal medicine and neurology at the Dartmouth-Hitchcock Medical Center, where he has been a faculty member since 1976, and acts as director of the Program in Clinical Ethics. Previously he served as assistant dean of clinical education at Dartmouth Medical School. He served for twenty-eight years on the American Academy of Neurology Ethics, Law & and Humanities Committee, with ten years as chairman. In 2011 he received the Presidential Award from the American Academy of Neurology for lifetime service to American neurology. He has authored more than two hundred articles and chapters on topics in neurology and clinical ethics.

Jacquelyn A. Burkell, PhD, is an associate professor of Information and Media Studies at the University of Western Ontario. She is interested in the impact of computer mediation on understanding, communication, and interpersonal relationship. Her research focuses on the empirical study of the interaction between people and technology, with a particular emphasis on the role of cognition. Burkell is a well-published researcher among the faculty of Communications and Open Learning at the University of Western Ontario.

The Canadian Paediatric Society (CPS) is the Canadian national association of pediatricians, committed to working together to advance the health of children. As a voluntary professional association, the CPS represents more than three thousand pediatricians, pediatric subspecialists, pediatric residents, and other people who work with and care for children and youth. Formed in 1922 and originally called the Canadian Society for the Study of Diseases of Children, CPS has evolved to represent all Canadian provinces and territories, and is governed by an elected board of directors.

Arthur L. Caplan, PhD, is the Drs. William F. and Virginia Connolly Mitty Professor and the founding director of the Division of Medical Ethics in NYU Langone Medical Center's Department of Population Health. Prior to working with NYU Langone, Caplan was the Sidney D. Caplan Professor of Bioethics at the University of Pennsylvania Perelman School of Medicine, where he created the Center for Bioethics and the Department of Medical Ethics. He is on the board of directors for a number of institutions, including the Franklin Institute and the American Association of University Professors Foundation. Caplan served as the codirector of the Joint Council of Europe/United Nations Study on Trafficking in Organs and Body Parts, and is currently the ethics advisor on synthetic biology to the Defense Advanced Research Projects Agency, an agency of the US Department of Defense. He has served on a number of national and international committees and is the recipient of many awards and honors, including the McGovern Medal of the American Medical Writers Association. Caplan is the author or editor of thirty-two books and over six hundred papers in peer-reviewed journals; he writes a regular column on bioethics for NBC.com and is a monthly commentator on bioethics and health care issues for WebMD/Medscape.

Alexander Morgan Capron, LLB, is a professor at the University of Southern California and the Scott H. Bice Chair in Healthcare Law, Policy and Ethics, as well as a professor of law and medicine with the Keck School of Medicine, and codirector of the Pacific Center for Health Policy and Ethics with the USC Gould School of Law. He spent four years as director of Ethics, Trade, Human Rights, and Health Law at the World Health Organization in Geneva. Capron was appointed by President Bill Clinton to the National Bioethics Advisory Commission and served as President of the International Association of Bioethics. He is a trustee of the Century Foundation, an officer of Public Responsibility in Medicine and Research, and an elected member of the Institute of Medicine with the National Academy of Sciences. Capron previously taught at Yale University, the University of Pennsylvania Medical and Law School, and Georgetown University. He has been extensively published.

Jennifer A. Chandler, LLM, is a professeure agrégée with the University of Ottawa's faculty of Law, and a member of the Bar of Ontario. She is the cochair of the Law and Ethics Group within the Canadian National Transplant Research Program. She is also a member of the Ethics Working Group on Organ Transplantation, within the Trillium Gift of Life Network. Chandler teaches Mental Health Law and Neuroethics and conducts research in relation to organ donation and transplantation as the holder of the 2012–2014 James Kreppner Fellowship. She also teaches Medical Legal Issues and Tort Law, Neuroethics, Bioethics, and Health Law and Policy.

Michael R. Charlton, MD, is a gastroenterologist in Rochester, Minnesota, and is affiliated with multiple hospitals in the area, including the Mayo Clinic and Mayo Clinic Health System in New Prague. He received his degree from Charing Cross Westminster Medical School in 1986 and is now director of an NIH-funded research program, where research activities are focused on a genomic and proteomic study of biomarkers of liver disease and on passive immunity in the prevention of viral hepatitis.

Frank C. Chaten, MD, is an internist specializing in pediatrics and critical care in Indianapolis, Indiana. He received his degree from the Medical College of Virginia and is a clinical associate at the University of Chicago, where he practices in Pediatrics and Pediatric Critical Care Medicine.

Winston Chiong, MD, PhD, is an assistant professor at the University of California, San Francisco School of Medicine in the department of neurology, specifically within their Memory and Aging Center. He received his PhD in philosophy from New York University and his MD from UCSF. His work at NYU focused on ethical issues in clinical research and medical education, personal identity, and brain death. Chiong's current research is focused on decision making and how it is affected by aging and neurodegenerative disease, as well as the ethical and policy implications of these changes.

Abdallah Daar, DPhilFRCSC, is professor of public health sciences at the Dalla Lana Faculty of Public Health at the University of Toronto, with a cross-appointment in the department of surgery. He is a senior scientist at the University Health Network and is director of ethics and commercialization at the McLaughlin-Rotman Centre for Global Health. He is also the Chief Science and Ethics

Officer and chair of the Scientific Advisory Board of Grand Challenges Canada. His major research focus is on the use of life sciences to ameliorate global health inequities, with a particular focus on building scientific capacity and increasing innovation in developing countries. Daar's academic career has spanned biomedical sciences, organ transplantation, surgery, global health, and bioethics. He is a member of the United Nations Secretary-General's Scientific Advisory Board and works in various advisory or consulting capacities with the UN, the World Health Organization, and UNESCO. He has received a number of international awards, holds the official world record for performing the youngest cadaver kidney transplant, and has published over 350 papers in peer-reviewed journals and six books concerning public health.

Gabriel M. Danovitch, MD, is a professor of clinical medicine in the University of California's Department of Nephrology: he is the medical director for the Kidney & Pancreas Transplant Program. His transplant-related research has focused on various aspects of clinical transplantation and particularly the development of new immunosuppressive drugs and innovative immunosuppressive protocols.

Francis L. Delmonico, MD, is a surgeon, clinical professor, and health expert in the field of transplantation. He is the medical director of the New England Organ Bank (NEOB) and Professor of Surgery at Harvard Medical School, where he is Emeritus Director of Renal Transplantation. He also currently serves as president of the Transplantation Society, an international nonprofit organization based in Montreal that works with international transplantation physicians and researchers. He has also been appointed as an advisor to the World Health Organization in matters of organ donation and transplantation.

Jennifer deSante, MD, MBE, is a pediatrician focused on the care of chronically ill children, particularly children with multiple medical diagnoses. Her research has spanned beginning-of-life issues, organ transplantation procurement, embryonic stem cell research policy, and vaccine ethics. She did her undergraduate work at Princeton University, where she majored in molecular biology, and upon graduating, she enrolled in Perelman School of Medicine at the University of Pennsylvania. She graduated with a combined doctorate of medicine and master's degree in bioethics in 2010. She recently completed her pediatric residency at the Children's Hospital of Philadelphia where she was an instructor in pediatrics at the University of Pennsylvania. In her work as a postdoctoral fellow in the NIH Department of Bioethics, she is focusing on issues related to children with special healthcare needs and the ethical challenges their caregivers face. She is currently exploring the limits on parental obligations and the role health care providers can play in assisting parents of chronically ill children.

Kristina Fiore is a health and science journalist living in New York. She reports from *MedPage Today* headquarters in New York, New York, with a focus on nutrition, diet, and exercise. She has written for newspapers and trade and consumer magazines and is a member of the National Association of Science Writers. Fiore holds a degree in Science, Health, and Environmental Reporting from New York University, and has bylines in a number of online media sources, including New Jersey Monthly, ABC News, and Newsday.

Robert D. Fitzgerald, MD, works in the Karl Landsteiner Institute for Anaesthesiology and Intensive Care Medicine, Wolkersbergenstraße 1, A-1130 Vienna. He currently lives in Vienna.

Elisabeth Furberg, PhD, is employed as a researcher and teacher with the Department of Philosophy at Stockholm University in Sweden. Her main areas of interests in philosophy are meta-ethics, applied ethics, and medical ethics, on which she has published extensively.

Ahad J. Ghods, MD, FACP, is a professor of medicine working in the Division of Nephrology and the Transplantation Unit of Hashemi Nejad Kidney Hospital, which is affiliated with the Iran University of Medical Sciences in Tehran.

Ronald D. Guttmann, MD, is emeritus professor of medicine and founding and former director of the McGill University Centre for Clinical Immunobiology and Transplantation. He is a cofounder, director, and executive vice president of Clinical and International Development, of BioMosaics Inc., a cancer biomarker company. Guttmann was the director of the first multidisciplinary transplant service in Canada at the Royal Victoria Hospital (1970). He is also a director of the Institute of Policy Research in Medicine and Emerging-technologies (IPRIME). Guttmann is an author of more than 310 original publications and has been an active consultant in the biomedical and biotechnology industry since 1985. He is a cofounder of and was the first president of the American Society of Transplantation, former vice president of the (International) Transplantation Society, president of the XVll World Congress of the Transplantation Society (Montreal 1998). His awards include the Distinguished Achievement Award of the American Society of Transplantation, Lifetime Achievement Award of the Institute of Kidney Diseases and Research Centre, Ahmedabad, India, and the Lifetime Achievement Award of the Canadian Society of Transplantation.

Scott D. Halpern, MD, PhD, MBE, received his BS in Psychology and Economics from Duke University, and his MD, PhD in Epidemiology, and masters of bioethics from the University of Pennsylvania. He has served as a consultant regarding ethical issues for the CDC, NIH, FDA, and UNOS. In 2008 he was selected as a Greenwall Foundation Faculty Scholar in Bioethics. His clinical interests include critical care medicine and the management of patients with pulmonary hypertension. His research interests include rationing of scarce medical resources, end-of-life decision making, behavioral economics, ICU ethics, ethics in HIV/AIDS, research ethics in pulmonary hypertension. He is currently affiliated with the University of Pennsylvania's Perelman School of Medicine.

Professor Sir Raymond ("Bill") Hoffenberg, MD, KBE, was an endocrinologist who specialized in the study of the thyroid. Born in South Africa, he was settled in the United Kingdom, where he was president of the Royal College of Physicians from 1983 to 1989, and president of Wolfson College at Oxford from 1985 to 1993. He was professor of medical ethics at the University of Queensland from 1993 to 1995, and was at one time president of London's Royal College of Physicians, as well as president of the International Society for Endocrinology and chair of the British Heart Foundation, among numerous other positions. He passed away in 2007.

Professor Sir Ian Kennedy, QC, LLD, FBA, FKC, FUCL, Hon.DSc, Hon.FRCP, is among the world's leading academics in the areas of the law and ethics of health. He is Emeritus Professor of Health Law, Ethics & Policy at University College London, a former dean of the Law School at King's College London, and founder of the Centre for Medical Law & Ethics. He chaired the public inquiry into children's heart surgery at the Bristol Royal Infirmary, chaired the Healthcare Commission, and chaired the Nuffield Council on Bioethics. He is a member of the board of the UK Research Integrity Office, chair of the King's Fund Inquiry into the quality of general practice in England, and is an Honorary Fellow of the British Academy, the Royal College of General Practitioners, the Royal College of Physicians, the Royal College of Paediatrics and Child Health, the Royal College of Anaesthetists, and the Royal College of Surgeons of Edinburgh. He is the author of seminal texts in medical/health law and ethics, and was the BBC's Reith Lecturer in 1980. Sir Ian was knighted in 2002 for his services to medical law and bioethics, and was appointed chair of the Independent Parliamentary Standards Authority in 2009.

Rachel Kohn, MD, is currently affiliated with the Center for Bioethics at the University of Pennsylvania's School of Medicine. She completed her residency in internal medicine at Massachusetts General Hospital in Boston, and though she specializes in internal medicine, her clinical interests include critical care, clinical epidemiology, and health outcomes.

Elysa R. Koppelman-White, PhD, is an assistant professor of philosophy at Oakland University in Rochester, Michigan. She has a PhD in philosophy from the University of Iowa,

MA in bioethics from Case Western Reserve University, MA in philosophy from Cleveland State University, and BA in philosophy from the University of Wisconsin, Madison. Her interests are in ethical theory, bioethics, professional ethics, research ethics, personal identity, and contemporary Jewish philosophy. She has served as a consultant in research ethics for the Online Center for Ethics in Engineering and Science and has created a website and online courses in the responsible conduct of research for the Cleveland Clinic Foundation. She also serves on the ethics committee and IRB of Pontiac Osteopathic Hospital.

Alan B. Leichtman, MD, is a board-certified nephrologist in Ann Arbor, Michigan. He is currently licensed to practice medicine in Michigan, where he is affiliated with University of Michigan Hospitals and Health Centers and VA Ann Arbor Hospitals. He is also a professor of internal medicine at the University of Michigan Medical School.

Michael Lock, MD, CCFP, FRCP, is the director and head of the Division of Radiation Oncology for the London Health Sciences Centre and an associate professor at the University of Western Ontario in London, Ontario, in the Schulich School of Medicine. He is cross-appointed as an associate professor in the Department of Medical Biophysics and professionally involved with the development of image-guided and radiobiologically guided radiotherapy for the London Regional Cancer Program. His current practice is focused on genitourinary cancers and breast cancers. Lock was the previous leader of the Breast Cancer Multidisciplinary Disease Site Team of the London Regional Cancer Program, and he is also an associate scientist at the Lawson Health Research Institute.

David C. Magnus, PhD, is Thomas A. Raffin Professor of Medicine and Biomedical Ethics, and Professor of Pediatrics at Stanford University, where he directs the Stanford Center for Biomedical Ethics. Magnus serves as president of the American Bioethics Program Directors, representing the leadership of sixty academic bioethics programs across North America. He received his PhD in philosophy from Stanford University and currently cochairs the Stanford Hospital and Clinics Ethics Committee. He serves as coeditor of the American Journal of Bioethics and is widely published on a range of topics, including health care reform, research ethics, end-of-life care, and genetic technology. His published journals include *Science, Hastings Center Report, Cambridge Quarterly of Healthcare Ethics,* and the *Journal of Law, Medicine and Ethics.* Along with his scholarly work, he has written a number of editorial pieces in prominent newspapers and has been quoted in *Time* magazine, *Newsweek,* the *Wall Street Journal,* and the *New York Times.* He has also appeared on many television shows including Good Morning America, CBS This Morning, FOX News Sunday, and ABC World News.

David Mayrhofer-Reinhartshuber, MD, works with the Ludwig Boltzmann Institute for Economy of Medicine in Anesthesia and Intensive Care, in Vienna, Austria. He is also associated with Vienna's Center for Healthcare Communication, through which he has published a number of articles regarding public health.

The Rev. Dr. James J. McCartney, OSA, is an associate professor in the Philosophy Department of Villanova University and adjunct professor in its School of Law. He received a PhD in philosophy from Georgetown University and also has graduate degrees in cell and molecular biology (MS, the Catholic University of America) and theology (MA, Augustinian College), as well as his bachelor's degree in philosophy from Villanova. He was formerly the director of Philosophy Doctoral Studies and chair of the Department at Villanova, and he teaches courses in bioethics, clinical ethics, bioethics and the law, the philosophy of medicine, and the philosophy of law. He serves on the editorial board of HealthCare Ethics Committee Forum, has coedited three books and published numerous articles, and has been invited to lecture and participate in workshops on bioethical issues on the local, national, and international levels.

Franklin G. Miller, PhD, is a senior faculty member associated with the National Institutes of Health, and their Clinical Center's Department of Bioethics. He serves on the Neuroscience Institutional Review Board of the NIH Intramural Research Program and the Ethics Committee for the Clinical Center. He received his degrees from Columbia University, and during the 1990s, he was part of the University of Virginia's faculty, where he taught various courses in bioethics. Miller has written numerous published articles in medical and bioethics journals on the ethics of clinical research, ethical issues concerning death and dying, professional integrity, and pragmatism and bioethics. Miller is a fellow of the Hastings Center, a faculty affiliate at the Kennedy Institute of Ethics, and associate professor of Public Health in the Division of Medical Ethics, Department of Public Health, at Weill Medical College. He co-leads a seminar for psychiatric research fellows on ethical issues in psychiatric research and coordinates the bioethics seminar for first-year fellows in the Department of Bioethics. Miller's current

research focuses principally on ethical issues in clinical research, including study design, informed consent, and the intersection between clinical research and health policy.

Barbara L. Neades, PhD, is a senior lecturer at Napier University's School of Nursing, in Edinburgh, Scotland. Her clinical background is in emergency nursing and law and ethics in health care, and she regularly presents in conferences on bioethical issues. She is a member of the Royal College of Nursing, the Royal College of Nursing Nurse Practitioner Group, the Scottish Resuscitation Group, the Royal College of Nursing's Ethical Advisory Committee, and a board member of Faculty of Emergency Nursing and Educational Lead. Her research interests include organ donation and emergency nursing.

Janis M. Orlowski, MD, is a nephrologist in Washington, DC, and is affiliated with MedStar Washington Hospital Center. She received her medical degree from the Medical College of Wisconsin and has been in practice for thirty-two years.

Janet Radcliffe-Richards, PhD, is professor of practical philosophy at the University of Oxford, and fellow, distinguished research fellow, and consultant at the Oxford Uehiro Centre for Practical Ethics. Formerly, she was lecturer in philosophy at the Open University, and then director of the Centre for Bioethics at the medical school at University College London. She is a philosopher who originally specialized in metaphysics and philosophy of science but has now for many years concentrated on the practical applications of philosophy, and has authored a number of works in the subject. She has been a frequent speaker at transplant conferences around the world and has sat on a variety of advisory and working committees in areas of philosophy and bioethics.

Amelie Raz graduated from Bryn Mawr College with a bachelor of science in biology, after winning first prize in an Undergraduate Biology Research Symposium in 2010, for her work on "Epigenetic Consequences of Sexual vs. Asexual Development in the Pea Aphid." She is currently a graduate student at the Reddien Lab, affiliated with the Massachusetts Institute of Technology's Department of Biology.

Michael A. Rees, MD, is the director of Renal Transplantation at the University of Toledo Medical Center, in Ohio, where he also works as a urologist and transplant surgeon. Additionally, he is the chief executive officer at Alliance for Paired Donation, centered in Maumee, Ohio, which has drastically changed the structure of organ donation in the United States.

Peter Reese, MD, is an assistant professor of medicine, assistant professor of epidemiology in Biostatistics and Epidemiology, and assistant professor of medical ethics and health policy with Penn Medicine in Philadelphia. He is a physician with board certifications in internal medicine and nephrology. Reese specializes in renal electrolyte and hypertension, and kidney and pancreas transplants.

Daniel P. Reid graduated from Villanova University with a bachelor of science in biology, and has previously published on the ethics and practicality of novel emergency medical services systems. He has both clinical and ethics experience at several New York–area medical centers, including NYU Langone

Medical Center under Arthur L. Caplan. Additionally, he served for three spring semesters as teaching assistant to James J. McCartney, helping with Ethics for Healthcare Professionals, which is an undergraduate nursing and philosophy course at Villanova University.

Michael Rey, MD, is a graduate of the University of Pennsylvania Perelman School of Medicine. Currently he is a third-year resident in the combined internal medicine and pediatrics program at the Children's Hospital of Philadelphia, a part of the PennMed Healthcare System. He has contributed to a number of contemporary bioethical publications, including *Informed Consent in Research to Improve the Number and Quality of Deceased-Donor Organs*.

Rosamond Rhodes, MD, is a professor of medical education and director of bioethics education at Icahn School of Medicine. She serves as a member of Mount Sinai's Ethics Committee and IACUC, and is also professor of philosophy at the Graduate Center, CUNY, and professor of bioethics and associate director of the Union-Mount Sinai Bioethics Program. Beyond the teaching setting, Rhodes serves as chair of the American Philosophical Association's committee on philosophy and medicine. She serves on the editorial boards of the international journals *Cambridge Quarterly of Healthcare Ethics, Bioethics,* and *Philosophy, Ethics and Humanities in Medicine,* as well as the MIT press Basic Bioethics series and the *Cambridge Dictionary of Bioethics*. She has published more than 160 articles and chapters on a broad range of issues in bioethics.

Alvin Elliot Roth, PhD, is the Craig and Susan McCaw Professor of Economics at Stanford University and the George Gund

Professor of Economics and business administration emeritus at Harvard University, and in the Harvard Business School. Roth has made significant contributions to the fields of game theory, market design, and experimental economics. In 2012 he won the Nobel Memorial Prize in Economic Sciences jointly with Lloyd Shapley "for the theory of stable allocations and the practice of market design." The best known of the market he has designed is the National Resident Matching Program, through which approximately twenty thousand doctors a year find their first employment as residents at American hospitals. He is one of the founders and designers of the New England Program for Kidney Exchange, for incompatible patient-donor pairs. He is the chair of the American Economic Association's Ad Hoc Committee on the Job Market, which has designed a number of recent changes in the market for new PhD economists. He is a fellow of the American Academy of Arts and Sciences and the Econometric Society, and has been a Guggenheim and Sloan fellow. He received his PhD at Stanford University, and came to Harvard from the University of Pittsburgh, where he was the Andrew Mellon Professor of Economics.

David J. Rothman, PhD, is an American author, and the Bernard Schoenberg Professor of Social Medicine and professor of history at the Columbia University College of Physicians and Surgeons, where he is director of the Center for the Study of Science and Medicine. He specializes in social history and the history of medicine. He received his BA from Columbia University and his PhD from Harvard University. He serves as the president of the Institute on Medicine as a Profession. Rothman's work has focused on the social history of American medicine and current health care practices.

His scholarship has also explored human rights in medicine, including organ trafficking, AIDS among Romanian orphans, and the ethics of research in third world countries. He has authored and coauthored a number of articles regarding medical professionalism, and has cochaired two task forces whose recommendations have appeared in the *Journal of the American Medical Association*. Rothman lives in New York City with his wife and frequent coauthor, Professor Sheila M. Rothman.

Shelia M. Rothman, PhD, is professor of public health in the Division of Sociomedical Sciences of the Joseph L. Mailman School of Public Health at Columbia University. She is also assistant to the deputy director of the Center for the Study of Society and Medicine at the Columbia College of Physicians & Surgeons at Columbia University. Trained in social history, she received her PhD from Columbia University. Her research focuses on the links between technologies and individual and group identity. One area of particular interest is the impact of genetic knowledge of group identity. Rothman recently received a Robert Wood Johnson Health Policy Investigator Award to study the policy implications of the growing reliance on live organ donors. Her most recent book coauthored with David Rothman is *The Pursuit of Perfection: The Promise and Perils of Medical Enhancement* (2003). Using historical and contemporary sources, it examines the development, promotion, and use of a range of hormonal therapies as well as the promise and current development of genetic technologies.

Jathan Sadowski is a PhD candidate in the "Human and Social Dimensions of Science and Technology," which is in the Consortium for Science, Policy & Outcomes at Arizona

State University (ASU). He mostly writes about the politics and ethics of technology, and he's currently researching a dissertation on "smart cities." Sadowski has published with a variety of both academic journals and popular media outlets. He has an MA in Applied Ethics from ASU and a BS in Philosophy from Rochester Institute of Technology.

Kannan P. Samy, MD, who completed his general surgery residency at Indiana University Medical Center, recently joined the Emory Transplant Center Lab, in Atlanta, Georgia, to conduct a two-year fellowship with Dr. Joseph Maglioccoa (2013–2015).

Shokoufeh Savaj, MD, is an associate professor of medicine and head of the Department of Internal Medicine in Firoozgar Hospital, which is part of the Iran University of Medical Sciences in Tehran.

Julian Savulescu, PhD, is an Australian philosopher and bioethicist. He is Uehiro Professor of Practical Ethics at the University of Oxford; director of the Oxford Centre for Neuroethics; fellow of St Cross College, Oxford; director of the Oxford Uehiro Centre for Practical Ethics; Sir Louis Matheson Distinguished Visiting Professor at Monash University; and head of the Melbourne–Oxford Stem Cell Collaboration, which is devoted to examining the ethical implications of cloning and embryonic stem cell research. He is the editor of the *Journal of Medical Ethics*, which is ranked as the top journal in bioethics worldwide by Google Scholar Metrics as of 2013. In addition to his background in applied ethics and philosophy, he also has a background in medicine and completed his MBBS (Hons) at Monash University. He completed his PhD at Monash University, under the supervision

of renowned bioethicist Peter Singer. His areas of research interest are extensive, but they include issues related to ethics of genetics especially, such as predictive genetic testing, preimplantation genetic diagnosis, prenatal testing, behavioral genetics, genetic enhancement, and gene therapy.

Thomas D. Schiano, MD, is a professor of medicine, a UNOS-certified Liver Transplant physician, and is board-certified in internal medicine, clinical nutrition, and gastroenterology. He is the medical director of Adult Liver Transplantation and director of Clinical Hepatology and Intestinal Transplantation at the Recanati/Miller Transplantation Institute, and has a clinical background in hepatology, gastroenterology, and clinical nutrition. He has expertise in the management of patients with cirrhosis and other acute/chronic liver diseases, as well as caring for patients prior to and after liver and intestinal transplantation. Schiano has varied clinical research interests including herbal treatments of liver disease, nutritional aspects of liver disease, living donor liver transplantation, and management of the complications of cirrhosis. In addition, he is member of the liver thrombosis program, which is an international referral center for adults and children with difficult to diagnose and unique blood clotting disorders affecting the liver and intestines.

Evan Selinger, PhD, associate professor in the Department of Philosophy at the Rochester Institute of Technology, received his PhD in philosophy at Stony Brook University in 2003. His research covers a range of issues in the philosophies of technology and expertise.

Robert A. Sells, MD, is a consultant general and transplant surgeon associated with the

Walton Centre for Neurology and Neurosurgery in Fazakerly, Liverpool. He is a fellow of the Royal College of Surgeons of England, a fellow of the Royal College of Surgeons of Edinburgh, and has contributed to the International Forum for Transplant Clinics, with the Renal Transplant Unit in Royal Liverpool University Hospital.

David Serur, MD, is a nephrologist in New York, New York, and is affiliated with New York-Presbyterian Hospital, where he is an associate attending physician. He is the medical director of the Rogosin Institute Transplantation Program, and an associate professor of clinical medicine at the Weill Medical College of Cornell University. He received his medical degree from State University of New York Downstate Medical Center College of Medicine and has been in practice for twenty-six years. He also speaks multiple languages, including Hebrew. His nephrology specialties generally fall under transplantation, and his clinical expertise includes kidney transplants and peritoneal dialysis.

Sam D. Shemie, MD, is a physician in the Division of Pediatric Critical Care and medical director, Extracorporeal Life Support Program at Montreal Children's Hospital, McGill University Health Centre. He is also professor of pediatrics, McGill University, and holds the Bertram Loeb Chair in Organ and Tissue Donation, Faculty of Arts, University of Ottawa, and was appointed Medical Director (Donation), Organs and Tissues, for the Canadian Blood Services. Shemie's area of specialty is organ replacement in critical illness. He is the former chair of the Donation Committee of the Canadian Council for Donation and Transplantation. His recent research interests have included the development and

implementation of national ICU-based organ donation strategies. He has contributed to a number of determinations in his field; most notably, in April 2003, he chaired a Canadian Forum entitled "From Severe Brain Injury to Neurological Determination of Death," which has developed new medical standards for brain death determination and organ donation in Canada for all age groups. In February 2004 he chaired a Canadian Forum entitled "Medical Management to Optimize Donor Organ Potential," which has developed national consensus guidelines to optimize organ donor function for the purposes of transplantation.

D. Alan Shewmon, MD, received his BA from Harvard University in 1971 as a music major. He went on to medical school at NYU, pediatric residency at Children's Hospital, San Francisco, and neurology residency at Loyola University Medical Center in Chicago. After a fellowship at UCLA, he has remained on the UCLA Medical School Faculty, with joint appointments in the Departments of Pediatrics and Neurology. Shewmon was director of UCLA's Pediatric Clinical Neurophysiology Laboratory and played a key role in the emergence of UCLA as one of the preeminent centers in the world for pediatric epilepsy surgery. He moved on to Olive View-UCLA Medical Center, a university-affiliated county hospital, as director of the Clinical Neurophysiology Laboratory and head of Pediatric Neurology. He later became chief of the Neurology Department there and vice chair of Neurology at UCLA. In 2011 he became Clinical Professor Emeritus at UCLA while continuing as chief of neurology at Olive View.

Nicholas Tilney, MD, is a general surgeon in Boston, Massachusetts. He is a Francis D. Moore Distinguished Professor of Surgery at

Brigham and Women's Hospital, where he completed his hospital residency in general surgery. He is a fellow of the American College of Surgeons, has been frequently published, and has taken part in the International Forum for Transplant Ethics.

Robert D. Truog, MD, is Professor of Medical Ethics, Anesthesiology & Pediatrics at Harvard Medical School and a senior associate in Critical Care Medicine at Children's Hospital, Boston. Truog received his medical degree from the University of California, Los Angeles, and is board certified in the practices of pediatrics, anesthesiology, and pediatric critical care medicine. He also holds a master's degree in philosophy from Brown University and an honorary master's of arts from Harvard University. Truog's major administrative roles include Director of Clinical Ethics in the Division of Medical Ethics and the Department of Social Medicine at Harvard Medical School; Director of the Institute for Professionalism and Ethical Practice at Children's Hospital; and chair of the Harvard Embryonic Stem Cell Research Oversight Committee (ESCRO). Truog has published more than two hundred articles in bioethics and related disciplines, and he lectures widely nationally and internationally. His writings on the subject of brain death have been translated into several languages, and in 1997 he provided expert testimony on this subject to the German Parliament. Truog is an active member of numerous committees and advisory boards, and has received several awards over the years, including the Christopher Grenvik Memorial Award from the Society of Critical Care Medicine for his contributions and leadership in the area of ethics.

Gunnar Tufveson, MD, is an adjunct professor in the Department of Surgical Sciences with Sweden's University of Uppsala. He specializes in the division of transplantation surgery.

Leigh Turner, PhD, is an associate professor in the Center for Bioethics, School of Public Health, and College of Pharmacy, associated with the University of Minnesota. Turner's current research examines ethical, social, and policy issues related to medical travel and the emergence of a global marketplace in health services. His research program includes ethical and social analysis of travel for unlicensed and unproven stem cell interventions, commercial organ transplantation, cosmetic surgery, and other procedures. In addition, Turner is conducting research on governance of stem cells and the proliferation of domestic and international clinics marketing stem cell products that have not received premarketing approval by FDA or other regulatory bodies. Turner's research draws upon methods and approaches from bioethics and social studies of medicine.

Charles Bradley Wallis, MD, is a consultant in anesthesia and intensive care medicine with the Scottish Intensive Care Society. A professional lead for critical care, Wallis is affiliated with the Western General Hospital in Edinburg, Scotland, in their Department of Anesthetics.

Staffen Welin, MD, is a consultant in the University of Uppsala's Unit of Endocrine Oncology in Sweden. He is affiliated with their Department of Medical Sciences.

Kyle Powys Whyte, PhD, is the Timnick Chair in the Humanities at Michigan State University and a member of the Environmental Philosophy & Ethics concentration. He is affiliated faculty for Peace and Justice Studies, Environmental Science and Policy, the Center for Regional Food Systems, Animal Studies, and American Indian Studies. He is an enrolled member of the Citizen Potawatomi Nation in Shawnee, Oklahoma. He writes primarily on environmental justice and American Indian philosophy, and has been extensively published. His most recent research addresses moral and political issues concerning climate change impacts on indigenous peoples. He is involved in the Michigan Environmental Justice Coalition, the Consortium for Socially Relevant Philosophy of/in Science, and a number of others.

Benjamin S. Wilfond, MD, is the director of the Treuman Katz Center for Pediatric Bioethics, chief of the Division of Bioethics, and attending physician at the Seattle Children's Hospital. Wilfond is also a professor for the Department of Pediatrics and an adjunct professor for the Department of Medical History and Ethics at the University of Washington School of Medicine. He conducts research on ethical and policy issues related to genetic testing, genetic research, and pediatric research. He recently has worked on issues related to newborn screening, disclosure of genetic research results, pediatric biobanks, and direct-to-consumer advertising of genetic tests.

He received his MD from UMDNJ–New Jersey Medical School and trained in Pediatrics, Pediatric Pulmonology and Medical Ethics at the University of Wisconsin. As a faculty member at the University of Arizona, he was the director of the Apnea/Bronchopulmonary dysplasia Clinic and the codirector of the Tucson Cystic Fibrosis Center. He has been on the medical staff at the NIH Clinical Center and the Pediatric Pulmonary Clinic and the Cystic Fibrosis Center at Johns Hopkins University. He is currently on Data Monitoring Committees for the Cystic Fibrosis Foundation, Therapeutic Development Network, and for National Heart, Lung and Blood Institute studies.

Dominic Wilkinson, MD, PhD, is director of medical ethics at the Oxford Uehiro Centre for Practical Ethics. He is a consultant neonatologist and Nuffield Medical Research Fellow, University of Oxford and John Radcliffe Hospital at Oxford. He trained as a doctor in Australia, as well as completing a master's degree in human bioethics at Monash University, Melbourne, before moving to Oxford to study for his doctorate and work as a consultant. He specializes in newborn intensive care and medical ethics but has worked as a doctor in neonatal, pediatric, and adult intensive care, and is currently consultant neonatologist at the John Radcliffe Hospital in Oxford. He is also associate professor of neonatal medicine and bioethics and consultant neonatologist at the Women's and Children's Hospital in Adelaide. He has an Early Career Fellowship with the NHMRC to investigate perinatal neuroethics and decision making. Wilkinson has recently completed a DPhil in Bioethics, looking at the ethical implications of the use of magnetic resonance imaging in newborn infants with birth asphyxia. He has written a large number of academic articles relating to ethical issues in intensive care. His research interests include end-of-life care, neuroethics, perinatal ethics, critical care ethics, and ethical questions associated with randomized, controlled trials.

Karol Józef Wojtyła, better known as Pope Saint John Paul II, served as Bishop of Rome from October 16, 1978, until his death on

April 2, 2005. He was the second-longest-serving pope in modern history, after Pope Pius IX, and has since been canonized as a saint. He accomplished a great deal during his papacy; notably, he supported a conservative interpretation of the Second Vatican Council and its reforms, and he contributed a great deal of writing in support of traditional Catholic doctrine.

Richard M. Zaner, PhD, is the A. G. Stahlman Professor Emeritus of Medical Ethics and Philosophy of Medicine at Vanderbilt University Medical Center. He is also professor of philosophy with Southern Methodist University and an editor with Ohio University Press. He began the first-ever clinical ethics consultation service with hospital appointment, published nine original books, and produced over 150 varied articles.

Kristin Zeiler, PhD, is an associate professor and docent of ethics at Linköping University in Sweden. She is also a Pro Futura Scientia Fellow at the Swedish Collegium for Advanced Study, with Uppsala University, and has previously been ethics fellow at Cardiff University and postdoctoral researcher at the World Health Organization in Geneva. Her research examines how medical treatment, the use of new technology, as well as experiences of pain and illness, can form our self-understandings and ways of engaging with others and the world.

Permissions and Credits

Editors' note: Previously published material appears as originally printed.

Chapter 1, "The Dead Donor Rule and the Concept of Death: Severing the Ties That Bind Them" by Elysa R. Koppelman, is republished with permission of Taylor and Francis, LLC ((http://www.tandfonline.com). © 2003 from *The American Journal of Bioethics*. The article can be found in *The American Journal of Bioethics* 3, no. 1 (2003): 1–9.

Chapter 2, "The Theoretical and Practical Importance of the Dead Donor Rule" by James McCartney, is republished with permission of Taylor and Francis, LLC (http://www.tandfonline.com). © 2003 from *The American Journal of Bioethics*. The article can be found in *The American Journal of Bioethics* 3, no. 1 (2003): 15–16.

Chapter 3, "The Dead-Donor Rule and the Future of Organ Donation" by Robert D. Truog, F. G. Miller, and S. D. Halpern, was originally published in the *New England Journal of Medicine* 369, no. 14 (October 2013): 1287–89. © 2013 Massachusetts Medical Society. Republished with permission of the Massachusetts Medical Society.

Chapter 4, "The Dead Donor Rule: Effect on the Virtuous Practice of Medicine" by Frank C. Chaten, was republished from *The Journal of Medical Ethics* 40, pp. 496–500. © 2014. With permission from BMJ Publishing Group, Ltd.

Chapter 5, "Brain Death without Definitions" by Winston Chiong, was originally published in the *Hastings Center Report* 35, no. 6 (2005): 20–30. © 2005 by John Wiley & Sons, Inc. Republished with permission from John Wiley & Sons, Inc.

Chapter 6, "Accepting Brain Death" by David C. Magnus, B. S. Wilfond, and A. L. Caplan, was originally published in the *New England Journal of Medicine* 370, no. 10 (March 6, 2014): 891–94 (first online February 5, 2014). © 2014 Massachusetts Medical Society. Republished with permission from the Massachusetts Medical Society.

Chapter 7, "Address to the International Congress on Transplants" by Karol Wojtyła (Pope John Paul II) was originally published in the United States in *National Catholic Bioethics Quarterly* 1 (2001): 89–92. © *Libreria Editrice Vaticana*, 2000. Republished with permission from *Libreria Editrice Vaticana*.

Chapter 8, "Brain Death: Can It Be Resuscitated?" by D. Alan Shewmon, was originally published in the *Hastings Center Report* 39, no. 2 (March/April 2009): 18–24. © 2005 by John Wiley & Sons, Inc. Republished with permission from John Wiley & Sons, Inc.

Chapter 9, "The Boundaries of Organ Donation after Circulatory Death" by James L. Bernat, was originally published in the *New England Journal of Medicine* 359, no. 7 (August 2008): 669–71. © 2008 Massachusetts Medical Society. Republished with permission from the Massachusetts Medical Society.

Chapter 10, "Should We Allow Organ Donation Euthanasia? Alternatives for Maximizing the Number and Quality of Organs for Transplantation" by Dominic Wilkinson and J. Savulescu, is an excerpt from *Bioethics* 26, no. 1 (2012): 46–48. © 2012 by John Wiley & Sons, Inc. Republished with permission of Blackwell Publishing, Ltd.

Index

Index

Index